Hausa Medicine

Hausa Medicine

Illness and Well-being in a West African Culture

L. Lewis Wall

Duke University Press   *Durham and London* 1988

© 1988 Duke University Press
All rights reserved
Printed in the United States of America
on acid-free paper ∞
Library of Congress Cataloging in Publication Data
appear on the last printed page of this book.

For

Helen, Jimmy, and Tom

Who else?

Contents

Figures and Plates

Acknowledgments

Zama da mutanen hankali shi ke raya zuciya.

(*The company of intelligent people keeps the heart alive.*)

HAUSA PROVERB

No one who writes a book of any length can accomplish the task without help from many different sources, both printed works and personal friends. While it is impossible to thank everyone who has played a part in bringing this project to completion, I offer my grateful thanks to everyone who helped me and especially to those people listed here.

The major resource I have used in writing this book is the data accumulated from personal experience over fifteen months of fieldwork. This has been supplemented by numerous references to the published material on Hausa society, which have helped me clarify my own thinking on what I observed. In locating these sources Salamone's extensive Hausa bibliography (1975a) has been most useful.

Hausa culture being a Muslim culture, it cannot be understood without an understanding of Islam. All quotations from the Koran have been taken from A. J. Arberry's translation, *The Koran Interpreted* (1964). In addition, two works by W. M. Watt have been very helpful: *Bell's Introduction to the Qur'an* (1970) and *Companion to the Qur'an* (1967).

Because of their pithy and enlightening nature I have made extensive use of Hausa proverbs (*karin magana*) throughout the text as a means of illuminating certain attitudes, situations, and beliefs that are important in understanding Hausa life and values. In this I have drawn on my own experience and the indispensable Hausa dictionaries by Bargery (1934) and Abraham (1962), as well as the extensive collections of Hausa proverbs compiled by various authors over the years (Merrick 1905; Rattray 1913, II; Whitting 1940;

Kirk-Greene 1966; Madauci et al. 1968; Skinner 1977b). Because of the great overlap in these collections I have not thought it necessary to give citations for the proverbs used. Whitting's collection (1940) is indexed by subject, which makes it somewhat easier to use.

I have used *'b, 'd,* and *'k* for the glottalized Hausa "hooked letters" throughout the text of this work, and my spelling of Hausa words has followed that found in Abraham's *Dictionary of the Hausa Language.* Since tones and vowel length are not normally indicated in modern printed Hausa (though indeed they are very important!), I have not indicated them in the body of the text. Readers seeking precise information on tone, vowel length, and the pronunciation of Hausa words are referred to Abraham's dictionary.

My largest debt is to the Hausa people who so generously gave of their time and interest in answering my questions. I could not possibly name all those who contributed to my understanding of their culture, but among them I must specifically thank Mallam Umaru Usuman, the Galadima of Malumfashi, the Makama of Bakori, Musa Kwantakwaran, Alhaji Audu Tela, Aminu, Kabulle, Ibrahim Bawa Mai-'Karfi, Ibrahim Nakakumi, Iro, Rabiu Bawa, Namale Mai-Goro, Mallam Sule, Tasu'u, Hassan, Bala Dam Barike, Mallam Goje, Mallam Barau, Rabiu Titi, Lawai Mai Toye-toye, Alhaji Audu Boka, 'Dam Baba, Uwarture, Damina, Uwale, Natakwibi, Mallam Hashimu, Muhammedu Mai-Shanu, Audu Mai-Magana, Tasallah, Garba Audu, Audu Dogon Boka, Mu'azu Sarkin Tasha, Yarima, Barguma, Mallam Idi Mai-Kama Aiki, Idi, Mairo, Binta, Yayi Sarkin Bori, Musa Mai-Komo, Nauyi, Musa Tari, Mallam Mato, Hajiya, Alhaji Mamuda, Alhaji Mada, Isa, Adamu, Buzu, and especially Ado, who touched me in a very deep and personal way. To all, I offer a heartfelt *na gode.*

My field research was made possible by generous grants from two sources. Initially, I received a Fulbright-Hays Fellowship from the Institute for International Education and the U.S. Department of State. I was fortunate to be able to supplement this and to extend my research with an International Doctoral Dissertation Fellowship from the Social Science Research Council in New York. The latter body also supplied funds to aid me in writing up this material. Further work in Oxford was made possible by a generous grant from the Rhodes Trust as an extension of the Rhodes Scholarship I held at Oxford from 1972 to 1974. I owe a special debt of thanks to Sir Edgar Williams of Rhodes

House for his many kindnesses in this and other regards. It was
through a conversation with him that the entire project got under way
in the first place. Additional support was given me by Dr. Robert Hudson of the Department of the History and Philosophy of Medicine at
the University of Kansas Medical Center, who awarded me a summer
research fellowship in that department in the summer of 1980 to aid me
in the completion of my research and writing.

In Malumfashi I owe special thanks to Dr. Andy Bradley and his
wife Jenny; Dr. Keith Plate and Carol; Dr. Nick Pugh and Jill; Father
Ceslaus Prazan; Richard Longhurst, with whom I shared many kindred
ties and concerns as a fellow "bush man" as a result of his own field
research in a village northeast of Malumashi; Mo, Frank, and the entire
Malumfashi Tuareg community; and finally, to Dr. Alan Williamson
and his wife, Jan. Alan in particular was an especially close friend, who
took a keen personal interest in my work. He died tragically of ful-
minant hepatitis a few months after I left Malumfashi. An obituary by
H. M. Gilles (1978) has appeared in the *Annals of Tropical Medicine
and Parasitology*. The Nigerian medical world is a far darker place as
a result of his passing.

In Zaria I received many kindnesses from Dr. Jerome Wells, Nancy
and David; Dr. Al Gray and Louise; Enefiok Essien; Professor Umaru
Shehu; Professor O. P. Verma; Dr. Leo Barrington and Liz; Dr. Henry
Troyer and Elsie; Jim and Barbara Murnane; Wes and Elaine Kroeker;
and particularly from David Pryor, whose door was always open when
I needed a place to stay.

In Funtua I received valuable help from the staff of the Funtua Agricultural Project.

In Kaduna Lillard and Betty Hill of the United States Information
Service were especially important contacts, good friends, and helpful
expediters of my problems.

In Jos I owe my thanks to Mallam Umaru Usuman and to Dr. Samuel
Rayapati and his wife, Joy, who shared their hospitality with me there
and also at the hospital compound in Garkida.

For various courtesies in several countries I owe my thanks to Paul
Lovejoy, Jerome Barkow, Murray Last, Ismail Abdalla, Robert Stock,
and John Janzen.

In Oxford my two principal advisors, A. H. M. Kirk-Greene and John
Beattie, have been extremely patient and helpful, particularly as so

much of the work on my doctoral thesis had to be discussed via the mails between England and the United States.

Mrs. Annilese Clarke gave me valuable help with German and Mrs. May Richards typed the final draft of my doctoral thesis swiftly, accurately, and with unfailing good humor. Jeanne Lee provided indispensable secretarial support in getting the final manuscript ready for the press.

At Duke I owe special thanks to Dr. Peter English, with whom I have had a stimulating and ongoing conversation about the history of medicine for several years. In the Department of Obstetrics and Gynecology Dr. Charles B. Hammond and Dr. Al Addison have provided me with financial, secretarial, and moral support throughout this project (even if they have remained somewhat bemused by it all). My editor at the Duke University Press, Reynolds Smith, has repeatedly steered me in the right direction when I started to take a different tack and has stayed with me during the long time it has taken to bring the manuscript to press. Editorial and publication costs have been greatly reduced by a generous grant from the Josiah Charles Trent Foundation, whose support I gratefully acknowledge.

My parents, Leonard and Evelyn Wall, and my brother Terry have been continual sources of support and strength in this as in all my endeavors. Finally, my wife Helen has provided enormous editorial help in the preparation of this work and has given me a warm and loving atmosphere in which to write it. In addition to helping produce this book, she has produced two wonderful sons (who may someday wish to read it), and although I met and married her after my return from Nigeria, she has become such an integral part of the entire experience that her absence from it I can no longer conceive.

September 21, 1987

Introduction

Irin da aka shuka ya kan tsiro.

(*The seed that is sown is the one that sprouts.*)

HAUSA PROVERB

In the preface to his novel *The Razor's Edge*, which I read in Malumfashi, Nigeria, shortly before moving into a rural Hausa village to begin my field research, W. Somerset Maugham wrote the following, which I copied down at the beginning of my field notes:

It is very difficult to know people, and I don't think one can ever really know any but one's countrymen. For men and women are not only themselves; they are also the region in which they were born, the city apartment or the farm in which they learnt to walk, the games they played as children, the old wives' tales they overheard, the food they ate, the schools they attended, the sports they followed, the poets they read, and the God they believed in. It is all these that have made them what they are, and these things are the things that you can't come to know by hearsay, you can only know them if you have lived them. You can only know them if you are them. And because you cannot know persons of a nation foreign to you except from observation, it is difficult to give them credibility in the pages of a book. (Maugham 1963:8–9)

These words are true for anthropology as well as for literature—indeed, they form the impetus for fieldwork—and as I now attempt to write a book about life in a rural Nigerian village, they seem more poignant than ever.

This work is an interpretive ethnography of rural Hausa life as I found it in one particular village in northern Nigeria in 1976–77. It is the product of one man working in a foreign culture through the medium of a foreign language among a remarkably gracious and hospitable people, who never fully understood what he was doing or why he was doing it. The picture that emerges is necessarily colored by these circumstances, but I hope that picture is a reasonably accurate one.

The main interest of this book is Hausa traditional medicine, but I have attempted to write a book that may also serve as a general introduction to Hausa culture for the uninitiated. Hausa medical practices make little sense unless set within the broader context of Hausa life, and as a result I have attempted to paint the background rather broadly before attempting any discussion of Hausa medicine per se. The reader may find this somewhat tedious; if so, I apologize, but I regard it as necessary. Without an understanding of the social setting and moral values that form their underpinning, any description of Hausa medical practices would be a mere catalogue of disconnected remedies, therapeutic techniques, and random medical facts that would give little insight into the workings of the Hausa medical "system."

It is hoped that this essay on rural Hausa life and customs will provide a deeper understanding of the wellsprings of that medical system, not only for those anthropologists who may be interested in the study of such systems, but especially for the non-Hausa medical practitioner—African, Asian, or European—who finds himself in Hausaland faced with treating sick and suffering patients from a foreign culture.

There are many studies of African medical systems by anthropologists (e.g., Field 1937; Turner 1968; Bryant 1970; Harwood 1971; Buxton 1973; Ngubane 1977; Buckley 1985) and some by physicians (e.g., Harley 1941; Gelfand 1956, 1964a, 1964b; Maclean 1971; Jansen 1973; Imperato 1977), but only a few that combine the insights of both disciplines in a fruitful way (e.g., Field 1960; Orley 1970; Janzen with Arkinstall 1978). This book is written by an anthropologist who has since become a clinician—a change largely catalyzed by the fieldwork itself.

"Research" is foreign to traditional Hausa culture. Hausa villagers do not go around with tape recorders and notebooks asking questions and writing down responses to their inquiries. The good graces with which they received me and my intrusions into their world never ceased to surprise me, considering that what I was doing was an intellectual exercise essentially irrelevant to their own lives and problems. The additional fact that I was interested in medical matters but was medically untrained at that time and unable to do much about their problems heightened this sense of irrelevance. The most lasting contribution I made in the course of my fieldwork, aside from whatever minor boost I may have given the local economy by my presence, was undoubtedly the time I took to arrange medical care for people at the hospital in Malumfashi and to transport them there for evaluation and treatment. To those who have witnessed the heartache of illness and disease among rural villagers there is no doubt that Africa needs caring, sympathetic practitioners of medicine far more than it needs anthropologists; indeed, it was this profound feeling of the essential irrelevance of academic anthropology to genuine human suffering that led me to abandon it for medicine—a decision I have not regretted in the least.

This book is not, therefore, a treatise on anthropological theory. I have become too wearied by the tribal warfare of Oxford anthropology to attempt such a thing, even if it were within my capabilities. Academic anthropologists will probably be dissatisfied with it as a result, and physicians will wish (as I do) that I had had medical training before I ventured off into the savannah to begin my sojourn among the Hausa. In any case, the press of clinical responsibilities has precluded the extensive revisions that would be necessary to make it completely acceptable to both camps.

There is theory behind this work, to be sure, but it is neither original nor, perhaps, profound. My main assumption is that Hausa behavior is understandable and their view of the world comprehensible if one takes the time to probe for the premises that lie behind their thought. It lies within the broad ethnographic tradition pioneered by the late Professor Sir E. E. Evans-Pritchard in his classic work on African thought, *Witchcraft, Oracles and Magic Among the Azande* (1937), but it makes no presumption to similar quality. The Hausa have reasons for what they do and for what they believe and they operate "rationally" from those starting points. This is not to say that they either behave or think "logically" in some strictly critical way comparable to a Western philosopher of science tackling a complex problem; but neither do we, and neither do the patients in our hospitals and clinics. They, too, have reasons for what they do and the more one comes to understand those hopes and fears and motivations, the better is the care that one can render to them.

The social anthropologist looks for "collective representations" and "social facts," whereas the clinician sees individual patients. However interested we may be in disease entities and disease processes, the final raw material with which medicine is concerned is the care of an illness in a suffering, individual patient. Social scientists who deal with medical matters often lose sight of this fact, and in the reification of social processes the reality of human suffering is obscured. The individual patient ought to be seen as a "system" for ethnographic study in her or his own right. As Houston pointed out nearly fifty years ago (1938:1417), the major difference between human medicine and veterinary medicine is the quality of the doctor-patient relationship. This fact is well known to traditional healers and no doubt contributes to their continuing popularity in African societies. Only those physicians who are willing to interact on a personal basis with the Hausa people themselves will be able to make the practice of scientific medicine in northern Nigeria anything more than a sophisticated veterinary medicine. The patients' personal concepts of life and health have a very real impact on what they choose to do about perceived illnesses.

The Hausa concept of *lafiya* may serve as a focal point in aiding our understanding of these thoughts and motivations. Through this lens many different aspects of Hausa culture may be brought clearly into view. *Lafiya* is a Hausa word, stemming from Arabic roots, which is often translated simply as "health"; but in reality *lafiya* is a much broader term that is more properly translated as "well-being," "balance," or "the right and proper relationship of things." The concept of "physical health" is better expressed by the Hausa phrase *lafiyar jiki*, "well-being of the body." Within the purview of Hausa medicine, *lafiya* refers to the correct, balanced, properly ordered state of the body. When that balance is upset *lafiya* is no longer present and illness results. If one is healthy he has *lafiya*; if one is ill *lafiya* is absent. The Hausa expression conveying this imbalance is *ba na da lafiya*, "I have no *lafiya*." *Lafiya* being a state of positive order, its absence is a pathological state to be corrected by the application of an appropriate restorative remedy.

When viewed from the social side, *lafiya* similarly refers to balance, order, and the right and proper relationship of things. Hausa rituals of greeting (which are often quite elaborate) stress the importance of *lafiya* as personal and social well-being. *Kana lafiya?* "Are you well?" *Kwana*

lafiya? "Did you sleep well?" *Gida lafiya?* "Is your household well?"
Ka zo lafiya? "Have you arrived safely?" The proper response to these
questions about social and personal order and tranquility is *Lafiya!*
"Fine!" or the more emphatic *Lafiya lau!* "Very well indeed!" If domestic relations are peaceful and orderly, then a man's household has
lafiya; but if social relations are disordered and tumultuous, if there is
strife in the household between co-wives, if there is tension in the village, if the crops are poor or disease is present, then the home or the
town is "spoiled" and *lafiya* is absent.

It is therefore easy to see that a mere medical treatment of concepts
of "health" is insufficient under these circumstances. While concepts of
anatomy, physiology, or the causation of illness are important in understanding bodily health, *lafiya* has profound social implications as well.
The Hausa concept of *lafiya* cannot be fully understood without reference to values of general morality, economy, and interpersonal relationships, not to mention the relationships of men and women to the spirit
world and to Allah. Hausa society is overwhelmingly a Muslim society,
and a major component of properly ordered social relationships is therefore a man's or woman's right relationship with God as defined by his
or her adherence to the social and religious requirements of Islam. Paramount among these requirements are proper dress, modest comportment, and performance of the required daily ritual prayers; but because
Hausaland has been thoroughly Islamic for less than 200 years and
because there are still large pockets of pagan Hausa in the rural countryside (not to mention secular influences percolating in from the cities)
even the correct Muslim balance of life is sometimes seen as threatened.
Public as well as private health involves religious, social, and biological
concerns, and the Hausa seek curative and prophylactic "medicines" in
all these overlapping spheres.

This book, which seeks an understanding of traditional Hausa medicine, must therefore take into account a great deal of information about
Hausa society in general. The broad meaning of *lafiya,* with its connotations of social and moral, as well as physical well-being, mandates
a broader approach to the topic than a mere cataloguing of medical
practices. The structure of this book, which at first may seem disjointed,
has an underlying logic that approaches medical problems from this
broader perspective.

The first chapter deals in general with the nature of village life and provides information on family structure, kinship, agriculture, and village economics. Against this background the second chapter describes the individual life cycle from birth to death and the rites of passage that accompany changes in social status. Chapter 3 then outlines the moral order provided by Islam and describes the virtues of moral excellence that are necessary for moral well-being. Having thus detailed the foundations of the social order, the fourth chapter describes those forces which threaten it: paganism, witchcraft, sorcery, spirit possession, and women. Consecutive chapters then proceed to more traditional "medical" concerns: concepts of anatomy and physiology and the causation of illness—which can be seen to arise from natural causes ordained by God or from the intrusion of evil influences, either spiritual or social—that disrupt bodily well-being. There follows an overview of the traditional Hausa medical practitioners who attempt to restore such disrupted order, including an in-depth look at two different styles of herbal practice. The final portion of the book attempts to delineate certain premises of Hausa medical thought and to explore the rationale of Hausa medicine and therapeutics within the overall framework of Hausa symbolism and the general concept of *lafiya*.

Readers will detect what can only be called a "male bias" throughout the course of this work. There are several reasons for this. The first is that Hausa society is firmly and unequivocally controlled by men, a situation that is underpinned by the strong masculine bias of Islam. Hausa women—while considerably freer than they first appear—are in general controlled by men and have few social options open to them. The "female question" is one that continually vexes Hausa men and it is no small surprise that women are seen as repositories of social discord and sources of potential illness. The second reason follows, unfortunately, from the first. Although as an outsider I was not so strictly bound by social convention and was able to have surprisingly cordial relations with a number of Hausa women, it was still extremely difficult for a male investigator to penetrate the obstacle of wife seclusion (*purdah*) and obtain detailed information about women's lives and thoughts. The seclusion of wives and the markedly inferior status of Hausa women are also major reasons why obstetrics and gynecology are such dismal aspects of Hausa traditional medicine. The medical condition of Hausa women is often truly appalling and the provision of adequate maternity services and gynecologic care remain among the largest un-addressed public health issues confronting the people of northern Nigeria. Let us hope that these aspects of Hausa medicine, at least, will not be long with us, whatever the other benefits of traditional practices may be.

Hausa Medicine

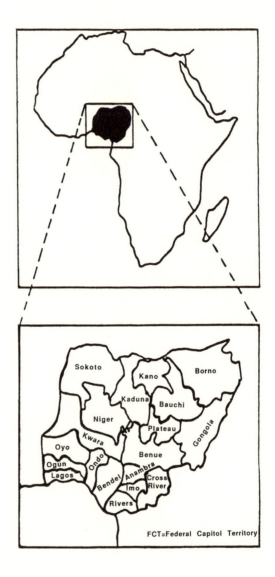

Figure 1   *The location of Nigeria and its constituent states.*

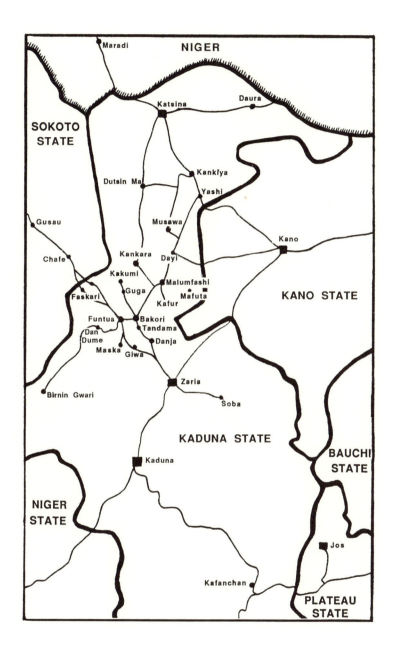

Figure 2 Kaduna State, Nigeria, showing details of southern Katsina.

I

The Nature of Village Life

Ana zaman 'karya, in ji Bamaguje.

("They can't really live here!" said the pagan Hausa man (when he saw the village).)

HAUSA PROVERB

■ Life's Dull Round

Before the sun comes up, when the sky is black and the air is still and clear, the faint sounds of *Allahu akbar!* "God is great!" begin to rise throughout a Hausa village. By the religious laws of Islam the first *salla* (prescribed prayer) is performed before sunrise, and the devout villager marks the beginning of his waking hours by facing Mecca and praising God. In short order the sounds of religious piety are mingled with the dull, rhythmic thuddings of the women pounding guinea-corn to prepare the early-morning *tuwo*—the doughy staple food that forms the backbone of the Hausa diet—for their compound. Men and boys kindle fires outside and huddle for warmth in the early morning chill, rubbing sleep from their eyes and pulling tattered blankets around them for comfort. Inside, the women have made their own fires and the *tuwo* begins to steam and bubble.

Throughout the village signs of life gradually appear. Small girls begin to make their way through the streets, selling cakes of fried millet or beans that their mothers have made. On a few selected corners the more enterprising have large, steaming pots of *koko* or *kunu*—thick, viscous gruel made from guinea-corn and other cereals and sweetened to pleasantness with tamarind juice and sugar—dipped out by the calabash into the omnipresent enameled metal bowls so characteristic of contemporary rural Hausaland. On their heads small boys carefully carry these bowls back home, where the hot liquid is drunk by the men from carved gourd spoons. The compound head drinks his fill and passes the remains on down to his young sons; or perhaps several neighbors or brothers will each suck down a spoonful in succession as they pass the bowl around from hand to hand in a spirit of friendship. The *tuwo* is brought—a brownish lump of hot, sticky dough not unlike an unbaked loaf of bread, covered in a vegetable sauce made of hot peppers, tomatoes, and okra, or the leaves of the baobab tree. After a brief invocation of *Bismillah!*, a shortened form of *Bismillahi-arrahmani-arrahim*, meaning "In the name of God the merciful," each man scoops off a portion of the pasty dough, dips it in the sauce, and pops it in his mouth, continuing until he has eaten his fill. He washes his hand, usually with water poured from a plastic teakettle of the kind widely sold in northern Nigeria—convenient vessels for carrying water for the ritual ablutions required before prayer. A bowl of cold well-water is handy for slaking thirst. The remains of the *tuwo* are left for the young children (who may have had their own bowl also) or they are distributed to the Koranic students, those continually hungry boys of eight, nine, or ten who have been sent by their families from other villages to study under a locally acknowledged religious authority and to live off the goodwill of the Muslim community. The women eat by themselves inside; although small girls and boys may eat together, only a prostitute (*karuwa*) would eat from the same bowl as a man.

The morning meal done, the business of greeting (*gaisuwa*) begins. Those families who have suffered the grief of death or the happiness of a marriage or birth are visited. Prior to a naming ceremony or a marriage the head of the family in question makes the rounds of his friends and acquaintances, telling them of the date and place for the celebration—always in the early morning around 7:00 A.M. The meal done, neighbors begin to file toward the house where the event is scheduled to occur, greeting the family head, receiving a kolanut or a sweet, and partaking in a brief communal recitation of the opening verses of the Koran while the marriage is completed or the child is named.[1] Men seat themselves outside the compound in the street while the proceedings are led by the officiating Muslim divine; women go inside to greet the wives and female members of the compound, while children run freely in and out. Such proceedings are brief, dignified, and on any given

1. The ritual cycle of such rites de passage is examined in more detail in chapter 2.

morning in a good-sized village as many as two or three such events may require one's presence.

By 8:00 A.M. in an agricultural season the men and their sons or hired laborers are setting off to the farms to cultivate the ground, plant their crops, harvest the produce, or merely check the progress of the fields. Such work usually lasts until mid-morning, when the sun comes out in full force, making continued physical labor unpleasant, and the field hands return to the village to relax until the heat of the day passes. At this time of morning large numbers of village children (but not all), dressed in green-and-white uniforms, are setting off for the village school, where they will absorb a rudimentary education.

By mid-morning the village is bustling. Bicycles are moving up and down the dirt roads throughout the settlement. Children are playing in the dust and running about, chasing the goats and sheep, which forage for greenery around the fences and less-traveled paths of the community. The clatter of treadle-operated sewing machines can be heard, making gowns, trousers, and shirts, accompanied by the sounds of Radio-Television Kaduna on battery-powered transistor radios in the more prosperous establishments. Shopkeepers are either tending their fields or relaxing in the shade outside their stores, selling soap for washing, sugar, salt, imported bouillon cubes, and other household items. Little girls not enrolled in school walk through the streets in groups or in pairs, playing together as they hawk the wares they have for sale: beancakes, *fura* (rolled, pounded balls of millet, mixed with sour milk and eaten as a porridge—the main midday meal for the Hausa peasant), roast groundnuts, mangoes, guavas, or kolanuts; whatever their mothers have given them to sell to earn the income they themselves cannot, being secluded inside the home by Islamic custom. Rattle-trap lorries, frequently loaded beyond capacity and driven beyond the limits of safety, screech to a halt at the lorry-park, unload goods and passengers, pick up the same for delivery to other near or distant locations, and move on. The odd motorcycle may roar past, to be lost in a blur of greasy blue smoke from its exhaust pipe. Donkeys, loaded with refuse to be taken to the fields as fertilizer or red laterite clay to be used in building, pass by. Neighbors stop to talk and gossip. Old women may be beating and winnowing grain outside. Young married women are rarely seen in public and only then on special occasions. Girls haul

water for washing from the main village well or from a well inside a
neighbor's compound. Fulani women from the cattle camps in the surrounding countryside appear in the village selling sour milk and butter
from large, carved gourd calabashes carried on their heads, bantering
with the village men in a spirit of independence rare in the more restrained village women.

The midday meal is informal—usually an individual responsibility—
and usually involves drinking *fura* sweetened with sugar and eating
beancakes or other light foods. The husband or compound head will
frequently buy a bowl of sour milk and send it inside for his wives and
family, keeping some for himself. Schoolchildren return home for a
meal as well, then straggle slowly back to class.

On market days, which take place on different days in the major
villages in a local area, people gravitate to the market by midday. Traders move their wares from their shops—a line of young boys with cardboard boxes filing from home to the marketplace transporting their
father's goods is a common sight. Bolts of cloth are unraveled in the
stalls. Men carry their pots for sale, their kolanuts, their plastic shoes,
and cheap perfumes and bars of soap. Craftsmen, leatherworkers, tailors, medicine sellers, sellers of used clothing from Britain and America,
purveyors of agricultural produce, all set up in their stalls. Girls carry
snack foods through the market, catering to the hungry. Grain is measured out and sold. Sellers of salt unload their cakes. The Fulani come
to look at livestock and have a day in the town—occasionally drinking
too much beer at the prostitutes' houses and getting into fights. On
market days in a village, except at the height of the agricultural season,
all the men are in the market visiting friends, taking care of business,
exchanging information, and making speculations about the state of the
village world.

In the early afternoon—at 2:00 P.M. by the reckoning of those villagers with wristwatches—*azahar* begins. This is the second *salla* of
the five daily required Muslim prayers and it is performed communally
by the men. The men and boys from neighboring compounds gather in
groups in the various quarters of the village to perform the prayers
together; but on Fridays (the major religious day in the Muslim weekly
calendar), they all meet at the Friday mosque for a communal performance of the *salla,* led by the officiating Islamic divine of the village.

As the afternoon progresses and the heat of the day dissipates, children come back from the village school; men move back to the fields to continue their work, returning toward late afternoon. The third *salla* takes place about 4:00 P.M. (*la'asar*) and again men and boys from neighboring households perform the rituals together. Women perform the *salla* individually, inside the compounds, and may be more or less devout, depending on personal inclinations, for Islam is a religion heavily dominated by men, in which women have a subservient role.

As sunset approaches the guinea-corn is pounded to make the evening *tuwo*. In an age of gradually increasing mechanization, motorized engines for milling grain have become increasingly popular—and for those wealthy enough to own them, quite lucrative. For a few *kobo* per calabash the strain of pounding by hand is avoided.[2] Long queues of girls with bowls of grain for grinding (both for the evening meal and for the following morning) can be seen at such locations, playing, laughing, and flirting. As the sun begins to set the evening *tuwo* is prepared. The men gather for the fourth *salla, magariba*. The work of the day is over and men who pray together at this time frequently eat together, small clusters of three or four or five neighbors gathered together near the doorways of their compounds, sharing *tuwo* and talking quietly. After sunset the evenings are generally spent in social activities. Men gather to talk to each other, and women are allowed to visit other compounds under cover of darkness (with their husband's permission). Young men go out in search of fun and adventure—and girls. Wilder members of the community will look for prostitutes to drink beer with or places to gamble at cards. Young girls will find their way to the "small market" where by the light of kerosene lamps people sell sugarcane, fruit, candies, and cakes. Here also people gather to greet friends and listen to village drummers striking up a beat for girls to dance to. More devout members of the community will gather to read the Koran or chant religious songs. In the dry season bonfires of guinea-

2. There are 100 kobo in a Nigerian naira. At the time of my fieldwork the naira was worth approximately U.S.$1.60 or £0.80. Throughout the course of the fieldwork the pound dropped dramatically. For Hausa purposes of calculation, based on the currency of the colonial period, one pound (Hausa, *pam*) equaled two naira, ten kobo equaled one shilling (Hausa, *sule*), and five kobo equaled sixpence (Hausa, *sisi*). The terms *pam, sule,* and *sisi* were commonly used in village economics.

corn stalks blaze away by the houses of noted religious teachers, where children can be found gathered around the fire loudly reciting the passages of scripture they are trying to memorize.

As the night wears on, the time for the final prayer of the day (*lisha*) approaches. This is performed either communally by groups of neighbors, or individually, depending on the circumstances at the time. Men who have been outside taking in the cool air of the evening gradually move inside their entry-huts to sleep, or retire to the hut of one of their wives. Children sleep where they find a spot—the entry-way of the household, with their mothers, or cuddled up next to brothers. The kerosene lamps gradually are turned out, the doorways to the houses shut, and late in the evening the village fades into the silence of night, broken in places by the faint droning of a radio playing popular Hausa songs by Alhaji Mamman Shata, or the boisterous shouts of a few rowdy youths.

■ Hausaland and the Hausa

The word *Hausa* refers, above all else, to a language, perhaps the most widely spoken in sub-Saharan Africa (Greenberg 1963:45). Over thirty years ago Westermann and Bryan wrote (1952:163): "The total number of Hausa-speakers cannot be estimated, in view of the enormous distribution of the Hausa and the great number of those who speak Hausa as a second language," a situation that is all the more true today. Hausa speakers are found in Nigeria, Benin, Togo, Ghana, Cameroon, Chad, and scattered through Sudanic Africa from Senegal to the Red Sea, from the Maghrib in North Africa down to the Zaire Basin, where their commercial interests as traders have taken them in quest of profits. The Hausa heartland, however, is that portion of the central Sudan located in the rolling savannah country south of the Sahel, bounded approximately by 10½ and 13½ degrees north latitude and by 4 and 10 degrees east longitude, roughly comprising the northern regions of modern Nigeria and the southern parts of Niger. Kirk-Greene (1967:84) estimated that there were some twenty million Hausa speakers in northern Nigeria alone.[3]

3. Linguistic maps showing the distribution of Hausa speakers may be found in Westermann and Bryan (1952), Prothero (1962), and Adamu (1978). Studies of Hausa communities outside the Hausa heartland proper include those by A. Cohen

The identification of Hausa with a language is so strong that it frequently is used as a synonym for "meaning" or for "language" itself. English, for example, may be called *Hausar Turawa*, "the *Hausa* of Europeans." It is not far from such a concept to that of *Hausa* as a way of living or a cultural system. A *Bahaushe* (f. *Bahaushiya*) is a native speaker of Hausa, one who is fully conversant with the distinctly "Hausa" ways of doing things that such linguistic competence implies—one who has internalized the cultural substructure lying behind the language itself.

Indeed, one can speak of a "Hausa culture" in a sense that transcends narrow tribal connotations. Hausaland is a culture area, not a tribal territory delimited by one small ethnic group. Central to Hausa culture is the Muslim religion. The presence of such a universalistic religion provides an identifying and unifying force that cuts across tribal-ethnic boundaries and allows for the incorporation of new members into Hausa society.[4] The nature of Hausa social organization also provides easy access to incorporation within the wider culture. In contrast to the tribal societies found throughout most of Africa, with their extensive networks of clanship and lineage ties, Hausa society is organized on principles of territoriality and residence, rather than kinship. The Hausa were organized at an early date in their history into a number of centralized kingdoms with territorial subdivisions, later united at the turn of the nineteenth century into a vast empire by the Fulani warrior and cleric Usman 'Dan Fodio. This fragmentation of local organization makes it easier for a stranger to be assimilated into Hausa ways, for the primary referent of social organization is the *gida* (household or compound) of the individual family, not their kin-relationship to the other members of the village. A man who speaks Hausa fluently, dresses in traditional Hausa garb, possesses a Muslim Hausa name, and espouses that religion, will be considered a *Bahaushe* if he claims to be one.[5]

(1969) on the Hausa of Ibadan, B. Winchester (1976) on the Hausa of Kumasi, Ghana, and J. Works (1976) on the Hausa communities in Chad.

4. The importance of Islam in becoming Hausa is stressed in Salamone (1975b).

5. "Taking into account the people often referred to as Hausa in written sources, and also the numerous oral traditions, particularly those which I gathered from many Hausa and non-Hausa informants in various *zangos* in West Africa, I have come to the conclusion that there can be no cut-and-dry definition of a Hausa person. This is because different criteria were, and still are, used by different people

Traditionally, there were seven "true" Hausa kingdoms, the *Hausa bakwai:* Daura, Kano, Zazzau (Zaria), Gobir, Katsina, and Garun Gabas. In addition, there were seven other states, the "worthless seven" (*banza bakwai*), not regarded as true Hausa, but linked to the others by common ties of kinship and custom and in which the Hausa language was spoken. Each of these kingdoms was characterized by a central fortified city called a *birni*, which dominated the surrounding countryside and from which the kingdom took its name.

The origins of these kingdoms are obscure. It is probable that the early social organization of the Hausa was a system of kinship ties and clans, as is generally the case in "stateless" African societies and as is presently found (in diluted form) among the pagan Maguzawa Hausa

---

at different times to define who was or should be regarded as Hausa. Some people used purely historical claims to Hausa ethnicity, others used cultural traits and social values as their yardstick, while others still used religion plus language. There are also people who on very rare occasions prefer to use occupational specialization in commerce. (Adamu 1976:75)

One basic cultural pattern dominates the social life and economy of the great majority of the peoples of Nigeria north of the Niger-Benue line. Its essential elements are Hausa speech, Moslem religion, and a blend of Hausa customs with the fundamentals of Moslem law and practice. It includes an ancient monarchical state organization, with a developed system of taxation: this generally takes the form of an emirate headed by a ruling dynasty of Fulani origin. There is a comparatively elaborate and often highly skilled agricultural technique whereby the rural communities provide both their own food and the surplus which maintains the urban aristocracy, merchants and artisans and the petty officials of the districts into which the emirate is divided for the purpose of administration. . . . the society and the economy of "Hausaland" and of the kingdom of Bornu to the east have an underlying uniformity. Here the local rural community, despite its self-sufficiency in food and in most other commodities, has long formed part of a wider administrative and economic framework. Tax-collectors and traders have for centuries been transporting the rural surpluses to the political capitals and the tradition of surplus production for distant centers of consumption, through trading, taxation and levies, is deeply implanted. At the same time, the continual ebb and flow of population and the large-scale transplantation of slaves to promote intensive cultivation in the vicinity of the capitals such as Kano, Zaria and Sokoto has emphasized the wider political and territorial framework of society at the expense of those ties of kinship and locality which bind the members of autonomous primitive communities". (Forde 1946:119)

of Nigeria and the pagan Hausa of Niger.[6] It is easy to surmise a period when individual households (*gida*, pl. *gidaje*), each under the authority of a household head (*maigida*), lived together in scattered clan-based hamlets ('*kauye*, pl. '*kauyuka*; or *unguwa*, pl. *unguwoyi*), perhaps under the nominal authority of a hamlet head (*mai-unguwa*). The major change might have come when a hamlet developed into a proper town (*gari*) with a headman (*mai-gari*) who relied for his position on the support of the hamlet heads of the surrounding hinterland. Immigration to the towns from outlying areas due to developing markets or their importance as cult centers in the old pagan religion could have caused them to expand. Gradually, a town could transform itself into a full-scale *birni*, a walled or fortified town, and thus become a prototypical "state" headed by a *sarki*, who could expand his dominions to include other towns and hamlets, eventually growing into a fairly substantial kingdom. These fortified cities probably would have been important centers of trade and commerce, a stimulus to immigration from outlying areas, and a source of military strength and protection from the predatory nomads and slave raiders who have plagued the Sudan throughout so much of its history. This gradual change—which probably occurred in numerous places in Hausaland over a long period of time—from a system of social organization based on kinship to one based primarily on the control of territory, constituted a political revolution of no small consequence in the central Sudan. The Islamization of these kingdoms in the fourteenth century and afterward paved the way for their incorporation into the wider world of Muslim culture and laid the foundations for the religious *jihad* ("holy war") of the Fulani warriors under Shehu 'Dan Fodio that cemented the kingdoms together into the more unified whole of the Sokoto Caliphate.[7]

As a result of these processes a hierarchical society emerged. At the

6. On stateless societies in Africa see Middleton and Tait (1958). On the Maguzawa see particularly Greenberg (1946, 1947a) and Krusius (1915). The pagan Hausa of Niger are discussed in G. Nicolas (1975).
7. This description of the growth of the Hausa kingdoms is based on the theories of Abdullahi Smith (1970), which supercede the less critical notions of M. G. Smith (1964a), H. A. S. Johnston (1966:xvi–xvii) and others who have relied on outmoded notions of "racial migration" that brought new forms of rule to Hausaland—even as the British brought their own colonial forms of government.

top was the sultan of Sokoto, who received the homage and allegiance of the emirs (*sarakuna*, s. *sarki*) of the kingdoms. Around the sultan and the emirs were grouped numerous officeholders (*masu-sarauta*) who depended upon their *sarki* (chief) for their positions, and were subject to removal by him for any reason. Among these courtiers were the district chiefs (*hakimai*, s. *hakimi*), who ruled the subdivisions of the emirates. Untrusted by the *sarki*, they lived under his watchful eye in the capital city, administering their domains through emissaries who conveyed instructions to the village headmen and returned the taxes collected at the village level to their overlords in the city. The *hakimi*, or district chief, was known as the *mai-'kasa*, "possessor of the land," and he appointed the village head, or *mai-gari*, "possessor of the town," subject to the approval of the *sarki*. These village heads in turn organized the village areas under them into wards or hamlet areas (*unguwoyi*, s. *unguwa*) and appointed their own subordinates to carry out their tasks. Alongside this structure was a system of Islamic courts presided over by an independent judge (*alkali*) who settled disputes according to Maliki Islamic law.

When the British conquered the Hausa states at the turn of the twentieth century they found indigenous governments with a developed bureaucracy and centralized authority, an efficient method of tax collection, and an established legal system. Rather than disrupt this system in favor of an untried creation of their own, they adopted the local structure of government to their own uses. The principal structural change made was the transfer of the *hakimai* from the capital city to residences in the districts under their charge, and the abolition of the system of emissaries as intermediates (this done not without considerable opposition from the emirs, who felt that their grasp over the countryside was thereby weakened).[8] This method of organization was incorporated into the Nigerian state under Lord Lugard and, with minor modifications, has remained the essential structure of local government in Hausaland ever since. Even the creation of new states by the post-independence Nigerian federal government has preserved the traditional polities of the emirates and the constituent subdivisions relatively

8. A summary of this process and the changes introduced may be found in Orr (1911), Perham (1937), Kirk-Greene (1965), and Nicholson (1969). The administrative history of Katsina Emirate is treated in Hull (1968).

intact, while adding new departments and consolidating administrative functions in other areas.

■ The Village World

The history and complex organization of the traditional Hausa kingdoms, with their kings and princes, viziers and court officials, feudal nobility and hangers-on, has gained the attention of many authors.[9] This titled elite, the *masu-sarauta*, has occupied a prominent place in discussions about Hausaland, but when one finally descends to the village level only the *talakawa* ("commoners") remain. Within the village domain there is only one real *mai-sarauta*, the village headman, called the *mai-gari*, "owner of the town," or *magajin gari*, the "elder brother" of the town. Only the *mai-gari* refers to the village as *garina*, "my town." Everybody else refers to it as *garimmu*, "our town." The village chief is the proximate arm of authority in village life, entrusted with the administration of the village and its surrounding village area, which is the smallest real administrative unit of the district.

The *mai-gari* is responsible for the organization of his territory, and, even as he is appointed by the *hakimi*, so he appoints his subordinates in the village: ward heads (*masu-unguwa*) who are his messengers and informants; a *sarkin tasha* or "chief of the lorry-park," who oversees the loading and unloading of vehicles arriving in the village; a *sarkin fawa*, "chief of the butchers." Additionally, he invests with his office the *limamin juma'a*, the congregational leader of the Friday mosque who is chosen by the *mallamai* (Koranic scholars) of the village. Other official functionaries exist in the village as well: a headmaster and schoolteachers sent down by the local education authority, perhaps a dispensary attendant or an overseer of an agricultural project. None of these people are traditional *masu-sarauta*, even though there is a tendency to regard government sinecures at any level as "modern chiefships." The performance of their duties depends heavily upon the cooperation of the village head, who must be regarded in practical terms as being their superior.

9. In particular see the works of M. G. Smith (1960, 1978), Hogben and Kirk-Greene (1966), Last (1967a), and Low (1972).

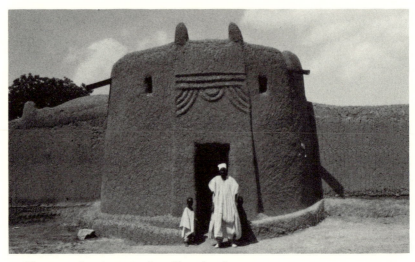

1. *The entry-hut* (zaure) *of a village headman.*

The headman is responsible for maintaining order in his village, settling minor disputes, collecting the taxes when they are due, and carrying out such directives as may be sent to him from the district headquarters and the *hakimi*. In this he has no judges or any police force of his own. Minor disputes are settled by his intervention; serious cases must be referred to the judge at the district level. Instances of serious crime are met through a spontaneous organization of villagers until the police can arrive from the district police station. In cases of violence such as a fight, the intervention of the populace serves as a deterrent; but in general a Hausa village is a peaceful place.[10]

For a rural villager the organization of the external world begins

10. During my stay in the village I witnessed only a few outbreaks of violence. One was an altercation between two laborers who worked on an agricultural project. It was a serious fight but nobody intervened until one of the men grabbed a large piece of wood and was about to bludgeon the man he was holding on the ground. Both men were then subdued and brought before the village head, who sent for the police and packed them off to the district *alkali*. In another case one of the notorious local troublemakers got drunk and, taunted by the village children, began throwing logs at them in the village marketplace. Several people subdued him and fastened his leg to a heavy log with a large metal staple (*gam*) designed for such a purpose. This *gam* was in the possession of one of the local healers who treated the insane and had frequent need for it.

with his family (*iyali*) and household or compound (*gida*), which may
contain the families of a father and his married sons, or the families of
married brothers. Beyond the *gida* are the neighbors (*ma'kwabta*) and
the neighborhood or quarter (*unguwa*) in which they live. The merging
of these *unguwoyi* forms the *gari*, the village. Surrounding the village
are the farms (*gonaki*), beyond which lies the inhospitable, uncultivated
bush (*daji*)—habitation of wild animals, spirits, a few scattered hamlets ('*kauyuka*) with their surrounding farms, and the Maguzawa
pagans (*arna*). In densely settled areas such as that around Kano, *daji*
may be virtually nonexistent, having been domesticated by the spread
of agriculture; but the polarity of thought between the civilized *gari*
and the untamed bush is an important one in Hausa thought.[11]

Beyond the village lie the neighboring towns. These form the market
links within which the village trader operates, different villages holding
markets on different days. Indeed, one of the primary marks of a true
gari is the presence of its market (*kasuwa*); a village without a market
is really just a hamlet in the eyes of its neighbors, even though it may
possess a village headman. Tracing the disperson of market days gives
a fairly good idea of the range of trading likely to be undertaken and
the consequent relationships of villages to one another (see Hill and
Smith 1972). Market days are often used as synonyms for the days of
the week, *ran 'Kwari*, " 'Kwari's day," being synonymous with Thurs-
day, the market day in the village of 'Kwari, for example.

In a wider sphere of organization the districts come into focus, each
being administered by the *hakimi* from his district headquarters. Although these districts have been grouped into divisions within the
states, rural villagers still regard themselves primarily as members of
a traditional emirate, for example, *Katsinawa* ("men of Katsina"), with
a correlative emphasis on traditional districts, rather than as inhabitants
of divisions or provinces—partly because the traditional demarcations
have survived while the organization of government above the district
level has often changed since independence.

At a still higher level of thought the villager will know he is an inhabitant of a state, such as Kaduna State or Kano State, but will feel
more at home as a *mutumin arewa*, a "man of the north," with its implication of belonging to the Muslim world. The Sokoto Caliphate

---

11. This is discussed in more detail in chapter 4.

unified the north into an empire and the sultan of Sokoto still bears the title *Sarkin Musulmi*, "chief of the Muslims," or, in its Arabic form *Amr al-mu'minin*, "commander of the Faithful." As such, Hausaland looks more toward Mecca than Lagos culturally, and frequently seems more a part of the Middle East than of sub-Saharan Africa.

Nonetheless, villagers know they are a part of Nigeria and part of the wider African world—uncertain though that knowledge often is. Many have traveled surprisingly widely within the country, on business, trading cattle, seeking dry-season work, or just out of wanderlust. Each year a handful of wealthy men depart from the village for Mecca, returning from the pilgrimage with the coveted title of *alhaji* and a wider experience of the (Muslim) world. Beyond this, however, knowledge is vague. America, Russia, England, France, Germany—for the rural Hausa these remain names associated with power and prestige, a vague world with which they are hardly familiar. Many conceive of Britain as south of Lagos and France as north of Katsina—the former because the British came up from the south during their conquest, the latter due to a confused notion of the status of Niger and Chad.[12]

For the vast majority of the people of Hausaland a rural village is the community by which their experience of the world is structured. The fascination of large metropolitan centers such as Kano, Katsina, or Zaria is there, but for the Hausa villager these are places to be visited and marveled at, not places to settle. The realm of everyday experience is bounded by the town and its surrounding countryside, the quarters of the village and the hamlets round about, the farmland where the crops are grown, and the wild, uncultivated bush. The nature of village life is, therefore, of crucial importance to an understanding of rural Hausa culture, for it forms the basic core of existence, the experiential and conceptual foundation on which many other perceptions of the world are based.

Three words are useful in defining the place of the village in relation to the hierarchical structure of society: *birni*, *gari*, and *'kauye*. Since the traditional emirates still form the benchmark from which the rural farmer takes his regional bearings, a *mutumin Katsina* ("man of Katsina") looks toward the great walled city (*birni*) of Katsina as the focal

12. Unfortunately, it is probably safe to say that the typical Hausa villager knows as much about Britain and America as the typical Briton or American knows about Africa or the Hausa.

point of his geographical identity. The *birni* is a great metropolis, a commercial center, traditionally a refuge in times of war or slave raiding, the home of nobility and important people, the seat of government, the repository of the great tradition from which the little tradition of his village taps its strength. A *gari*, on the other hand, is merely a village or a town, of secondary importance. These terms are relative— what is *birni* to some is *gari* to others, and what is *gari* to some, to others is merely *'kauye*, a "hick town" or a tiny hamlet out in the bush. The *birni* is the capital: *birnin Katsina* is the great city of Katsina, at the head of all the *Katsinawa*; Lagos is *birnin Nijeriya*, the most important city in the country, the headquarters for the government and the home of the rulers of the entire land. To a man who lives in Kano or Katsina, the *gari* par excellence is his city—all the others are *'kauye*, "out in the sticks." To a Hausa peasant living in a modest village of 3,000 souls with a market twice a week, the *gari* is his village, and the *'kauyuka* are the scattered hamlets roundabout containing only a handful of families. He is the sophisticated urbanite; they are "bush." The *birni*, viewed in local terms, is the major administrative and commercial center nearby, where markets go on all the time. Villagers in southern Katsina used to refer to the town of Funtua, with its twenty-four-hour electric power, cotton ginnery, government hospital, administrative offices, railroad station, and secondary schools as *birnimmu*, "our [local] *birni*," as opposed to Katsina, which was the *birni* for the whole emirate. Funtua was the *birni*, their village outlying it was the *gari*, and the hamlets still further out were the *'kauye*.[13]

The *gari*, then, is the principal Hausa referent to the social world. To be a *'dan gari*, a "son of the village," is to be a man informed about what is going on, an active and influential participant in affairs, a true "son of the soil" or a "man about town." As such, the term is used as an expression of approbation, a compliment. Contrapuntally, to be a *'dan duniya*, a "son of the world," or a *'dan iska*, a "son of the wind," is to be a rootless drifter, a wastrel, one who goes away and leaves the village to travel and seek after adventure and engage in suspect and riotous living, neglecting his proper role as a respectful, stable member of the village community. At the other end of the scale is the *'dan*

13. For a discussion of urban influences on the rural Hausa see Miner (1965). Patterns of labor migration to Funtua in particular are discussed in Olofson (1976).

'kauye, a "son of a hamlet," a country bumpkin who lacks sophistica-
tion, proper manners, and is ignorant of the way the world really runs.
Both the 'dan duniya and the 'dan 'kauye are extremes opposed to the
ideal status of being a 'dan gari.

As the village is the usual limit of everyday experience—many girls
reach puberty and marry without having been more than a few miles
from their natal village, and boys may reach advanced youth before
they have any travel experience—it is not surprising that the noun gari
has connotations such as "everybody," "the whole world," "the sphere
of human affairs."[14] To say of a man ganin gari gareshi (literally "seeing the town is with him") is to say that he is clever, perceptive in
observing the world, that he knows what's what. To say something like
gari ba da'di ("the town is unpleasant") or gari ya lalace ("the town
has spoiled") means that the general state of affairs is not good, that
times are hard, or that morals and proper behavior have declined. To
"know the town" is to know how things are going, to participate fully
in communal affairs, to fit in smoothly with the functioning of village
society. In general living, the village world and the moral order are
synonymous.

The typical Hausa village is a closely settled concatenation of compounds, joining each other in a maze of walls and fences with entry-
huts opening onto the street.[15] Most Hausa construction in rural areas
is done with sun-dried mud-bricks. A shallow foundation is cut in the
ground and from this base a wall is built with bricks and a sticky mortar of clay and straw until it reaches the desired height. For a dwelling,
the roof is made by laying large pieces of wood obliquely on the corners
of the walls, working in from the sides toward the center, then covering
these with woven grass mats or pieces of cardboard until the whole is
closed over. This rough roof is then encased by several inches of thick
mud plaster and allowed to dry. Needless to say, such work is only done
in the dry season before the coming of the rains and must be repeated
every year in order to insure a leak-free roof throughout the wet agricultural season. The very wealthy can afford roofs of corrugated sheet
metal and plaster walls covered with a thin veneer of cement. The poor
members of the community must be content with conical thatched roofs,

14. The connotations of the noun gari in Hausa are dealt with in two excellent
articles by Dalby (1964, 1975).
15. On traditional Hausa architecture and town planning see Moughtin (1964).

usually set on a hut made from cheaper materials—lashed bundles of guinea-corn stalks set in the ground and plastered over with mud—buildings that are not unpleasant to live in, but are fearful fire hazards at the height of the dry season.[16]

The compounds of a neighborhood are arranged in lines down the streets. These may be of varying size and shape, usually two compounds deep with a street on each side so that if one were to enter a compound, scale the rear fence into the neighboring household, and go out his neighbor's front entryway, he would be back on another street. In more complicated arrangements access is provided by a narrow alleyway, which branches in and out within the settled area, emerging again onto the main thoroughfare. Frequently, too, there are gates from compound to compound inside so that women who are secluded from public view by the rules of Islamic *purdah* marriage (in Hausa, *auren kulle*, "locked-up marriage") can have access to friends and neighbors without exposing themselves to the common gaze. The exact demarcation of one household from another depends upon the character of the compound head, his relations with his neighbors, and the mode of construction employed—solid mud-brick walls are much more imposing than a sagging fence of cornstalks, which always deteriorates within a season or two.

Thus, walking down a village street one is faced with what appears to be a nearly continuous wall of mud-bricks, interspersed with guinea-corn fencing, and with numerous doorways piercing the exterior facade. Many of these doorways will have mud-brick benches built up alongside them, where men gather to chat and idle away the hours in the

16. In communities as densely settled as Hausa villages, fires (*gobara*) are frightening things, and some occur in every village each year. Since the dried stalks of guinea-corn, the major food source, are widely used in building (this is also a major reason for the reluctance to raise shorter-stemmed but larger-yielding varieties), the fire potential is enormous. A fire out of control in one compound can quickly spread to those surrounding it in a rapidly rising conflagration that destroys all a man's possessions, leaving him completely destitute in the space of a few short minutes. Some of the saddest sights I have seen in my life have been isolated compounds out in the bush destroyed by fire, or a section of a village blackened and burnt out. In such cases a man's neighbors will collect as much money as they can to help tide the unfortunate victim over. The Hausa proverb, however, expresses the situation better: *Gida biyu maganin gobara*, "Two houses are medicine for fire."

shade. Some doors will open into houses, others will give access to a shop where a tailor (or perhaps several tailors) will be hard at work sewing for customers, or a store where a merchant will have his wares displayed: salt, sugar, batteries, perfume, bicycle parts, cheap earrings, candies. Along the sides of the street in the shade of trees men will have set up small tables selling mangoes, kolanuts, candy, bits of coconut, or sugarcane. Old women, past the age where wife seclusion is regarded as necessary, may be sitting in the shade selling vegetables, yarn, or cooked foods. Under a tree farther along, a bicycle mechanic may have his place of business. Scrawny goats and sheep commonly forage for food around the walls of compounds and in the road. Ducks may be seen picking with their bills for food in the wet patches where the water from compound washing places and urinary latrines runs out through small holes in the walls into rudimentary (or nonexistent) gutters by the street. Chickens squawk and cackle in the dust, searching for seeds.

■ Household, Family, and Kinship

The entry-hut (*zaure*) opening to the street is the social focus of a man's household. The *zaure* is the place where a man greets his friends, receives social calls, and conducts his business. It is where men gather to discuss the state of the world, and where many—particularly the boys in the family—sleep at night. The inside of the compound (which cannot usually be glimpsed from inside the entry-hut due to the presence of an L-shaped wall designed to ensure privacy) is off-limits to all except the most intimate friends of the family. Children, of course, can and do enter almost any compound at will—they are welcome everywhere and serve as intermediaries between the women of various households who have no other means of communication with each other; but men do not enter the inner recesses of their neighbors' homes except under extraordinary circumstances—a feast on the naming day of a child, to help with funeral arrangements, to aid in construction of a new building, or to replaster a roof or wall, etc. This is usually true even of intimate companions, who will send a child inside to inquire if their friend is at home. It simply is not proper for a "strange" adult male to be in the company of another man's wives.[17]

17. Even after fifteen months of friendly residence in a village of some 3,000 people comprising nearly 600 separate households, there were only about a dozen com-

Within the compound proper there are several different areas. In a household where a man has more than one wife, each wife will have her own hut. The husband will frequently have his own room as well, perhaps communicating with the *zaure* by a separate door. In the middle of the compound is a central cooking area, marked off by the three stones (*murfu*) used to support the cooking pots. While there may be more than one wife, there is only one *murfu*, for the wives alternate in preparing the food for the household or work in conjunction with each other. An ideally situated household will have its own well, further minimizing the necessity for the women of the family to go out in public. Total seclusion of women is not only deemed desirable from a religious point of view, but also shows that the compound is sufficiently well-off economically to afford to keep its women inside. Adjoining the compound wall, to one side of the courtyard, is a place used for washing and bathing. In the back of the compound is the latrine (*bayan gida*, "behind the compound"), a deep well-like pit covered over except for an opening (usually a large clay pot with the bottom broken out) where household members can defecate or urinate.[18] This opening is covered with a clay pot when not in use. If the compound has goats or sheep there is usually a shelter for them inside, as well. A man wealthy enough to own cattle (used for plowing fields) will either build a separate compound in the village to use as a corral or will leave them in the bush under the care of a trusted Fulani cattle-herder.

This *gida*—a word best translated as "household" or "compound"— is the basic unit of social organization, the small domain that each man rules as his own. As the proverb says, *Mutum a gidansa sarki ne*, "A man in his *gida* is a chief." The head of the *gida*, the *maigida* (literally "owner of the *gida*") is the senior male, usually the husband of the women and the father of the sons who may be living with him. In gen-

---

pounds that I would not have hesitated to enter—and allowances were made for the fact that I was a European and not totally bound by local Hausa strictures of behavior.

18. The location where one urinates is not quite so important as where defecation takes place, if for no other reason than urine is liquid and evaporates to dryness leaving no traces, whereas feces do not. A man would always go inside his compound to defecate, but would not hesitate to go off by the side of the road and urinate in the grass or against a wall or fence. Women, of course, take care of both bodily functions inside.

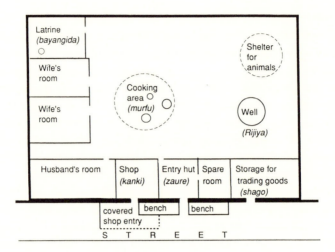

Figure 3   Sketch plan of the compound of Alhaji Audu Tela,
a prosperous village trader.

eral usage, however, any man who gets married is referred to as *mai-gida*, even though he may be living with and economically dependent on his father, who is recognized as the senior authority in the compound. Similarly, an old man who is no longer able to work and is living with his son is called *maigida* out of respect, even though it is obvious that the real authority now lies with his son. Sometimes a father and several older married sons will all live together, in which case each family (*iyali*) within the compound is recognized as having a *maigida* within the larger *gida* as a whole. In these cases a question such as "Who is *maigida* here?" will elicit a response like "There are three *masugida* here." In extraordinary circumstances the *maigida* may even be a woman, a widow living alone, for example. In the case of one disreputable village reprobate—a slacker and a wastrel who lived in his father's old compound with his widowed mother—only she possessed sufficient moral standing in the community to be regarded rightly as the *maigida*.[19]

19. This fellow's father had been killed in an automobile crash several years before and he had promptly squandered his inheritance. His fields were never well tended; he merely planted them and harvested what came up at the end of the season. He

The *gida* itself is composed of the wives (*mata*) and children (*yara*) of the household head, his sons and their families, unmarried daughters, older relatives who are no longer able to support themselves, and any other people who may be living more or less permanently with them, such as a hired laborer who is working the fields of the household head and is also taking lodging with him, or patients who have come for prolonged treatment at the compound of a healer (*boka*). In cases such as these, the persons in question would be reckoned as members of the household (*gida*), but probably not as members of the family (*iyali*). For most purposes, however, the *gida* and the *iyali* are synonymous. The primary term of reference is the *gida*, for it refers to a residence and a location (the actual buildings of the compound), as well as the members inhabiting it; the *iyali* is usually coterminous with this, but as this is more a term of blood relationship, not necessarily so.

Hausa kinship organization does not extend beyond these conceptions of the *gida* and *iyali*. There is no pyramiding segmentary kinship system encompassing the whole social order such as those found among the Nuer or other East African tribes. The most important unit of social organization is the household. In daily living broader ties of kinship are relatively unimportant.[20] Muslim village-dwelling Hausa have no system of clanship, which exists even among the pagan Maguzawa Hausa only in rudimentary form.[21] There is no Hausa word that may properly be translated as "clan." *Dangi* is the only word that approximates such a sense, and it is best translated by the more general term "relatives." The word *iyali* refers primarily to the husband, his wives, and their

---

spent most of his time with prostitutes (and always complained of having gonorrhea), gambling, drinking beer, or traveling to other villages in search of excitement. Although he had been married, his wife had left him, taking their child with her. His half-brother, on the other hand, was one of the nicest men I have ever met, and was widely regarded as a man of excellent character (*mutumin kirki*), as opposed to his brother, who was variously described as a *shegen banza* (worthless bastard), a *'dan iska* (son of the wind, that is, having no proper responsibilities) or a *'dan bura* (son of a penis).

20. "Indeed, it would appear to be perfectly possible to consider the structure of a Hausa town or village without paying any attention at all to the operation of kinship principles, although these do in fact play a small part, though mainly only in the allocation of offices" D. P. L. Dry (1950:180).

21. See the discussion of this subject in Greenberg (1947a).

children. *Dangi,* on the other hand, is used to refer to more distant relatives, the family of the mother's brother or the father's brother, etc. Two brothers, for example, each married and living in a separate *gida* would be considered *iyali daban,* "of different families," but *dangi duka 'daya,* "of the same *dangi*" (that is, relatives of each other). If one were discussing both brothers in relation to their father, they would be *iyali 'daya,* "of the same family," since he begat them both.

The only Hausa word for kinship relationships at a level higher than *dangi* is *kabila,* or "tribe," which is used only in reference to different ethnic groups such as Ibo, Yoruba, Nupe, Tiv, Gwari, and so on. In general speech a construction such as *mutanen Ibo,* "Ibo people," or *Yarabawa,* "Yorubas," would probably be used in place of *kabila.*

The terminology of Hausa kinship *(dangantaka)* describes and organizes the wider field of relationships that surrounds the basic family *(iyali).*[22] The Hausa reckon descent bilaterally, and a man may trace relationship through his father's kin *(dangin uba)* or his mother's *(dangin uwa),* but in practical matters such as residence, inheritance, marriage negotiations, etc., the agnatic side is more important. The nomenclature of kinship describes the pattern of blood and affinal ties within which the individual is placed, and gives a clue as to the proper behavior expected from an individual so situated. Relationships of seniority and youth are an important aspect of the structure of this system.

An individual has two biological parents: a father, *uba,* and a mother, *uwa.* Together they are the "ones who gave birth to an individual," *mahaifa.* These are terms of reference, not address. To use them to the individual in question would be impolite; rather, a child addresses his father as *baba* (or perhaps *alhaji,* if he has made the pilgrimage to Mecca), and his mother as *inna.* There are, however, other individuals to whom these words are also applied. *Baba* is a term referring to the father's brothers, husbands of the father's sisters, and by polite extension, to older men of the father's generation as a term of affectionate

22. Other discussions of Hausa kinship terminology may be found in D. P. L. Dry (1950, 1956), M. F. Smith (1954), M. G. Smith (1954:21–27, 1955, 1965a, 1978:46–50), Madauci et al. (1968:25–80), Faulkingham (1970:131–42), Nicolas (1975), and LeVine and Price-Williams (1974). There are some regional variations in terminology through Hausaland.

respect.[23] *Inna* is used in addressing sisters of the mother, the mother's brother's wife, and the mother's co-wives in the compound. Two other words, *gwaggo* and *baba*,[24] are sometimes used to describe the father's sister or the wife of the father's brother. *Kawu* refers to the mother's brother and may also be used to address the husband of one of the mother's sisters. The word *iyaye*, "parents," which is related to the word for family (*iyali*) often is used to include various of these other members of the biological parents' generation. The generation above that of one's parents consists of *kakani*, "grandparents," and the term *kaka* is used for any grandparent, male or female, and collateral relatives such as great-uncles, great-aunts, etc. Great-grandparents are also included in the term *kaka*. The term *kakanin kakanimmu*, "our grandparents' grandparents" is a general term for ancestors.

With reference to the generation of his parents, a child stands in a situation of discipline and respect, particularly regarding the paternal side. Since there is a patrilateral bias to Hausa society due to residence, marriage, farming obligations, and so forth, it is not surprising that those relatives denoted *baba* ("father") should be treated with deference and respect as persons of authority, while simultaneously there is an easier relationship with the *kawu* (the maternal uncle) which often borders on affectionate friendship, even though such an uncle still has the right of discipline. Women, occupying positions of little power in society (as perpetual minors in Islamic law) but entrusted with the preparation of food and most of the day-to-day tasks of raising children, are sources of more affection and comfort than are the men, even though they, too, must discipline the children. Grandparents, however, one generation removed and often past positions of active economic responsibility in the household, stand in a playful status to their grandchildren, and are regarded as proper "joking partners" (*abokin wasa*) for them.

Within the child's own generation there are several categories of relationships. The most basic distinction is that between children of the same father and mother, *'yanuwa* (literally "children of the mother"),

23. I was often called *baba* as a term of respect, particularly by women old enough to be my grandmother—a situation that never ceased to amuse me.
24. Here *baba* is a different word from the above, being high-long, low-short tonally, in contrast with the low-long, high-short tones of "father."

and children of the same father but different mothers, 'yanuba (literally "children of the father"). This is a distinction of some significance in a society where polygamous marriages are commonplace. In general, the term used for brother is 'danuwa, "son of the mother," and that for sister is 'yaruwa, "daughter of the mother." Attention is not drawn to the difference in parentage among brothers and sisters unless someone is looking for trouble. For social purposes full consanguinity should always be emphasized. As the proverb says, 'Danuwa rabin jiki, "A brother is half of the body." Additionally, there are terms of age grada-tion among siblings: wa means "elder brother," 'kane means "younger brother," yaya refers to a senior sister, and 'kanwa designates a junior sister. These terms are all used for cousins, patrilateral or matrilateral. With all of these people the child has an easy, playful relationship, even though elder children may be entrusted with looking after the younger ones. These relationships form an important part of the child's social development: Mafi da'din rai 'danuwa, "A brother is dearer than life itself," in the proverbial wisdom.

In the generation below oneself the kinship designations are straight-forward: 'da means "son," and 'diya or 'ya means "daughter." These terms are used for nephews and nieces as well, and may be extended to others with whom one has a similarly close kind of relationship.[25] The first child born to a marriage is referred to as 'dam fari, "the first son" if it is a boy and 'yar fari, "the first daughter" if it is a girl. The firstborn child is never addressed by name by the parents, this transi-tional relationship being an object of "respectful shame," (kunya). In contrast, the youngest child is called auta and an especially affectionate relationship with his parents may develop. When parents get too old to work they will often take up residence with their youngest son. Grand-sons are called jika, granddaughters jikanya; great-nephews and nieces are included as well. Great-grandchildren and great-great-grandchildren may be included in the above classifications, or the terms ta'ba kunne or 'dan jika, and tatta'ba kunne may be used, respectively. All one's descendants are referred to collectively as zuri'a.

Within the household itself the compound head is addressed as mai-

25. Several older members of the community with whom I was quite close adopted me as their "son." On occasion I have even heard people say ya haife ni, "he begat me" in playful terms of such people, with whom no blood relationship existed.

gida, or perhaps *alhaji.* He commands a position of respect, as does his senior wife, the *uwargida,* "mother of the compound." The youngest wife is called *amarya,* "bride," and often may be treated as if she were a servant by the other, older women of the household. Wives may adopt the kin terms for sisters in their dealings with each other, or they may call each other by name. Husbands and wives may also call each other by name, depending on their relationship. The interaction of husbands and wives is subject to individual variation. The relationship may be affectionate and close, or it may be formal and more distant. It is always complicated by the addition of another wife.

By its very nature plural marriage is a diplomatic challenge, the success or failure of which depends upon a judicious balance among husband and co-wives. While a second wife may be welcomed by her senior as a friend and helpmate, the equipoise between them is one of the most precarious in Hausa society. The word for co-wife is *kishiya,* which translates literally as "the jealous one," from *kishi,* "jealousy." It also has the connotation of opposite, as in *ba'ki kishiyar fari ne,* "Black is the opposite [literally co-wife] of white." In a polygamous society where one man has several wives and separate sets of offspring from each one, the politics of the household can be very treacherous. A man must treat each wife equally, provide her with a room and clothing equivalent to her rivals, and provide for her children on an equal footing with the others. To develop an imbalance in his domestic politics, to create a favored wife (*mowa*) and a wife who is scorned (*bora*) is to invite disruption, quarreling, perhaps adultery or divorce (*kashen aure,* "killing the marriage"). Such internal politics affect the children and their interrelations as well. The word *'danubanci,* "the ways of half-brothers" is a Hausa synonym for "malevolence."

Hausa proverbs provide a wealth of commentary on wifely rivalries: *Kishiya mai-ban haushi,* "Co-wife, bringer of vexation." *Ba na gasa gado 'dan kishiya ya hau,* "I will not make a bed for my co-wife's son to use." *Ba kukana ba, uwar kishiya ta mutu,* "It's not my sorrow— my co-wife's mother died." *Da alheri, uwar kishiya ta hau kura,* "Goodbye and good luck, the mother of my co-wife has ridden off on a hyena." *Na ta'ba ki da alherin Allah, kishiya ta ta'ba kishiya da bakin wuta,* " ' I've touched you with God's blessing!' cried the co-wife as she stuck her rival with a firebrand." In Hausa folklore the treacheries of co-wives are legendary,[26] and in talking about sorcery (*sammu*) the subject of rival wives invariably comes up for discussion.

Marriage creates a whole new set of affinal relationships (*surukuta*), which are assimilated to the kinship terminology. Male in-laws, particularly the father of the bride, are referred to as *suruki;* female in-laws, particularly the new wife's mother, are called *suruka.* These relationships with the father and mother of one's wife, with her elder brothers and sisters, and with the father's other wives, are all marked by rigid behavior and "respectful avoidance" (*kunya*). A man's dealings with these people will be dignified, polite, and formal, and they will be addressed (at least early in the relationship) by the terms *suruki* and *suruka.* Some time later, depending on the individuals involved, he may refer to them by other terms of kinship reference: a man referring to his father-in-law as *baba,* his mother-in-law as *inna,* his brothers and sisters-in-law as *wa, 'kane, yaya, 'kanwa,* etc. With his junior in-laws, however, the case is much different. His wife's younger brothers and sisters assume the status of younger brothers and sisters to him and joking relationships are formed between them. The wife's younger sisters may be playfully called "wife" by her husband. Similarly, her husband's brothers will refer to her as "our wife" and a good deal of banter will be exchanged between them.

Although the Hausa have no clans or lineages extending kinship beyond the family (*iyali*) and immediate circle of relatives (*dangi*), kinship terminology pervades much of social life. The imagery of blood relationship is frequently used in situations where one wants to minimize the social distance between two people, to create a feeling of intimacy and personal closeness. The terms *'danuwa* and *'yaruwa,* "full brother" and "full sister," are often extended to include anyone who resides in the same village, emirate, or state, belongs to the same tribe, or comes from the same country. *'Da,* "son" is used to mean somebody coming from a particular area, such as *'Dan Kano,* "a Kano man," or one who has an intimate relationship with a particular item. Policemen are called *'dan sanda,* "sons of the cudgel" for example. Terms such as *'dan gari,* "son of the village," and *'dan iska,* "son of the wind," have been discussed previously. Terms such as *uban gida,* "father of the

26. See particularly Tremearne (1913), Johnston (1966), and Skinner (1969, 1977a) for examples of the treacheries of co-wives in Hausa folklore.

compound," and *ubangiji*, "father" or "master," are used by subordinates, laborers, and similar dependents in reference to their superiors, who should assume a fatherly, caring, protective attitude toward them. As such, these terms are frequently used by beggars, who by employing the terminology of kinship hope to create a sense of moral obligation in the person addressed. A beggar will frequently claim to be an orphan (*maraya*) in addition to using the vocabulary of kinship, hoping to further his cause by suggesting that only the person to whom he is appealing can meet his needs. Hence the proverb *In ka ji maraya, rago*, "If you hear [a man plead he is] an orphan, [mark him as] a loafer."

If the use of kinship terminology in non-kin settings serves to minimize the social distance between two people, denial of kinship, or the more pointed implication that someone lacks legitimate ancestry, maximizes the social distance between them and puts (or tries to put) the other beyond the moral pale. Almost all Hausa insults and obscenities are based around this notion. A *shege* is a "bastard," and *shegentaka*, "bastardliness" refers to a whole range of mischievous, immoral, or criminal behavior. One Hausa proverb which is an exhortation to stop useless tasks states *Bari neman uba ga shege, Allah bai yi masa uba ba*, "Stop looking for the father of a bastard; God didn't make one for him." *'Dan karuwa*, "son of a whore," has similar implications. In both cases a man is defined or described as lacking decent family, with all the behavioral expectations that encompasses. The obscenities *ubanka!* ("Your father!") and *uwarka!* ("Your mother!") sometimes loosely translated in Hausa dictionaries as "damn you!," carry similar connotations.[27] Actually these are shortened forms of *ka ci burar ubanka!*, "You eat your father's penis!" or *ka ci uwarka!*, "You motherfucker!"[28] —truly outrageous expressions in almost any culture. *Kafiri*, "unbeliever," goes beyond kinship in placing a man outside the entire moral order of Islam.

---

27. On one ocassion the young daughter (she was only three or four years old) of one of my neighbors had been naughty and had angered her father. He grabbed her by the arm, shook her, scolded her and said "*uwarki!*" to her several times, sending her inside the compound crying. The incongruity of a man saying *uwarki*, "your mother!" to his own daughter has never left me.
28. Even as "gosh!" is a more acceptable expression than "God!" or "darn!" than "damn!" in English.

■ Agriculture and the Cycle of the Seasons

The economic basis of rural life is agriculture, and the fundamental
farming unit is the family (*iyali*). The village forms a central area of
habitations, around which are scattered farm plots (*gonaki*) of varying
shapes and sizes that give the countryside the ragged patchwork appearance it has when seen from the air. Each family head has his own
personal farms, called *gayauni*, which he cultivates for food and to
raise cash crops for hard currency. If he is fortunate his land will all
be closely grouped; if not, his labor will be increased as he spreads his
efforts in varying sectors of the countryside. Title to land is not absolute—the community, through the village chief, ultimately has some say
in how unused or abandoned land is apportioned[29]—but in practice the
usufructuary rights to land use are permanent and heritable, unless
modified by other dispositions such as lease (*haya*), loan (*aro*), sale
(*saye*), gift (*kyauta*), pledging against a loan (*jingina*), placing in trust
(*ajiya*) while an extended journey is made, or a sharecropping arrangement (*kashi mu raba*) in which, for example, a man aids another in
raising groundnuts on his own land, in return for which privilege and
assistance the crop is divided after harvest.

In addition to these *gayauna* farms a man may be in *gandu*. *Gandu*
is a voluntary economic relationship between fathers and sons (or more
rarely between brothers) in which the son enters into an agreement to

---

29. "Land tenure in Hausaland has a double ancestry, in traditional African concepts of communal ownership and in Islamic land law which recognized individual tenure. The basis of the present system was communal, whereby it was recognized that members resident within the village community had the right to use as
much of the land of the community as they required, but in no sense could the
land be alienated from the community. Little is known of legal conditions under
the Hausa rulers, but after the Fulani conquered Hausaland during the nineteenth
century they arrogated to themselves ownership of land. However, the customary
rights of the individual farmer to occupy and use a portion of the land of his community survived. Rights to land were held by the family whilst the village head
maintained the traditional community control of land. Land was allocated by him
to immigrants settling in the community and reverted to the community in the
events of migration, fallow land being left beyond a recognized number of years,
and the death of an heirless cultivator. Normally at death, land was transferred to
the heirs of the cultivator". (Goddard et al. 1971:27) On land tenure see also
Luning (1965) and McDowell (1969).

cultivate a large family farm under his father's supervision and control, in return for which the father provides food for the son's family, pays the tax (*haraji*) for the adult males in the *gandu*, and looks after the housing needs of the entire compound.[30] Sons in *gandu* will also have *gayauni* farms to cultivate for their own benefit in the afternoons after the *gandu* work of the morning is finished. The *gandu* arrangement makes it easier for a newly married son to establish his household and also provides security for the father as he ages by binding together his own welfare with that of his sons. The proverb says *'Dan mai-gona wanda ya fi 'dan mai-gayya, ko da da nuna iyaka*, "The son of the house is better than a hireling, whatever work you want him for."

Since the economic foundation of rural Hausaland is farming, the rhythms of nature dictate the ebb and flow of economic activity. Although the European calendar is used for governmental and administrative purposes, and the uncorrected Muslim lunar calendar (which rotates through the European calendar over the course of time) is used to keep track of ritual events such as the fast of Ramadan and the month of the pilgrimage, it is the cycle of the seasons that determines the passage of social time and the economic preoccupations of village life. Since nearly all rural Hausa men are farmers first and pursue other occupations secondarily, their activities must follow the course that nature dictates, farming when the weather mandates it and undertaking other enterprises when agricultural activity is not feasible.

The climate of Hausaland is tropical savannah with distinct wet and dry seasons.[31] The mean annual rainfall around Zaria is about 43 inches, decreasing steadily to about 30 inches in the vicinity of Sokoto or Katsina; the dry season is perfectly rainless. This marked disparity in the distribution of rain throughout the year manifests itself in the vegetation of the surrounding countryside—blasted, brown, and withered throughout the dry season, but springing into lush verdancy when the rains descend. The dry season (*rani*) lasts roughly from October through April or May and is followed by a wet season (*damina*) lasting from June through September, although there may be considerable

30. On *gandu* arrangements among the Hausa see Greenberg (1964:17–19), Buntjer (1971), and especially Hill (1972:38–56).
31. See Buchanan and Pugh (1955:21–40) and Hore (1970) on the climate of northern Nigeria.

variation in these dates. The Hausa recognize subdivisions in these seasons, giving a yearly cycle of four seasons, each with its attendant characteristics.

The beginning of the dry season corresponds to the ripening of the crops and is known in Hausa as *kaka,* the harvest. The days are hot but the nights begin to cool. The relative humidity begins to drop, and dust and haze accumulate as the land dries out. December and January are the months of *hunturu,* the harmattan wind that blows down from northeastern Africa bringing masses of dust and grit, which cloud the air up to heights of 5,000 feet, giving the sky a gloomy, overcast look which may be mistaken by foreigners for approaching rain. Visibility may decrease notably—a factor that often results in the closing of Kano airport. Days when the haze is slight may be very hot, but the nights are often cold, and fires are built in the early morning in the villages for heat. The harvest marks the end of agricultural activities and with it dry season occupations are undertaken—crafts, repair of buildings, and occasional migration in search of wage labor. The cotton harvest occurs during harmattan but this is finished by late January or early February, and then several slack months follow. *Bazara,* the period of mounting humidity and heat prior to the rains, is probably the most miserable time of the year. The days are often oppressively hot and there is little alleviation at night. Many people sleep outside to gain relief from *zuffa,* the overbearing heat, humidity, and their own constant sweating, which is intensified by the mud-brick houses, with their lack of lighting and poor ventilation. In this period farmers begin to prepare for planting, rooting out old cornstalks and burning them in the fields. More prosperous farmers haul compound sweepings and dung from the village to their fields to use as fertilizer (*taki*). Early in the morning one can see strings of laden donkeys heading for the fields, where scattered little mounds of refuse mark their progress across the landowner's domain.

In April or May the first relief from the heat comes in the form of the early light rains. Once the first spatters have started to soften the ground the village farmers begin to prepare for planting. If the field has been fallow it must be plowed with ridges raised to receive the seed. Unless the farmer is wealthy enough to have his own team of oxen and metal plow, or to have enough money laid aside to hire them, this must be done by hand. The *galma,* a large, flat-bladed hoe which is

almost more like a shovel, is used for such work. If the field was cultivated the previous year it may not need much reworking, only weeding
in preparation for the seed. After three or four showers the land is
ready for planting. The principal Hausa foods are *dawa* (guinea-corn,
Sorghum vulgare) and *gero* (millet, *Pennisetum typhoideum*), but fal-
lowing, rotation, and intercropping are common and a wide variety
of other foodstuffs are grown: cassava, okra, red peppers, sweet potatoes, yams, tomatoes, rice, sugarcane, sweet corn, onions, cowpeas,
koko-yams, and groundnuts.

Guinea-corn and millet are planted early in the agricultural season.
When the land has been prepared the farmer takes his hoe and a bowl
of seed and begins walking up and down his field. Every two steps or
so he digs a small hole with the hoe or with his foot, throws down a
small portion of seed, covers it over, and moves on until the entire field
has been sown. This done, he hopes for rain to come and water the
seeds until they sprout and push through the soil. If the rains are contrary and stop inexplicably, the young shoots may die and replanting
will be necessary. The period from planting to the onset of the daily
showers of the full rainy season is a time of some uneasiness. Some
men, however, are fortunate enough to hold farmland near a river. This
land, called *fadama*, is valuable for it has ready access to water and can
be irrigated to sustain crops the year round. A dike can be made in the
riverbed to gather water for raising into the field by bucket and lever.
Onions, peppers, tomatoes, and the like can then be grown throughout
the seasons. Some men of exceptional energy may maintain such a
garden close to the village by digging a well next to it and hauling water
out to keep their small plot of vegetables moist enough to survive; but
most farmers can only wait and hope: *Damina mai-ban samu,* "Season
of rains, giver of wealth."

Once the sprouts have broken through the soil the arduous work of
cultivating begins, for with the shoots of guinea-corn come weeds. The
care with which the young plants are tended has a direct relation to the
success of the crops. Farmers who are diligent and work hard do well
if the weather remains favorable; wastrels who plant and then idle their
time away come off badly when the harvest is brought in, and numerous proverbs exhort people to industry using the farming motif: *In ka
ga yabanya ta yi kyau daga noman fari ta samu,* "If you see young corn
doing well, it is the result of the first hoeing." *Noma da tsambare*

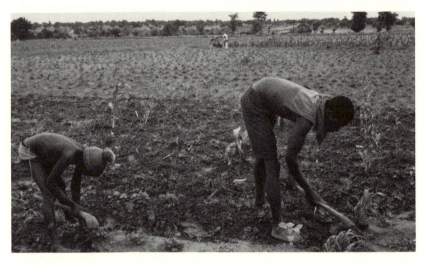

2. *Cultivating the fields by hand.*

wahala ne sai ya kara ciyawa, "Farming without weeding means trouble as the grass grows." *Kowa ya yi noma ya huta da awo*, "he who farms is spared buying corn." The agricultural season is a period of constant labor. As soon as the morning meal is over, men and boys leave for the farms, breaking at midday, then returning to the fields in the afternoon. Growing crops do not wait on the farmer's leisure. *Bawan damina, baturen rani*, "slave in the rains, 'white man' in the dry season"—only when the harvest is in can a man relax. Until the crops ripen the farmer must rely on his stored grain or whatever he may buy in the market-place. It therefore comes as a relief when the harvest is fully ripe and ready for gathering.

When the crops stand tall and fully grown the countryside is com-pletely transformed. Whereas in the dry season one could see for miles when standing in the fields, now the crops are high and almost jungle-like in places. Hausa guinea-corn grows quite tall, up to eight feet or higher at times.[32] These tall cornstalks are prized commodities for fenc-ing and building and are an integral part of the harvest—a fact that has worked against attempts to introduce higher-yielding but shorter-

32. A situation in which it is easy for the neophyte anthropologist to get lost in the countryside.

stalked varieties. Normally, the stalks are cut down with a small hand sickle and left in the fields. The heads, laden with grain, are then cut off and tied into small bundles for transport back to the village, where they are placed in elevated mud-and-cornstalk granaries until they are needed. When all of the crop has been carried to the village and stored, the cornstalks are gathered up and stacked in the field or are carried in for use in other activities such as building, fuel for cooking, or bonfires to provide light for nighttime Koranic schools. A bundle of corn is threshed by piling it on mats laid on the ground, flailing it, then scooping it into large gourd calabashes and pouring it out to winnow in the wind. The threshed grain may be stored in enameled basins or large sacks until pounded for making *tuwo*.

In addition to foodstuffs such as guinea-corn, farmers grow cash crops for sale: tobacco, henna, hemp, groundnuts, and cotton. Southern Katsina lies in the heartland of the Hausa cotton-growing region, and cotton forms the main cash crop for farmers there. Groundnuts are also grown, but village farmers often remarked that it took more effort to raise them than cotton, and they preferred the latter.[33] Cotton seed is provided by the Northern States Marketing Board, which also serves as the only buyer for cotton—a monopolistic arrangement designed to ensure a constant price for cotton in the face of fluctuating markets, although as Hill has noted (1972:289): "the original aim of stabilizing the producer-price over a term of years, by building up reserves in years when world prices were high, and deliberately depleting them when world prices fell, has been forgotten, and Marketing Boards have increasingly been used as convenient devices for taxing farmers, by means of export duties and other similar taxes."

Cotton is planted in the middle of the rainy season after careful plowing of the fields, in the same manner as guinea-corn or millet. Those able to afford it have their fields plowed by oxen, use commercial fertilizer bought in the market or from one of the agricultural development projects, and may even try to spray their crops with insecticides. The crop is weeded several times in the course of its growth. When the harvest time approaches, the cotton board sends its representatives to establish the cotton market on the outskirts of the village. Scales are

33. The fact that the 1975 groundnut crop was a failure all across Nigeria may have something to do with this attitude.

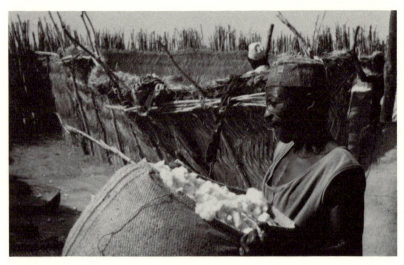

3. At work in the village cotton market.

erected, covered stalls for grading cotton are built, and lorries are hired to transport the raw cotton out of the village. When the cotton is ready the farmers turn out in force, and even women are taken to the fields to work—the harvest of cash crops such as cotton and groundnuts being one of the few times when, out of economic necessity, the restrictions of closed marriage may be lifted. The cotton is bagged, loaded on donkeys, and taken to the market, where each load is spread out on grass mats and graded as either Grade I or Grade II. Grade I (*lamba wan*) is higher quality than Grade II (*lamba tu*) and commands a higher price.[34] The farmer's load is then carried inside to the scales and weighed, and he is paid in cash for what he has brought in.[35] The cotton is stuffed into large bags, which are sewn shut and stacked for

34. The Hausa terms come from the English "number one" and "number two," respectively.
35. Since many of the men working in these markets are illiterate, the bookkeeping is often confused and haphazard, and charges of dishonesty can easily arise out of error. One man of sterling character and impeccable honesty—although illiterate—was accused of such a misappropriation of monies by a political rival in the village, who had recently seen his faction soundly defeated in the recent local government elections. The error eventually was resolved, but not without engendering more bad feeling between the two men.

transport to one of the ginneries in Funtua, Malumfashi, Gusau, or Zaria.

■ Secondary Occupations and Trading

The idiom of farming pervades rural Hausa culture,[36] but the rural economy is a mixed economy. While the major source of livelihood is agriculture, many men pursue an additional occupation (*sana'a*). These occupations may go on all year as a supplement to their income from farming, but invariably they take on added importance in the dry season when the agricultural labors are finished. The range of crafts and trades that may form a man's *sana'a* is extensive: drummer, crier or praise-singer, butcher, leatherworker, blacksmith, barber (*wanzami*), healer (*boka*), tinker, bicycle or motorcycle mechanic, carpenter, tailor, schoolteacher in a government school, Koranic scholar (*mallam*), laborer, market broker, weaver, or trader.[37] Some men pursue several trades at once in search of the elusive naira.

The proverb says *A san mutum a kan cinikinsa ko shan giya ta ke,* "A man is known by his occupation, even if it's just drinking beer." The Hausa particle *mai*, meaning "possessor of" or "owner of," is applied to personal characteristics: for example, *mai-'karfi* is "the strong one" or "possessor of strength"; *mai-kama aiki,* "the industrious worker"; the village head is *mai-gari,* "holder of the town," and so on. Such appellations are particularly important in business and trading,

36. A good example of this is a view that was taken of my work. One close friend of mine always referred to the village as my "farm" (*gona*) and my ballpoint pen as my "hoe" (*fartanya*). When I went out to stroll through the village and chat with people he always said I was "out checking on my farm."

37. Probably the most interesting occupation I came across was that of the *welda*. Several West African companies now make cheap rubber shoes and sandals which are very popular as footwear in rural Hausaland. The durability of these items is not very great. The thongs of the sandals tear out and holes are worn through the bottoms of the rubber slippers in a short time. The job of the *welda* is to take miscellaneous scraps of soft plastic and use hot irons to patch holes and reattach torn thongs on rubber shoes. The Hausa word comes from the English "welder."

Descriptions of these Hausa occupations may be found in Taylor and Webb (1932), Madauci et al. (1968) and in the anonymous work in Hausa *Labaru Na Da Da Na Yanzu* ("News of Then and Now") (1968). On the interesting occupation of praise-singing, see M. G. Smith (1957).

for they serve to identify people with particular items or occupations and, hence, to locate them in the structure of village life. *Namale mai-goro* is "Namale of the kolanuts"; *Ibrahim ma'dinki* is "Ibrahim the tailor" ("Ibrahim who sews"); *Lawai mai-toye-toye* is "Lawai the fried-food seller," etc. In market barter one asks for *mai-albasa*, "the onion man" or *mai-zuma*, "the honey seller." The Katsina word for a small market trader is *mashimfi'di*, "one who spreads out a mat [on which to show his wares]." In a society where rules of naming by family are as yet ambiguous (if they may be said to exist at all), identification by trade, residence, or personal characteristics are important in the fabric of daily living. If sons pick up and follow their father's occupation, these identifications take on more permanent meanings, and such continuity is approved.[38] *'Dan asali ya fi shigege*, "A son of pedigree is better than a newcomer"—one born to the job is best.

It cannot legitimately be said that there is a class stratification within Hausa village society.[39] There are differences in wealth, to be sure, between a trader who has accumulated enough money to buy a lorry and a poor wage-laborer who works in the fields of his neighbors and does odd jobs for his keep. But in practical reality the vast majority of villagers regard each other as belonging to the same social group: the *talakawa*, or society of peasant farmers. They all are part of the slowly changing rural agricultural world. Where everyone lives in houses made of mud-bricks or plastered cornstalks, enormous differences in the standards of living are unlikely; those that do exist are manifested mainly in the acquisition of consumer goods such as wristwatches, metal beds, transistor radios, and flashy clothes.

There are, however, gradations in status and prestige, particularly with regard to occupations. The village headman and the *limam* of the Friday mosque stand at the head of the list, followed closely by Koranic scholars of high standing. Prosperous farmers and traders come next, their wealth and commercial success being seen as a special favor of God. Craftsmen such as tailors, smiths, potters, and weavers hold an

38. The origins of English names such as Smith, Carpenter, and Baker are parallel cases.
39. M. G. Smith implied such class distinctions in his article on Hausa social status (1959), but was clearly straining reality in so doing. He has been criticized by Yeld (1960), and more trenchantly in "The Absence of Class" in Hill (1972:175–88). His reply to Yeld is in M. G. Smith (1961).

intermediate position, while the bottom spaces are occupied by butchers, barbers, drummers, praise-singers, and laborers. But even so, no one occupation is seen as "better" than another—a *sana'a* is a *sana'a*—and a person's position in society is determined by far more than his occupation alone.

Farming aside, the most common village occupation is trading. The Hausa are a commercial people and have been so for centuries. The early prominence of Katsina and Kano was due largely to their position on the trans-Saharan caravan routes. While not operating on such a grand scale, the rural Hausa villager is nonetheless a market venturer. The Hausa word for business or "trading," *ciniki*, is practically a synonym for *sana'a*, "occupation." *Cinikin duniya*, "trading of the world," is an expression used in the sense of "the way of the world," the manner in which fate wheels and deals with the lives of men. Nearly everybody trades in something, if only on a small scale, and the constant interchange of kolanuts and small coins in the process of greeting is but one manifestation of the deeply rooted economic transactionalism of Hausa culture.[40] It might be said with only slight exaggeration that the Hausa man's two activities are farming and trading, for each is favored in its turn by the dichotomy of the seasons. In the wet season people are detained by the imperatives of agriculture and the difficulty of traveling in the mud and rain; in the dry season they are free to travel as they please and the harvest of the cash crops means there is ready money for trade goods. As a result, wet-season markets are less busy than those of the dry season, and trade is sluggish.

Village markets are not held every day.[41] Usually they take place once or twice a week, the market day varying from place to place within a given locality to permit people to attend all the nearby markets and spread the economic activities over a broader area. Markets are generally set on the edge of town, next to the road, allowing free

40. This economic interchange extends to children, who early pick up commercial interests, buying and selling things for their mothers, who are secluded inside the houses. Children also branch out on their own, selling toys they have made to their friends, etc. One enterprising lad, a neighbor of mine, asked if he could have my old magazines, which I bought in Zaria from time to time. Since he liked to look at the pictures I let him have them, only to discover that he was doing a lively business among his friends, selling them for ten kobo a copy!
41. On Hausa markets see particularly M. G. Smith (1955, 1965), and Hill and Smith (1972).

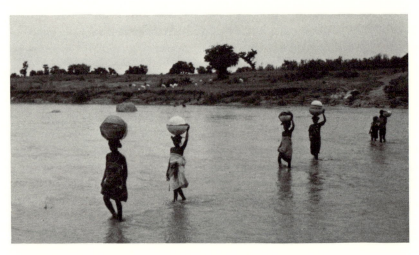

4. *Fulani women crossing the river to come to the village
in the wet season.*

access for lorry traffic and permitting the market to expand if necessary.
Throughout the marketplace are large numbers of open-sided sheds
covered with either thatch or a sheet-tin roof. These are the market
stalls where traders display their wares, paying a nominal monthly fee
to the local government authority for a license. It is not necessary to
have such a stall; a position can be taken up under the shade of a tree
or out in the sun with wares spread out on a grass mat; alternatively, a
trader can simply walk through the market displaying goods for sale on
a tray or in a basket—a practice called *talla* in Hausa. There are various
sections of the market where people engaged in similar trades congregate—a section reserved for the sale of animals, a section devoted to
the vending of snack food by women, an area for trading in grain, a
section for the sale of roasted meats, and another for the sale of freshly
slaughtered meat.

On nonmarket days there is always some activity in the marketplace—a few old men or women selling vegetables, children playing, a
lorry occasionally discharging passengers—but on market days the
place is crammed full of people and wares of all descriptions. The activity begins about 8:00 in the morning, when the butchers set to work
slaughtering animals at the nearby abattoir for the meat they hope to

sell in the market that day. Gradually, others begin to drift in from the countryside. Fulani women come with their sour milk. Maguzawa men and women arrive with produce from their farms and thick fermented beer, which they will sell to the less devout members of the Muslim community. Large-scale traders from the village begin to move their goods to market by about ten o'clock and the marketplace is booming by noon. Lorries and the ubiquitous Ford vans arrive and depart at frequent intervals, doing a vigorous business in shuttling buyers and sellers from the larger, more distant villages and towns on the main roads. Bicycles from nearby villages arrive in abundance, their drivers often balancing precarious loads of trading goods on their heads as they navigate the paths through the surrounding farmland.

The village as a whole is busy, not just the marketplace. If the market day happens to be Friday, many additional people will arrive from outlying areas to take part in the communal prayers at the village mosque. Others will wander through the streets to greet friends and relations. Herbal healers (*bokaye*) who have consulting practices in their compounds always do bigger business on market days. Disputes and problems from the hamlets are brought before the village headman for advice or settlement. And, not unexpectedly, the village prostitutes (*karuwai*) do a brisk business in prepared food, freshly brewed beer, cigarettes, and sex.

Trade in the market is done by barter: offer and counteroffer. A prospective buyer inquires and is given a price that is invariably too high. The customer counters, usually to receive the reply *Albarka!*, ("No sale!") But, as the proverb says, *mai-neman rangwame ba shi hana ciniki*, "He who bargains for a reduction does not prevent trading." After a few minutes of haggling something approaching the "true market price" may be reached, below which the seller makes no profit, and a deal is struck. This procedure can make markets a trap for the unwary and maximizes the necessity to be wily and shrewd. Much traditional wisdom seizes on this point: *Kasuwa ba gidan kowa ba*, "The market is nobody's home." *Fatauci ba gayya ba ne*, "Trading isn't 'mutual help'." *Ko a Makka riba 'daya ta ke*, "Even in Mecca profit is profit." The clever man who manages to maximize his position as a trader is a respected fellow; indeed, a trader who prospers is seen as having *arziki*, "special fortune," a blessing of God upon his activities. For the others who do not profit as much, there is always hope for better luck next time: *Ciniki goma maganin mai-gasa;* "Ten deals is the medicine for [market] envy."

The contents of Hausa markets, even rural ones, are limitless in variety. Articles of trade range from plastic shoes and teapots, cheap perfumes, herbal medicines, bars of soap, agricultural produce, and homemade rope to sophisticated consumer goods like wristwatches, transistor radios, and tape recorders. Metalworkers sell axeheads and hoes. Retailers of cloth sell Nigerian products from the textile mills in Kaduna and imported goods from Europe that have made their way through the distribution system to reach the rural countryside. Both Hausa men and women are fond of good clothing. Women like brightly colored prints, and men envy sleek, elegant materials that speak of affluence. Pilgrims returning from Mecca nearly always bring back bolts of expensive material to use in gowns for themselves and their families. Kolanuts are ubiquitous in Hausa markets and form an integral part of life. One of the few stimulants permitted to devout Muslims, they are given and exchanged in greeting and form an integral part of the etiquette of behavior. The trading networks from the south are old and extensive;[42] and there are kola brokers in every village. Large markets have a special area for selling cattle, where cattle brokers dicker with Fulani herders, examine animals, and try to outwit each other. Often a man never has actual physical possession of the animal he buys, it being sold again before he leaves the market; or he may entrust it to a Fulani herder to tend for him until he can resell it at a profit.[43] Salt is brought in from Bornu, agate necklaces from Arabia, and fish from the Niger River.[44] Secondhand clothes from the United States and elsewhere are inexpensive and sell readily.[45] Almost anything can be purchased in a Hausa market if one is willing to look hard enough, wait long enough—and pay the price when he finds it.

Most of the business in the market is transacted between about ten

42. On the kola trade in Hausaland see Cohen (1966) and Lovejoy (1971).
43. See Cohen (1965) for a discussion of a Hausa cattle market.
44. The salt trade in Hausaland is discussed in Lovejoy (1978a).
45. Items of clothing I have seen include a "Wheeling West Virginia Little League Baseball" T-shirt on a grubby village boy, a T-shirt from the College of Northern Iowa, and a remarkable ragged sweatshirt which proclaimed in bold print: "Bitch Bitch Bitch." When I saw a pair of underwear emblazoned with the comic book figures of "Batman and Robin," I knew it was a small world indeed.

o'clock in the morning and four in the afternoon. People stay around until their business is done and they are satisfied with having "eaten the market" (*cin kasuwa*). *Ko yanzu kasuwa ta watse 'dan koli ya sami rabonsa*, "Whenever the market breaks up the trader has made his bit," says the proverb. As late afternoon approaches, those who have come from hamlets out in the countryside or villages farther away start heading toward home. Traders like to have their goods sorted and packed away again before evening, so by the time the sun starts to sink to the position for the *la'azar* prayers the market has begun to fade. As evening comes the market is nearly deserted. People have gone to their compounds to say the sunset prayers (*magariba*) and to eat their *tuwo*. Only a few sellers of food and snacks, travelers waiting for the last lorry out, and those getting drunk in the compounds of prositutes remain. *Da'dewa a kasuwa shi ya kawo ganin fa'dan mahauta*, "Loitering in the market only makes you witness the butchers' fights."

Secluded women are not seen in the marketplace. The only women one is likely to encounter there are the poor, the old, Fulani women, prostitutes, pagan Maguzawa, or women traveling through to other destinations; but this does not mean that the women of the village who are kept in *purdah* are excluded from economic activities. An extensive and prosperous trade is carried out among secluded women via intermediaries from their compounds, usually children. The *maigida* of the household is responsible for providing food for the people who live there. This food comes out of the grain stores from his farm, or from grain purchased in the market. He provides his wives with *cefane*—money for daily housekeeping expenses, the purchase of condiments for cooking, and so on. The household head is similarly responsible for providing the members of his family with decent clothing and adequate shelter. Beyond this, however, the women of the household are on their own. For niceties and spending money they must depend largely upon their own initiative. As a result, they are vigorous traders who work diligently to build up a store of wealth that belongs to them alone. They may be assisted by their husbands, who often provide starting capital (*jari*) for their wives' enterprises, but the profits remain separate from the income of the husband.

The goods carried in this household trade are varied but consist mainly of prepared foodstuffs. Hausa custom is to eat only two meals per day, generally *tuwo* cooked in the morning and evening. This is supplemented by snack meals during the day, the arrangements for which are loose and informally structured. Often one must fend for oneself. Consequently, women do a large business in the sale of ready-to-eat morsels that fill this gap, and the household trading network is largely oriented around the sale of these food items: fried groundnut cakes, balls of ground millet for mixing with sour milk, various sorts of beancakes, sweet Hausa "taffy" candy, mangoes, locust-bean cakes for making soup, kolanuts, roasted groundnuts, prepared rice, spicy morsels made from cowpeas, gruel of various types, steamed leaves from the horseradish tree, and a whole range of condiments for cooking—groundnut oil, salt, pepper, baobab leaves, tomatoes, okra, and so forth. These items are readied each morning and placed on trays, which are given to the children—especially girls—to carry with them around the village. As these items are sold—at a price, for example, of one kobo per beancake—the children collect the money and when all the items are sold they return home with it to their mothers (usually minus a little for "expenses") to get a new load and start again.

This results in what Polly Hill has called (1969:396) "the honeycomb trade" of Hausaland—entrepreneurial women sitting secluded in their compound "cells" carrying on a thriving business with the women in other such "cells" via their intermediaries.[46] Not only does this system generate income for the women involved, it also works to break down the isolation imposed by wife seclusion, which prevents all but the most financially depressed (such as widows with no family) or morally profligate women from going from house to house and provides a system of communication that ties the women together in their own social network, separate from that of the men.[47]

The structure of rural Hausa life is based around the village—its households and compounds, and the circle of the family, friends, and resident kinfolk—looking out into the wider world of local markets

46. One interesting case in the village in which I worked was that of the sole Yoruba woman who lived in the village. Although a Muslim married to a Muslim Yoruba man, she was not restricted by wife seclusion, which is generally not practiced by the Muslim Yoruba. As a result, she carried on a thriving trade in the house-to-house sale of cloth, turning both her religion and her ethnic heritage to commercial advantage.
47. It also allows shrewd women to build up enough money to be partly independent of their husbands.

and the traditional structure of the Hausa kingdoms, modified by time and governmental innovation. The economy rests on the dual foundations of farming and trade, in which cash crops and seasonal occupations play a major role. The bifurcation of the year into wet and dry seasons provides a steady point of reference for local activities, dividing the year into agricultural and nonagricultural spheres of concern. Within the structure of this basic setting the individual moves along "life's dull round," progressing through the cycles of his life—the subject to which we now turn.

Stages
on Life's Way

Mai rashin yau, shi ne
mai samun gobe.

(*He who lacks today*
will gain tomorrow.)

HAUSA PROVERB

The collective representations that form the foundations of Hausa society and culture endure, with modifications, from generation to generation. It is this constellation of assumptions about the world and the interrelations of individuals within it that gives structure and order—and ultimately meaning—to the lives of the Hausa people. But this is not a static process, nor does the individual experience it as such. Life is movement, a series of transitions from one status to another, some clearly defined and socially recognized, others more subtle, dependent upon the individual's characteristics and abilities. The structural realities of social organization and the postulates of the moral order form the stage on which he plays out his life, the benchmarks from which he gauges meaning as he progresses from infancy and childhood to maturity, old age, and death. In order to understand the world in which the Hausa villager lives, the general structure of this process must be appreciated.[1]

■ Birth and Naming

The encounter with the world begins at birth, when the village baby is born into a network of social relations which begin to influence him immediately, and in which he himself exerts no small influence. The Hausa proverbs state *Haifuwa maganin mutuwa,* "Birth is the medicine for death," and *Haifuwa maganin takaici,* "Birth is the medicine for frustration," for the incorporation of new life en-

1. The best general discussion of the Hausa life cycle is still Mary F. Smith's (1954) translation of the autobiography of the Hausa woman Baba of Karo.

sures growth, security, prosperity, and the perpetuation of one's name
and lineage.

A compound in which a birth has just occurred is a busy place. Not
only does the mother of the child need attention—for labor in Hausaland is frequently traumatic and often complicated by Hausa obstetrical
practices[2]—but preparations must be made for officially recognizing
the child and giving him or her a name. The mother is confined inside
her hut for a week following delivery, baking in the heat of the fires
thought to impart strength to her and drinking medicinal gruel loaded
with potash, which is believed to have a similar effect. Older women
from her compound or neighboring compounds lend a hand, while the
men make arrangements for the naming ceremony. Word spreads of
the new child's arrival and the father takes pains personally to mention
the event to his close friends and to invite them to the naming ceremony. Women receive the news through their own special network of
communications.

The naming day comes seven days after the birth. As with most
Hausa ceremonies, the formal declaration of the child's name takes
place in the morning, usually about 7:00, allowing enough time for the
morning *tuwo* to be prepared and eaten in the compounds around the
village.[3] As the time approaches, men begin strolling over to the entry-
hut of the compound. The *maigida* and his family have placed rows of
grass mats on the earth around the entryway, and the male guests come
and seat themselves, chatting quietly and greeting friends. Groups of
two or three women may be seen coming toward the compound, which
they enter, segregating themselves inside with the mother of the child
and the other women of the compound, away from the men. Male
members of the family or praise-singers deputed by the household head
move among the assembled guests, passing out kolanuts or the popular
cheap hard sweets in their brittle cellophane wrappers. When the *limam*
arrives with his party, events may proceed.

As the principal religious functionary of the village, the *limam* enters

2. These practices are discussed in more detail in chapter 4.
3. Hausa naming practices are also described in Rattray (1913, II:188–90), Taylor
and Webb (1932:14–41), Trimingham (1959:154–58), Hassan and Na'ibi (1962:63),
Madauci et al. (1968:6–10), and Ferguson (1973:249–54). Details of names and
their meanings are found in Abraham (1959:189–93) and also in Madauci et al.
(1968).

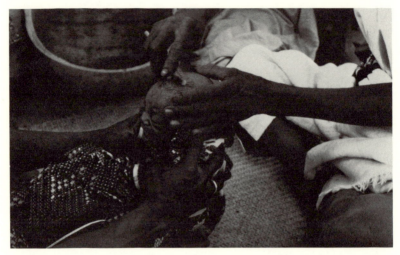

5. Muhammadu, seven days old, gets his head shaved on his naming day.

the hut along with those who are to be in immediate attendance at the naming of the child. The naming itself is brief and formal. As the ceremony begins inside, a praise-singer (*maro'ki*) takes up his position outside the doorway. The *Fatiha*[4] is recited three times, with the crowd sitting outside covering their faces in prayer as the verse is repeated. As the name of the child is pronounced inside, the *maro'ki* calls it out: *Allah shi raya, Muhammadu Salisu! Allah shi raya!* "God grant you life, Muhammadu Salisu! May God grant you life!" From inside the compound the high shrill ululations of the women respond to the men, and the crowd begins to break up. All this time the praise-singers are calling out blessings on the child and blessings on selected individuals

4. The *Fatiha* is the opening sura of the Koran:
    In the Name of God, the Merciful, the Compassionate
      Praise belongs to God, the Lord of all Being,
        the All-merciful, the All-compassionate,
          the Master of the Day of Doom.
  Thee only we serve; to Thee alone we pray for succour.
        Guide us in the straight path,
      the path of those whom'Thou hast blessed
    not of those against whom Thou are wrathful,
      nor of those who are astray.

in the crowd, angling for a few kolanuts or coins as recompense for their services.

As the bulk of the crowd of neighbors and casual friends disperses, the closest friends of the family remain. Inside, the chief butcher, one of his subordinates, or a male member of the family cuts the throat of a ram—providing the family in question is wealthy enough to afford one—and butchers it for roasting. Portions of the ram are usually reserved for the midwife who cut the umbilical cord, the barber who shaves the baby, the butcher, and perhaps a few honored guests. Hot steaming *tuwo* has been prepared, with the luxury of a meat sauce (finances again permitting). Additional fare may include rice, beans, sweet gruel, and chicken fried in oil and covered with a hot, peppery sauce. This repast is served to the honored guests, who eat with high pleasure, and the leavings are put out for the Koranic students who are living in the village away from their own homes and subsisting on the goodwill of their teachers and the Islamic community. As the bowl is set out and the word is given, a veritable stampede of boys with flying hands devour the sticky dough or rice in an instant.

The ceremony of shaving the baby's head now takes place. From birth the child has been in possession of a head of soft, curly hair. Now that he (or she) has been named, this shaving of the head completes the child's incorporation into Muslim society. If the baby is a boy this will be the first of many such shavings, for Muslim men traditionally wear their heads clean-shaven.[5] The child is brought out, either in front of the compound or into the courtyard inside the compound, where the *wanzami* (barber) and his assistant have prepared themselves on a grass mat. Serviced by a bowl of water, a bar of hard soap, and his straight razor, the barber nestles the well-wrapped child in his lap, lathers the baby's head with soap, and deftly shaves away the locks of hair. It is unusual for the infant to remain impassive throughout the course of this ordeal, and the cries of the child are met with injunctions to be quiet and greetings of praise from the *maro'ki*. At the finish, the barber will often chew a bit of kolanut in his mouth and rub the crum-

5. More sophisticated "modern" Hausa—the younger men with more secular education and experience in the world of towns and cities—prefer cropped or styled hair rather than the more provincial shaven heads. Such influences penetrate the villages as well in this younger age group.

bling pieces over the child's head as an aftershave poultice before tendering him back to the charge of the women.

When the shaving is done it is customary for the child's "tribal markings" to be made at the same time.[6] These follow the pattern of the father and may be very simple or quite elaborate. Tattooing is done with a straight razor, the cuts being made and then rubbed with soot from the bottom of a cooking pot or a solution of ink. Girls usually have additional tattooes around the mouth and frequently will add to their markings in later life for cosmetic purposes, while men eschew them. Uvulectomy is generally performed three or four days after birth.

■ Infancy and Childhood

There are two Hausa words for the period of infancy: *jariri,* and the more descriptive *na goyo,* "the carried one."[7] Until a child learns to walk on his own he is his mother's constant companion, carried on her back, held firmly in place by a long cloth tied around her waist. The proverb *Jariri bai san gari da nesa ba,* "The baby doesn't know the town is far away" is definitely true! As the newest member of the household, the infant is everyone's favorite, and although there may be some jealousy from a displaced sibling, he is an object of pride to his parents, an investment in the future. Inarticulate, helpless, and dependent on the family for all his needs, the baby can express himself only by crying. One Hausa proverb succinctly states *Jariri bai san babu ba,* "A baby does not know 'No.' " An infant's cries are reproaches to his mother, who hurries to comfort him by giving him a breast to suck: *Uwa ita ta ke maganin kukan 'danta,* "The mother is the medicine for her child's crying."

The relationship between the child and his mother in this period is

6. A selection of northern Nigerian tribal markings is given in Tremearne (1913: 518–35).

7. The verb *goye,* meaning "to carry a baby on one's back," has been extended into the motorized world to have the additional meaning of carrying someone behind the driver on the rear seat of a motorcycle. The driver is the "mother" who decides where to go and supplies the means of doing so, and the rider is the "baby" who merely tags along. It is instructive in this regard that although many men in the village in which I lived had motorcycles, whenever the village headman needed to go somewhere (not having a motorcycle himself) I was the one deputed to carry him, it being beneath his dignity to be carried by a subordinate.

very close. *Yankan uwa ya isa ma 'da,* "Killing the mother suffices for the child," as a proverb puts it. The mother's milk is regarded as a bridge between her and the nursing baby. Something wrong with the mother may affect her breasts so that ingestion of her milk leads to withered limbs, infantile paralysis, later development of leprosy, or general ill health in the child, even though the mother may appear to be in perfect health. The phenomenon of *wabi*—a mother who bears children only to have them all die in succession at an early age—is sometimes attributed to bad milk (*nono ba kyau*), and the wide variety of herbal nostrums found in the traditional pharmacopoeia (based mainly on the white, milky sap of fig trees and other plants) attests to the importance of this relationship in Hausa thought.[8]

As the infant gradually learns to walk his social world enlarges, and he is now free to move about the compound, wander outside, and make his way to the compounds of neighbors, watched over by his elder brothers and sisters. This emancipation from his mother's back is

---

8. Hausa possesses two words for milk: *madara,* which refers to sweet milk fresh from the cow or to commercial preparations available in tins, used mainly for putting in tea; and *nono,* which refers to the sour milk sold by Fulani women and universally preferred by the Hausa for drinking. *Nono* is also the word used for the breast milk of the mother. This usage of *nono* has some interesting medical relationships. *Madara* is almost never drunk by adults, who complain that it makes them sick. Because infants relish and thrive on the milk of their mothers' breasts, the word *nono* is used for it, even though it is sweet, not sour milk.

The reason for this disparity is that the Hausa suffer to a large degree from adult-onset lactase deficiency. The newborn in all mammalian species are almost never deficient in lactase, the enzyme (a beta-galactosidase) responsible for the hydrolysis of the glucose-galactose bond in the disaccharide milk sugar lactose— a major component of human milk. This allows the absorption of the two hydrolyzed sugar moieties across the intestinal mucosa and their subsequent degradation to produce energy. Kretchmer et al. (1971) have demonstrated that the Hausa show a high proportion (76 percent) of adult lactose intolerance due to a lack of this enzyme, as compared with a relatively low incidence (22 percent) among nomadic Fulani cattle-herders, who utilize large amounts of dairy products in their diet.

I vividly recall making a visit to a Fulani camp with a Hausa friend from our village and being asked by the Fulani herders if I would like a calabash of *madara.* Fresh milk being something of a rarity, I eagerly assented, and they were delighted. As I gulped down the milk I offered some to Ibrahim, my friend from the village. He declined, saying he hadn't had any *madara* since he was an infant, and wouldn't take any now because it was sure to make him sick. The Fulanis laughed and we shared the milk together with relish.

marked by a gradual change in his eating habits and the substitution of adult foods like *tuwo* as the child is weaned (*yaye*). The Koran exhorts mothers to suckle their children for two years, (Sura II, 233) a practice the Hausa try to adopt. This is coupled with the precept that women nursing children should not have sexual relations for fear of producing another pregnancy, thereby spoiling their milk and injuring the nursing child.[9] Needless to say, such an injunction is difficult to endure, and many Hausa men state candidly that they ignore it.[10] The rule, interestingly, possesses enough force as a moral absolute that Hausa men use it as a justification for both plural marriages and the existence of prostitutes, for how can men live without a sexual outlet?

As the child begins moving in wider circles, new obligations are placed upon him.[11] By the time he is two or three, new standards of decorum begin to be applied, and he is expected to have learned stricter rules of toilet training and modesty. He must defecate away from the dwellings, behind the compound, although in a hot climate it is of little

9. The old Hausa woman Baba of Karo explained it thus (M. F. Smith 1954:148):
   A mother should not go to her husband while she has a child she is suckling. If she does, the child gets thin, he dries up, he won't get strong, he won't be healthy. If she goes after a year, the child won't get strong; but if she goes after two years it is nothing, he is already strong before that, it does not matter if she conceives again after two years. If she only sleeps with her husband and does not become pregnant, it will not hurt her child, it will not spoil her milk. But if another child enters in, her milk will make the first one ill. If she must go to her husband, she should take a kolanut and sew it up in leather into a charm and wear it round her waist; when she weans her child that is that, she throws away the charm and does as she wishes, then there is another child. It is not sleeping with the husband that spoils her milk, it is the pregnancy that does that. But if her husband desires her, then in the day she carries her child, at night she carries her husband—this is what pleases Allah. He does not like argumentative women. But it is not right that she should sleep with her husband for two years; if he insists she should wear the kolanut charm. As you know, there is medicine to make the pregnancy "go to sleep," but that is not a good thing.
10. Violations of this principle are not necessarily as daring as one might expect, since the constant neural stimulus of the nursing child at the mother's breast results in prolonged lactational amenorrhea and prolonged anovulation, which serves as an effective form of contraception (Konner and Worthman 1980; Short 1984).
11. On the social development of the Hausa child see E. Dry (1956) and LeVine and Price-Williams (1974).

consequence precisely where he urinates, as it dries quickly.[12] At an early age girls are expected to cover their genitals with an apron or body cloth and to wear a head-tie; boys begin to wear short pants or trousers, although in both cases their bellies are so rotund that nothing stays on for long.

When children reach the age of four or five they are able to perform simple tasks, like bringing items requested by a parent or sibling or carrying items on a tray for sale. Little girls in particular are given a few beancakes or groundnuts to sell as they wander around the village with their playmates, bringing the few coins they earn to their mothers when they return home. Little boys may be given similar responsibilities, but in neither case is it really a matter of assigned work; rather, it is an activity to be carried out at one's leisure, in the midst of more pressing activities such as following one's elder siblings around, meeting friends, and visiting the compounds of neighbors and relatives.

With advancing age and understanding these tasks become more complex and responsible, such as tending sheep or goats in the countryside, minding the shop for their father while he is away, and following the chores of the agricultural cycle—planting, cultivating, and harvesting. Boys and girls may both branch out into their own financial activities, gathering grass along the footpaths outside the village to sell as fodder or selling kolanuts on a commission basis (10 percent is a common figure) for one of the men who acts as a kola broker. These activities are generally unstructured. The Hausa child has a childhood unrestrained by rigid sets of duties to perform. They are not yet fully functional members of society and consequently are allowed a latitude in their activities that adults do not have. Children may enter and leave almost any compound freely, whereas adults would not do so (men will rarely enter the interior of the compounds of even their best friends). Children are thus great carriers of news and information among the women of the village and are welcomed as such.

Recreation takes many forms for the Hausa child, often in imitation of adult activities. Girls play house, carry younger brothers and sisters strapped to their backs or, when no sibling is available, may replace

12. One never sees females (except little girls) urinating in public, but it is commonplace to see a man stroll to the side of the road, the edge of a fence or a compound wall, squat, and relieve his bladder.

him with a long, thin gourd carefully tied in place. Boys build models of lorries from patiently whittled cornstalks or roll an old bicycle wheel down a dusty village path. They may perform impromptu prayer (*salla*) or join in with the men, to everyone's delight. Cheap rubber balls are very popular toys and many an impromptu game of football has been arranged in the yard of the village school. In summer one can always go swimming in the river, and nighttime finds the flowering of the "small market"—a section of the village on one of the main thoroughfares where people meet to talk by the light of kerosene lamps amidst the sellers of kolanuts, purveyors of fruits and candies, and hawkers of roasted meat. Most nights a drummer can be found in front of somebody's compound, beating the *kalangu* or another type of drum for the young girls to dance to, and where there are girls dancing boys are sure to be found as well. These dances are a very important social event for the mingling of the sexes, especially under the cover of darkness, where more interesting activities can be arranged. Market days bring new faces and a whirl of activity to the village *kasuwa*, where there is always something to do and friends to meet. Occasionally, one can find a ride on the lorry going to market in a neighboring village. And, above all, there is the indefatigable ingenuity of childhood in finding entertainment through mischievous outlets.[13]

With the exception of Koranic instruction the traditional education of the village child is mainly informal. In large part it consists of the observation of elders and their behavior. Simple tasks are taught by example as the occasion arises, but formal instruction in work and duties is sporadic. Emphasis is placed on knowing correct behavior and assuming one's proper place in society. The child should be deferential and helpful to adults, and should show respect and modesty. Failure to know correct behavior is a source of embarrassment met by admoni-

13. I have one vivid memory of hearing strange noises out on the street late one night that prompted me to leave my compound to investigate. There was a partial moon, which cast a pale, whitish light up and down the walls of the neighboring houses. Suddenly, with a fit of ghoulish laughter, an enormous man over ten feet tall came careening toward me out from under the trees. Startled, and somewhat frightened, I jumped back as he went lunging past. Then I noticed a pack of laughing boys running after him. They had made a large cross out of cornstalks, covered it with a flowing gown and set a hat on top of it. One boy ran along underneath it, waving it up and down in the air, while his friends ran after him full of excitement.

tions and quick reproach. Reprimands almost always suffice for punishment. The tone of society is such that a harsh word from an adult is usually enough to set an errant child in line, and it is rare to see an adult strike a child except for a gross infraction of conduct.[14] In a setting such as this, in which change is slow and technology still fairly rudimentary, inculcation of moral values takes precedence over technical skills.

Introduction of Western-style education and the establishment of primary schools in rural villages has changed this picture somewhat. The admirable object of the government is to provide universal primary education for all Nigerian children and an attempt is made to teach the fundamentals of reading and writing in romanized Hausa script, some English, basic mathematics, Nigerian history, geography, and some hygiene, as well as Islamic religious values (in Muslim parts of the country). The schools are open to both sexes alike, and during the school term boys and girls may be seen trooping to the outskirts of the village in their green-and-white uniforms. The importance of such education has yet to be appreciated by most. For the vast majority it is another world, of little or no relevance to village life. The boys enrolled far outnumber the girls, who are sent (so it seems) largely because education will perhaps enhance their value when it comes time to negotiate marriage payments. The quality of teaching is poor and is based on rote memorization rather than the development of thought. It is not unusual to walk past the school and see one small child in front of the class pointing out words on the chalkboard with a stick while the teachers congregate outside in the courtyard washing the headmaster's motorcycle. The child who perseveres and fights his way out of a rural classroom to gain a place in secondary school is unusual indeed—and only one or two succeed in any given year. Many fathers would still prefer their sons to master Koranic scholarship rather than pursue a secular education.[15]

14. The Hausa proverb *Bugi da ka ga fa'dan uwar tasa,* "Hit a child and quarrel with his mother" holds some striking truths. On one occasion I remember a boy who had been whipped by the headmaster of the village school for some infraction. Upon returning home he told his mother who, outraged, grabbed a heavy piece of wood and set out to give the man a thrashing. She was prevented in this only by being physically restrained until her temper subsided.

15. The Hausa term for "government school" is *makarantar boko—boko* meaning

Religious education is important both for boys and girls, and begins at an early age. Much of the proper ritual behavior is learned through observation of adults performing the mandatory prayers (salla), and children are encouraged to follow suit. Formal training takes place when children are sent to study the Koran and learn rudimentary Arabic. Particularly during the dry season, large groups of children can be seen at night gathered around large cornstalk bonfires, attempting to memorize selected portions of the Koran that have been laboriously written out for them on wooden slates. It is important that girls learn the fundamentals of religious duty, but much more emphasis is placed upon the education of males. This religious training is accelerated when the boy reaches the age for circumcision.

■ Circumcision

Circumcision (in Hausa, kaciya) is not mentioned specifically in the Koran, but Muslims regard it as essential to the faith of Islam (Levy 1957:251). In West Africa circumcision widely antedates the introduction of Islam, but has been transformed into an Islamic custom that marks the transition from child to youth (Trimingham 1959:161–63). Usually, when a Hausa boy has reached the age of seven or eight he is ready to be circumcised, but many boys are circumcised earlier, at the age of five or six, and nothing is quite so galling to a lad as to be the only one of his playmates still wandering around with his foreskin intact. The event itself, though traumatic for the child involved, is not an elaborate ceremony; rather, it is a task that must be done and is essentially a family matter, not a communal one.[16]

As with other ceremonies, the circumcision takes place in the morning. Only very close friends and relatives are invited—the crowds are never as big as for a naming, wedding, or funeral. The event may take place inside the compound or out front, depending on the particular arrangements of the household. The cutting is done by a barber (wanzami) who is asked to perform the service by the boy's father. First, a

---

"book" and also "deceit"—as contrasted to makarantar alkur'ani, "Koranic school." Alkur'ani is a word frequently used synonymously with "truth" in Hausa.

16. On circumcision among the Hausa see also Rattray (1913, II:192–98), Taylor and Webb (1932:40–45), Trimingham (1959:161–63), Madauci et al. (1968:11–13), and Ferguson (1973:256–60).

sharp digging stick is brought out and a small hole is dug in the ground, approximately five inches in diameter and nine inches deep. The earth is removed and carefully cleared off to one side. Grass mats are placed around the hole, which will receive the blood from the operation. The grass mats ensure greater comfort and if the ground is damp they will serve to prevent cold (*sanyi*) from penetrating the vulnerable body of the boy and causing illness. A large tub of cold water is readied while the barber sharpens his razor (*aska*), the same kind as is used to shave the head.

This done, the boy is brought out. He is stark naked, with a freshly shaved head, looking quite pitiful, with anxiety marked on every feature. It is a mark of courage and maturity not to show fear, but this is hard to do. The procedure is terribly painful. The boy is taken over to the mats and seated, his legs spread out on either side of the hole, his penis dropped over the center. One man sits behind him, throwing his legs over those of the boy to hold them firmly on the ground. The child's arms are pinned behind his back, holding him immobile. The barber then throws his legs over those of the man who is holding the boy, facing him. The child is thus held fast by the concerted efforts of two full-grown men, one behind him and one in front. The actual business of cutting is done in quite close quarters.

The circumcision can now begin. First, the barber washes the penis with cold water from the tub. This ensures cleanliness and also induces vasoconstriction, which reduces bleeding in the course of the operation. While the barber washes the penis he carefully arranges the foreskin to his liking before proceeding to the actual cutting. Then he sets to work. Using deft motions of his hand, drawing the blade toward him, he slices the foreskin away in five or six strokes, washing off the blood as necessary to obtain a clear view of what he is doing. The process appears immensely painful and the boy writhes considerably. Although the boy is supposed to steel himself and "take it like a man," it is rare for a circumcision not to be punctuated by the cry of *Wayyo Allah! Wayyo Allah!*, a common Hausa ejaculation when in physical or emotional pain. All the while, of course, the *maro'ka* are busy and the entire operation is marked by the hyperbole of praises like *Abdul Basiru ya zama mutum!* ("Abdul Basiru has become a man!") or *Muhammadu Salisu ya yi girma!* ("Muhammadu Salisu has grown up!"). The women of the compound respond from inside with ululations of joy.

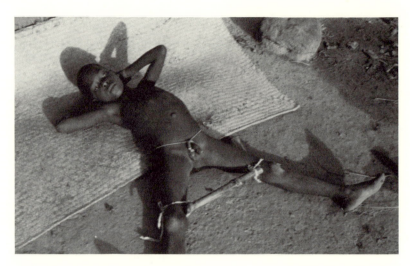

6. Circumcision: The healing process.

The actual cutting takes only a few minutes, though it must seem like an eternity to the boy involved. When it is over the barber continues to wash the penis with cold water to reduce the flow of blood, which gradually slows as coagulation begins. By this time it is probably unnecessary to hold the boy down any longer and he is left sitting on the mat, his penis dripping blood into the hole in the ground, tears streaming down his cheeks while he struggles to control himself. When the flow of blood has slowed considerably the barber will take out a small bag of *magani* (medicine), usually powdered grasses (*haki*) or similar substances, and pour them over the wound to aid in the clotting. All the while a continual stream of praise for the youth (who is no longer a "little boy") is poured out by the *maro'ka*, announcing to the world that *gyara ya yi kyau!*—"He's really been fixed up now!"

The men now come and give the barber coins in appreciation for his work, a standard Hausa practice on any occasion of significance, an elaboration of *ku'din gaisuwa* ("money of greeting") or the giving of kolanuts (*goro*). While this is going on, the feast inside has been readied and bowls of hot *tuwo*, steaming rice, beancakes, and meal will be brought out for the participants. The boy himself will be fed well for several days to allow him to build up his strength after the ordeal.

The hole into which the blood has flowed is filled with the dirt taken from it originally, no particular precautions being taken in the process. When the food has been distributed and eaten the festivities are over. The compound head pays the barber a sum ranging from three to five naira, disperses some coins to the *maro'ki* and his companions, and the company departs.

All in all, circumcision is a fairly informal process. The Hausa are not an elaborately ritual people and this particular ceremony is more a family celebration than anything else. Indeed, in the case of one circumcision the boy's grandfather, who was the chief *limam* of the village mosque, did not even arrive until the circumcision was completed.

In theory, the wounds should heal in about two weeks, although from personal observation it appears that a month is a more reasonable amount of time—and this, of course, varies with individual circumstances and the amount of care taken to ensure that the penis is not reinjured. The boys go around naked at this time—pants would only aggravate their discomfort—and the newly circumcised penis is nestled in a triangular sheath made from cornstalks to keep it from bouncing against the thighs. At night a forked stick (*karkiya*) is tied between the knees to prevent the youth from rolling over, breaking the scab, and reopening the wound. During this period boys wear their injuries as a badge of honor as they saunter spraddle-legged around the village, and many can be overheard to remark that the women had better watch out for they are now ready and primed for action![17]

Circumcision is a sort of rite de passage, but it does not mark the transition from boy to man, from childhood to adulthood—only marriage and the arrival of the first child stamp a man as socially complete. It does, however, entail a change in status and the introduction of new responsibilities as the boy becomes a youth. Foremost among these changes is the assumption of a more rigorous attitude toward religious obligations. By the time a boy is old enough to be circumcised he should be mature enough to observe the five daily times of prayer, to make a conscientious effort at keeping the fast at Ramadan, and to begin seri-

17. In areas where medical facilities are available hospital circumcision is becoming more popular, and on any given day one can usually see some small boys with bandages on, walking bow-legged down the road away from the hospital with their fathers.

ous study of the Koran. For many boys circumcision marks the beginning of their period as an *almajari* (Koranic student) sent to study with
a learned *mallam* outside the village.

■ Courtship and Marriage

For girls there is no ordeal such as circumcision,[18] but by the time they
have reached the age where their male counterparts are circumcised,
sexual role differentiation is well developed. From an essentially gen-
derless infancy they have emerged into a world where sexual differences and discrimination are an increasingly important part of their
lives. Young boys and girls are treated as equals, but as they age the
differences between them assume more importance. Girls continue to
sleep in the hut of their mother, whereas boys gradually begin to sleep
with their brothers in the entry-hut of the compound. Younger children
eat together irrespective of their sex, but as they approach six to eight
years of age, brothers begin to eat by themselves or with the men, and
girls begin to eat separately or with the women inside the compound.
Girls begin to have more domestic tasks to perform, selling their
mother's wares around the village, running errands, carrying messages
to other compounds. Boys frequently have more freedom.

These tasks accelerate as the girl's physical maturity begins to show.
The most general word for a girl is *yarinya* (pl. *'yam mata*), the feminine form of *yaro* ("boy"). A more specific word, *bera*, refers to a
young girl before her breasts begin to develop. During this period a girl
is only an incipient woman and has a large degree of freedom, mixing
easily with boys and men. As she matures and her breasts begin to develop, this status starts to change. Initially, these changes are objects
of much merriment and teasing among the men of the village, and the
girls throw back quite spirited replies. As the girl blooms into a
budurwa with fully formed breasts, however, she stands on the thresh-

18. At birth or shortly thereafter, so my barber friends told me, hymenectomy or
clitorectomy is sometimes performed, usually for medical reasons similar to those
advanced for the practice of uvulectomy: fear that the appendage in question will
grow large and obstruct a passageway in the body. In preparation for childbirth
certain cuts (*gishiri*) are sometimes made inside the vagina; but there is no practice of female circumcision comparable to that undergone by boys.

Rattray, however, gives a text describing female circumcision (1913, II:200–202).

old of marriage and adulthood and must conduct herself with proper modesty *(kunya)* and deference—qualities of maturity frequently lacking in boys of a similar age. Since girls marry shortly after the onset of menstruation *(haila)* at thirteen or fourteen—much earlier than do the *samari* (male youths) of the village—their progress in accepting the adult role of their sex in society accelerates at a much more rapid pace.

While a girl at puberty prepares to enter the role of wife—with motherhood following soon after—a boy merely becomes a *saurayi*, a youth or young man. A girl's time as a *budurwa* is relatively short; she then becomes an *amarya*, a bride. The youth, however, remains single until he is about twenty, and thus spends a considerable portion of his life in his father's household as a sexually mature but unmarried man. During this portion of his life a youth will take on more responsibilities for the family's agricultural lands and other economic activities. During the agricultural seasons he will be actively engaged in planting, cultivation, or harvesting. If his father is wealthy enough to own cattle the youth will spend considerable amounts of his time tending them. In all likelihood his father will have given him some farmland of his own, which he can tend with an eye toward saving money to get married. During the dry season he may hire himself out as a laborer, repairing roofs and walls, or he may go off to another part of the country to "eat the dry season" *(cin rani)* as hired labor. If his father is a trader he will asume new responsibilities in the running of his father's shop, or, if his father is a tailor, he will spend much of his time sitting behind a foot-powered sewing machine, turning out caps, shirts, and pants. Those few who have managed to leave the village to attend secondary school will have a very different sort of life, spending much of their time in the larger towns gaining experiences and developing attitudes that are often at variance with the village world of their childhood. This time is often hard, for the youth is no longer a child but neither is he a man. As the proverb says: *Gaba mai wuya, baya mai takaici,* "To be in front is hard, to be behind is frustrating."

There are, however, compensations. Although the youth is struggling toward full manhood, his responsibilities are not yet very burdensome and there is still considerable time for the enjoyment of life. Not surprisingly, a major interest is *'yam mata,* girls, and courtship plays a significant part in how he spends his time. In the evenings, after the evening *salla* has been performed and the *tuwo* eaten, time remains to meet with friends, converse, stroll around the village "drinking the night air" (*shan iska*), and locate girls to flirt with.

Village youths and village girls are well aware of each other's presence as they carry out their daily tasks. In the course of things a young man will find some particular girl (or perhaps several) who excites his interest. When a likely opportunity presents itself, he will seek her out as she walks through the village on some errand and declare his interest to her. If she expresses similar feelings he will try to arrange a rendezvous with her during the evening, so that they may converse more intimately. If she agrees he will give her a few kobo or a shilling as a token and continue on his way, full of expectations. If she is truly interested she will turn up to meet him, otherwise she will pocket his gift and go her own way, adding to his frustrations.

Conversation (*hira*) is an art which is highly valued among the Hausa, and it is a major form of social activity. The conversational banter of courtship (usually called *ta'di*, but also *hira*) between a youth and the girl he is pursuing is no exception. The girl will show up with her best friend (*'kawa*) to meet the youth who has expressed his interest. Likely he will be in the company of one of his best friends. They will find a secluded place inside an entry-hut or on a bench in the shadows outside a compound to talk quietly, tease each other, and develop their friendship.

If the girl is willing and the youth is persuasive enough, after some time they may retire elsewhere to engage in more physical expressions of affection, caressing each other or masturbating. This practice, known as *tsarance*, is not regarded as immoral provided actual sexual intercourse does not occur. It is a normal part of growing up, the early exploration of sexuality that culminates in marriage and family. A slightly more discerning view of things, however, is given by the cognate word *tsaranci*, which refers to illicit intercourse between young people, and the proverbial expression *Tsarance madakin zina*, "Masturbation shares a room with fornication," shows the not infrequent outcome of this practice. Ideal moral precepts are expressed in such sayings as *Kekyawar 'kwarya tana ragaya da faifanta a rufe*, "The best calabash stays hung up with its cover on top," exhorting girls to stay home—but no young girl is to be denied the excitement of the village at night and the experiences it has to offer.

When a youth and his girl part, he again gives her some money as *toshi*—money given to cement bonds of affection—or *goro*, a small present given in politeness. This is not payment for sexual services, nor is it regarded as degrading. It is one of the many forms of monetary interchange that occur in Hausa etiquette. Not to do this would be impolite and insulting. This *toshi* need not be much—a few kobo, three or four shillings—but if a young man is seriously seeking a wife, not to do this would be fatal to his aspirations.

The process of courtship is beset by many vagaries. Because girls marry so much younger than do men there is always a surplus of suitors flocking around them. Unless there is some striking flaw in the girl's character or appearance she will not lack for attention. Consequently, there are plenty of village girls who will string a youth along only to collect his *toshi* and leave him dangling. A Hausa *budurwa* can be just as fickle and capricious as her European counterpart. Hausa proverbs contain many sentiments on this subject: *Duniya ce. Idan wata ta ki ka, sake wata,* "Such is the world—if one girl spurns you, take up with another." *Son masoyin wani 'koshin wahala,* "Loving one who loves another is a bellyful of trouble." *In ka ga budurwar bana da kyau, ta ba'di ta fi ta,* "If you think this year's girls are pretty, next year's will be better!" Even, perhaps, *Zamanka kai kadai ya fi zama da mugunyar mace,* "Living by yourself is better than living with a bad woman!" But in the course of time deeper relationships are formed, and the serious business of *neman aure,* "seeking marriage," is begun.[19]

19. There are several types of marriage in Hausaland, some of which are no longer practiced. By far the most common is *auren so,* a "marriage of affection," in which the two partners find each other through the processes of courtship described in this chapter. *Auren zumunta* is a "marriage of kinship," which is fairly common as well. This is a marriage between cousins, usually the children of two brothers. *|| cousins* If this can be arranged it is highly prized, for as the proverb says, *Zuma zuma ne,* "Kinship is honey." A third type is *auren sadaka,* an "alms marriage," in which a girl is given as a bride to a Koranic scholar, taking no *ku'din aure* (marriage payments) in return. This is prized as a form of charitable giving. Many of my friends told me this was by far the most praiseworthy type of marriage to make, but few would be willing to pass up the marriage payments that would come to them on the marriage of a daughter. Other types of marriage may be found mentioned in the literature, but would be regarded as anachronistic today.

On Hausa marriage customs see Rattray (1913, II:150–84), Tremearne (1913: 74–92), Taylor and Webb (1932:3–15), Dry (1950:158–70), M. F. Smith (1954:85–118), M. G. Smith (1955:56–68), Trimingham (1959:163–78), Hassan and Na'ibi (1962:55–62), Madauci et al. (1968:13–21), and Ferguson (1973:275–84).

A youth who has undertaken to get himself a wife must first of all be sure that the girl he desires is interested in him. Undoubtedly, they have talked and become acquainted with each other. If he has told her that he is truly fond of her, and if she reciprocates, he will tell her to let her parents know that he would like to stop by their compound to greet them on such-and-such a day. This message will be conveyed to her parents and the girl will then let her youth know that they are apprised of his upcoming visit. Then, on the day in question, the youth will dress in his best clothes and, together with his best friend, will go to the girl's compound to greet her parents. This is a formal visit marked by no small amount of apprehension and embarrassment (kunya) on the part of the youth.

Upon arriving, the youth and his friend will enter the compound and greet the women, especially the girl's mother, inquiring if her father is at home. He will receive them and they will exchange greetings, although not much conversation will ensue—the reason they are there is obvious enough. This done, they will sit in silence for five or ten minutes and the nervous youth will then take his leave of the father, giving his friend fifty kobo or one naira to give to the father and mother of the girl as goro. Then he and his friend will depart for their compound to discuss and reevaluate the events of the day. This is not a formal proposal of marriage—if events are to take such a course a long process of negotiation will take place between the two families involved—but it is a formal meeting with the girl's father, which serves to identify the youth as a suitor interested in the girl as a potential wife.

Although the boy has visited her parents and made himself known to them, he is still a long way from getting married to her. Indeed, although she has consented to his visiting her parents she may be interested in several other village youths, who may also have made such visits. Her parents may also have their eyes cast upon some friend or relative as a potential husband for her. The youth, therefore, must press his case with the girl and continue the process of courtship. If he is truly serious about her, he will inform his father of his interest and hold a conversation with him about "that girl from Alhaji Audu's compound." Fathers, being possessed of some faculties of observation of their own, likely have noticed these goings-on for some time and may broach the subject themselves with their sons.

One way of making a serious declaration of interest in a girl comes at *Sallah* (*idi*), the major religious festival in the Muslim calendar.[20] At *Sallah* everyone gets new clothes, dresses up in their finery, and enjoys a festive spirit. To make the most of this a serious youth will collect his resources and prepare a *kayan Sallah*, "basket of presents for *Sallah*," for his girl. This will include such things as soap for washing, perfumes, talcum powder, cosmetic creams, and body lotions of the type manufactured in Kano and elsewhere, a pair of fine sandals, a *kallabi* (head-tie) and similar items of dress, together with several naira. He will place all of these things in a large bucket or basket and take them to the girl's compound, where he will give them to a senior member of the household, telling them that this present is for the girl to make herself beautiful (*yi kwalliya*) for the upcoming festival. It will be gratefully received and carried in to the girl, who should be more than a little flattered.

By this time, it being obvious to all that the youth is serious in his quest for the girl, a deputation of two or more men from his family will be sent to visit the girl's father with a proposal of marriage. This deputation usually consists of the boy's father and one of the father's brothers or close friends. After the customary greetings a brief discussion will be held. The girl's father will tell them that the girl seems to be interested in marriage to the youth and that he will consult with her and her mother to see what should be done. The men are told to return in a week for the family's reply. The boy's father and his companion at this point will present the girl's father with ten naira or so as *toshi*, money of persuasion that also serves as a pledge of their honorable intent and good faith. They will then take their leave and return home to tell the expectant young man what has happened.

When the allotted time has passed, the father of the prospective bridegroom and his companion will return to the girl's house to receive the reply to their proposal of marriage. Assuming that the reception has been favorable, the girl's father will then tell the men how much money they will have to pay as *ku'din aure*, "marriage money." This is not a "sale" of the bride in any sense of the word; it is rather a compensation to her family for having raised the girl to womanhood and is part of a more general process of forming a bond between two families, not just

20. These are "Big Sallah" (*Babban Sallah*)—the Festival of the Sacrifice (*Id-el-Kabir* in Arabic)—and "Little Sallah" (*Karamar Sallah*)—the festival at the end of the fast of Ramadan (*Id-el-Fitr* in Arabic).

between two individuals. The amount of money involved can vary considerably, depending on the status of the family involved and the characteristics of the girl. A figure of thirty or forty naira as *ku'din aure* would be fairly typical, but it could be somewhat less or considerably more. This money is divided with the girl's mother. If the father of the prospective groom has brought a sufficient amount of money with him in anticipation, he will hand it over to the girl's father. Otherwise, he must return home and bring it at a later date. Once this money has been paid, the girl's family tells the boy's family that they may prepare the *kayan sa rana*, "gifts for setting the date" or *kayan baiko*, "betrothal gifts," and bring them to their compound. After this is done the date for the wedding ceremony will be set (*sa rana*).[21]

The family of the bridegroom set about collecting the *kayan sa rana*. Precisely what this entails is subject to considerable variation, but a typical list might be as follows: 1 mattress, 1 blanket, 4 boxes of sugar, 1 large grass or plastic mat, 2 large enamel bowls suitable for washing, 2 smaller enamel bowls suitable for holding drinking water, 4 *tiya*[22] of millet, 4 *tiya* of guinea-corn, and a large sack of salt. When these have been collected the women of the groom's family will carry the goods through the village in a long procession to the compound of the girl's family and will deposit them with the women there. This presentation having been made, they will carry word back to their household as to when the men may come to set the formal date for the wedding.

It is obvious from the preceding discussion that the preparation of

21. Sometimes these arrangements can get quite complicated. One notorious case in the village in which I lived involved a wealthy alhaji, close friend of the village headman, who had a lovely young daughter attending secondary school outside the village. This alhaji had arranged a marriage for her with one man from a large city who had gone so far as to pay him considerable *ku'din aure*. In the interim, a better offer of marriage was made by another man from another city, who paid substantially more *ku'din aure*. The marriage with this latter man took place and the girl was taken away. In the meantime the other man found out what was afoot, went to the courts, and got an injunction against the marriage. The poor girl was shuttled among various relatives until the case was settled, at which time her marriage was annulled, the *ku'din aure* was returned to the second suitor, and she was married to the first claimant.

22. A *tiya* is an enamel bowl used for measuring grain in Hausaland, and is subject to some local variation in size.

a Hausa marriage involves a considerable outlay of money. *Toshi,*
ku'din aure, the *kayan sa rana,* not to mention the later wedding presents (*kayan aure*), require a substantial amount of money. This is one
reason why some Hausa youths marry late—their family cannot afford
the cost of a wife. As the proverb says, *Ana wahala neman aure ba*
ku'di, "Looking for marriage without money is trouble," and also *Ba*
neman aure ke da wuya ba, bidan ku'di, "Arranging a marriage is not
difficult—it's paying the money!" This also explains why so many
marriages take place in January and February, after the cotton harvest
is in—families then have the money to make marriage payments and
to buy the necessary goods.[23]

At the agreed-upon time the formal fixing of the marriage date takes
place. This is a formal process that takes place in front of the village
headman (*maigari*), the *limam,* and the representatives (*wali,* pl.
waliyyai, usually paternal uncles) of the two families. The groom's
family brings kolanuts to distribute among the assembled men of the
village, as well as money (one naira is a common amount) to be paid
to the *limam,* the *maigari,* and the *wali* of the bride.[24] Prayers are said,
the date is fixed a month or two in advance, and the crowd disperses.

As the date for the wedding approaches, the groom's family prepares
the *kayan lefe* or *kayan aure* for the bride. This consists of cosmetics
and fine clothing to be used in dressing the bride for her wedding day.
About ten days before the wedding these articles are taken to the
bride's compound and presented to the women there for safekeeping.

When the morning of the wedding day arrives, the friends and
neighbors of both families gather at the house of the bride. Men sit on
the ground outside the entry-hut, women enter the compound to be
with the women of the household. Kolanuts supplied by the groom's
family are passed out to all the visitors. The *maigari* and the *limam*
are both present, as are the *waliyyai* of the bride and groom. Inside the
entry-hut the formal union of the two young people takes place with
their family representatives as proxies. The *maigari* is given one naira

23. In any discussion about marriage a great deal of time is spent on elaborations
of the things a man must gather in order to get a wife. This is obviously of great
practical importance to the unmarried youth who is seeking a wife—sometimes
painfully so if his family's finances are strained.
24. This money, paid to the *wali* of the bride, is called *rigar uba,* "gown of the
father" in Katsina.

for the official registration of the wedding (*ku'din takarda*, "money of the paper") and the *limam* is given one naira for officiating. After the prayers which formalize the proceedings have been said, the crowd drifts away. The actual "tying of the marriage" (*'dauren aure*) lasts only a few minutes.

The night before the wedding there may be drumming and dancing at the compound of the bridegroom, particularly if he lives in a different village; but in any case, on the afternoon and evening of the wedding all of the girls and women from both compounds will gather with the drummers at the compound of the bride's family. Outside the entry-hut there will be drumming and dancing and all of the girls of the village will come to celebrate. The party from the groom's household will call out to be given the bride, for they have come for her. This may go on for several hours, after which time the bride's family will finally give in to their demands. The party of the groom will pay *ku'din wanka*, "washing money," and *ku'din kunshi*, "henna money," to the girls attending the bride for the pains they will take in preparing her.

The bride—a nervous and frightened young girl—will be taken from her room into the compound courtyard. She will be given a kolanut to prevent her from crying out and will then be bathed and dressed in her finery. Then she will be taken to the front of the compound and given into the custody of the groom's friends, one of whom will have a bicycle. The bride will be balanced on the handlebars—a common mode of transportation in Hausaland—and carried to the household of the groom, where her own room has been readied for her. She will spend the first night of her married life in this room in the company of her best friend or perhaps with a younger sister from her own compound.

The following morning the girl's parents will come to see her new room and inspect her surroundings. After a short visit they will return to their home. That afternoon the groom's family will prepare a feast of *tuwo*, rice, *fura*, and other delectables to be sent to the bride's family; the bride's family will reciprocate the following morning. Then, in the afternoon, another procession will form, carrying all of the bride's possessions, including the *gara* (presents and foodstuffs given her by her parents), from her parents' compound to her new home. A bed, mattress, sacks of rice, salt, pepper, millet, palm oil, butter, enamel pots and basins, tables, benches, chairs—all can be seen bobbing up and down on the heads of brightly dressed women as they make their way to the bride's new home and spread her wealth out before her.

Later that evening the bride is again washed and prepared to look her best. As night wears on and the bride is left alone in her room, the groom makes his appearance with one or more of his friends. They bring gifts of their own—kolanuts, perfume, candies, and money, all neatly arranged in a small box. They meet the bride and greet her, but she says nothing—a few words at best. With much effort they attempt to get her to break her silence and start laughing, and all of them enjoy discussing the events of the past few days. After a while the groom's friends take their leave and he sees them on their way, returning at last to his bride to spend the night with her; and, as one villager put it: *Shi ke nan. Sai 'ya'ya.* "That's it. Now children!"

The transition from village girl to married woman is abrupt, and may be traumatic. This is not simply because of the normal anxiety that might be felt with any change in status. There are enormous differences in behavior associated with this change. Prior to marriage a *budurwa* has enormous freedom. She may come and go in her father's compound as she pleases. She is free to wander the streets of the village in the company of her best friends, to flirt with the village boys and banter with the men. On market days she may travel to other villages. Her activities and sphere of movement are only modestly circumscribed. With marriage, however, her behavior must change dramatically. No longer is she free to come and go at her own discretion. Her movements are limited by her husband's wishes. If it is economically feasible she will be secluded in his family's compound. As the newest wife of the compound she will be subject to the commands of the other women and cut off from the friendly support of her own family in day-to-day affairs. If she happens to be the junior wife of a man who is already married she may encounter the hostility of her senior co-wife, who regards her as a rival. Nothing is more striking to the observer who has lived in a village for some time than the sudden and complete disappearance of the village girls he has seen every day and chatted with in the course of his daily tasks.

There are many compensations for this change in status, however. The girl is at last starting to fulfill her function in life as her society defines it by becoming a wife and, soon, a mother. This step toward maturity brings new prestige, especially among the circle of girls she has left. If she is not free to wander the village streets with them, they at least are still able to come to visit her; and if she is married in the same village in which she grew up there will be plenty of familiar children running in and out all the time. Most likely the women of her new compound will look forward to having a new member in their group to lighten the work and share in the gossip. The family that receives the bride must welcome her and provide for her: *Tilas a gyara ma amarya daki,* "A bride must have a room prepared for her." Ill-treatment of their daughter would not be long endured by her family.

The new husband, too, undergoes a change in status. He is still called *ango,* "bridegroom," but now that he has a wife the proud title of *maigida,* "owner of the house" is applied to him as well. He will still be a junior member of his father's household. His father will be the senior *maigida* with whom the real power lies; but the son will be given the title now as a courtesy indicative of his new status.

The behavioral changes associated with a young man who has taken a wife are not as great as those imposed upon the girl. He will still have the freedom to come and go as he pleases, going out to greet his friends, strolling in the night air. He still may flirt with the village girls, who will make much of his new status and tease him unmercifully (as will all his friends). The most important change, however, is the assumption of new economic responsibilities. Now, having a wife, his duties to the *gida* and to his father (who has undoubtedly financed the marriage) have grown considerably: *Kekketa auren so ba abinci,* "A marriage of love with no food soon splits up." His labors now have a somewhat different meaning.

■ Maturity

Gandu is the Hausa word referring to communal farming, usually between a father and his sons. This sort of relationship probably existed between the father and his son prior to the marriage. The youth was given responsibilities on the family land, and in return the father maintained him in the compound, paid his tax (*haraji*), and looked after his welfare. In addition, the boy was given his own farm (*gayauna*) to work separately. In spite of this, however, most young men are not in a financial position to set out on their own at the time of marriage and, hence, a young man will remain in *gandu* with his fa-

ther, supplying labor under his father's supervision and authority while
laying the foundations of his own family. The produce from his own
farm and any work that he may do on the side as hired labor or in pursuit of a trade remains the bridegroom's, to be set aside in anticipation
of improving his future and supporting his family.

The birth of the first child marks the final transition to adulthood
for both husband and wife. The man truly has a family now, of which
he is the head. The child is his own.[25] Likewise, the wife has realized
her purpose in life—becoming a mother—and, God willing, will continue to produce children: *Haifuwa 'daya foran gindi ne,* "One birth
trains the womb." Due to the pivotal position of this child in the social
growth of his parents, direct reference to his name is avoided. The first
birth is an event marked by *kunya* ("modesty") and the firstborn child
merits special demarcation from those who follow.

After the naming ceremony the new mother will return with the
child to her father's home to be with her mother. She will remain there
for some months, learning from her mother the proper ways of treating
an infant and undergoing a series of hot baths (*wanka*) to ensure that
she regains her strength. In subsequent births she will remain in her
husband's compound and the responsibility for these therapeutic washings will lie with her.

Through the birth of his children a man truly becomes a *maigida,*
learning in the process the meaning of the proverb *Aikin gona da
wuya idan ya 'kare da da'din ci,* "Farm-work is hard, but when it's
done how pleasant it is to eat!" When he has reached a state of prosperity he may decide to leave his father's *gandu,* taking his share of
the farmland with him, perhaps purchasing another farm from money
he has saved or borrowed. If he does not leave—and there is a sense
of moral propriety associated with staying—he will certainly spend
more time on his own *gayauna,* proportional to his mounting responsibilities. Many sons remain in *gandu* until their father's death. Increasingly, *gandu* is seen as a temporary state of affairs allowing a man
time to stabilize himself economically before setting up his own com-

25. This is legally true. If for some reason divorce occurs before a child is born to
the marriage, the bridewealth paid in compensation for the bride would be returned. If a divorce were to occur after the birth of children, the child would remain with the father while the divorced wife returned to her father's compound.
The child is the profit (*riba*) collected off the investment of the *ku'din aure.*

pound.[26] As one man of about thirty with two wives and several children remarked when asked if he was in *gandu* with his father and
brothers, *A'a. Mun yi girma!* "No. We've grown up!"[27]

If a man prospers at his trade and in his farming he may choose to
take a second wife. This will increase his prestige and also his economic
liabilities, for a second wife means more children and more expendi-
tures. Similarly, though he may rely upon his father and his father's
income to provide his first wife for him, the financial arrangements for
any subsequent marriages must be borne by himself. The co-wife
(*kishiya*) that he obtains, therefore, is a status symbol, a mark of his
prosperity and a measure of his importance (*girma*). Not everyone
prospers enough to undertake such obligations and still fewer manage
to become wealthy enough to marry a third or even a fourth wife. Two
women—one older, one younger—can become close friends; with three
or more wives factions can easily arise which destroy the domestic
tranquility a man seeks in his household. Many men aspire to marry a
second wife; few aspire to marry more.

With success a man comes to occupy a larger place in the wider
village community. Age, experience, a reputation for truth (*gaskiya*),
moral excellence (*kirki*), and sterling character (*hali*) give his opinion
weight in local matters. Friends will seek his counsel and respect his
advice. If this moral force is coupled with economic power his influence
will be greater still. He can become one of the real molders of local
sentiment—a fact that will be of increasing importance as Nigeria in-
troduces more democratic forms of local government.[28] One Hausa

26. See the discussions of this subject in Buntjer (1971) and Goddard (1973).
27. This does not, of course, mean severing family ties. The family in question
lived, essentially, in one huge compound—the father, three married sons, and their
families all together. The brothers shared a common tailor shop. They were quite
close and helped each other considerably, even though they kept their resources
separate.
28. One example demonstrates this clearly. While I was living in the village, elections were held to select electors in each village area to choose a local government
council for the division in which the village was located. Six electors were to be
chosen from our village area. Two separate slates of candidates emerged, one
backed by the village headman, the district chief, and some of the wealthier villagers who were known to be the "*maigari's* men"; the other composed of independent men of the community. All of the former group were suspected of being
more interested in *sarauta* (official positions) than in the welfare of the com-

proverb states: *Babba juji ne; kowa ya zo da shara, ya zuba,* "An influential man is a trash heap; everybody comes with sweepings and dumps on him"—the village elders are the repositories for everyone's troubles.

As a man grows older his children mature, and he has the pleasure of seeing his sons and daughters pass through the stages of growth he has traversed. Guiding and directing them, and fulfilling his obligations as defined by his society and his religion, occupy his time. If he becomes a wealthy man he may undertake the pilgrimage to Mecca and become an *alhaji*—the highest rank of social distinction open to the common man. The cycles of the seasons, the agricultural rhythms, form the pattern of his years—patterns that endure in rural Hausaland and set the tone of life even if one has branched out into commerce beyond the confines of agriculture. Village life, in general, is slow and predictable; it is easy to gauge the passing of time.

■ Old Age and Death

Women have much more freedom of movement when they reach menopause and their children are grown. They may now attend the Friday prayers at the village mosque, sitting outside together, removed from the body of men. They can sell their own wares in the markets, visit friends during the day, and perhaps establish some location under a tree in the village where they set up each day to sell beancakes or other delectables. If they have large families—many sons and daughters living in the same village—there are always plenty of family matters (and plenty of grandchildren) to keep them occupied. But if they are widows and all their family is gone they may be forced into continuous, petty trading to obtain enough income to survive, or they may move in with kind-hearted neighbors or friends. In many villages there are numerous broken-down huts on the outskirts of town occupied by widows struggling to get by. The lot of the aged, single woman is not easy.

Men watch their daughters marry and move elsewhere. Their sons grow older, enter into *gandu* with them, and later establish their own

---

munity. The latter group comprised six prosperous men (several of whom were good friends of mine), all of whom were men of outstanding personal character and integrity. The "antiestablishment" ticket easily swept all six places in the election.

compounds. At some point the father will become too old to work in the fields and must rely more and more on his sons or hired labor to do the work for him. At length he may cease agricultural work altogether, relying on his sons for support. He will then spend his days weaving mats, perhaps visiting old cronies, trading in the market, or simply taking his ease in the sun on a grass mat in front of the compound, keeping watch on the village activities that he surveys.

At some point in the cycle of life death intervenes. It may come very early—the under-five mortality rate reaches 50 percent in many parts of Hausaland—or it may be after a fuller, more productive life. By and large the Hausa are not a particularly emotional people, but truly noteworthy expressions of emotion by young and old alike are associated with death. *Ranar mutuwa so ya yi kunya*, "On the day of death love is ashamed."

When death has been ascertained by the family no speed is lost in preparing the body for burial.[29] Hausa burial customs are more for the disposal of the corpse than the commemoration of the dead. Within a few hours of death the body will be interred; only a death occurring late at night will delay the process very much. The body is laid out inside the compound and washed; men wash the bodies of men, women wash those of women. Someone will be sent to inform a tailor, who will busy himself sewing the shroud. Word will spread to the neighbors. Someone will be dispatched to the village mosque to bring the collapsible bier kept there for the transport of corpses. When the body has been washed, dressed, and covered in the shroud, it will be brought out in front of the compound; perhaps it will be covered with a colored body cloth as well. The men will gather behind the body, facing Mecca, and pray, led by the *limam*. Then a procession will form, led by the *limam*, with the corpse following on the bier. This funeral procession will make its way to the burial ground on the outskirts of town.

The grave will have been dug by others by the time the party reaches the graveyard. Hausa graves are shallow, usually two and one-half to three feet in depth, with the longitudinal axis in a north-south line and the face turned east toward Mecca. The deepest part of the grave is a

29. On Hausa death and burial customs see Rattray (1913, II:204–20), Tremearne (1913:103–7), Taylor and Webb (1932:136–47), Trimingham (1959:178–83), M. F. Smith (1954:passim), Hassan and Na'ibi (1962:63–64), and Madauci et al. (1968: 23–25).

long, narrow trench in the middle in which the corpse is laid. Higher up there is a step-like shelf on both sides of the trench. Upon reaching the graveyard the corpse is unstrapped and taken from the bier, then lowered by several men into the trench. Only the shrouded body is placed in the grave. Stout sticks are taken and placed over the top of the corpse, resting on the edges of the shallower pit in the grave. Once this has been done potsherds are placed over the sticks, forming a subterranean roof over the body that prevents earth from falling on the corpse. This completed (in the midst of constant, if solemn, advice from the members of the funeral party), the chinks between the potsherds are plastered together with hard lumps of earth and mud plaster. The earth from the pit is then heaped on top of this structure by the members of the funeral entourage, leaving a shallow mound perhaps eighteen inches in height. No marker is placed on the grave. The procession then re-forms and returns to the village. The bier is returned to its place in the village mosque.

For those who remain in this world (*duniya*), not yet having passed into the next (*lahira*), life must go on. The dead one is commemorated in prayers said on the day of the death and on the third, seventh, and fortieth days thereafter. These take place in the morning, in front of the entry-hut of the dead man's compound. Women whose husbands have died must undergo a period of ritual uncleanliness and mourning (*iddar takaba*) as prescribed by Islamic law, lasting some four months and ten days, during which their activities are curtailed. Women cannot marry again until this period has passed; men may remarry at any time. For the members of the *gida* in which the death has occurred there is the ongoing grief and sense of loss which must be overcome. To aid in this the family will receive a stream of visitors coming to greet them and express their condolences for some time after the tragic event has taken place. *Kwanta, ka mutu, ka ga mai-'kaunarka*, "Lie down and die and you'll know the one who loves you."

After death, and grief, the rest of the world goes on. One Hausa proverb expresses the idea that life contains certain unavoidable risks that must be faced: *Rai kasko ne. Wurin bi da shi ke rushewa*, "Life is a clay pot—it breaks where you take it." Fragility and impermanence are inherent characteristics of living in this world. The "clay pot" of life is carried through the stages that have been described here: birth, infancy and childhood, puberty, courtship and marriage, maturity, old age, and finally, death—whenever it may occur. This chronological process takes place within the structural organization of Hausa society, but its ultimate significance must be measured by the standards of the Hausa moral order that determine the meaning of life for those who accept them.

Islam
and the
Moral Order

*Allah shi ke da rabo, da
mutum ya ke da rabo
ba zai ba wani ba.*

*(God apportions; did
man apportion he would
not give to anyone.)*

HAUSA PROVERB

■ Muhammadiyya: Islam, The Way of the
Prophet

The fundamental starting point for understanding Hausa culture is Islam, for it is
upon Muslim foundations that the Hausa
worldview is based. Indeed, as Dry has written (1952:3): "To be a Hausa is to be a
Muslim, and a man who is not a Muslim is
not considered, regardless of all other cultural
criteria, to be a Hausa in any significant sense
of the term." In fact, the Hausa language is
so heavily indebted to Arabic for its philosophical and abstract vocabulary that it
would be virtually impossible to reconstruct
many "*Ur*-Hausa" concepts separated from
their Islamic contexts.[1]

The religion of Islam stems from the revelations given to the Prophet Muhammed that
took place in the towns of Mecca and Medina
in west-central Arabia in the early part of
the seventh century A.D.[2] In Hausa the Islamic
religion is known as *Lislama*, "Islam,"
Musulunci, "the ways of Muslims," or most
commonly simply as *Muhammadiyya*, "the

1. On Arabic loan words in Hausa see Greenberg
(1947b) and Hiskett (1965). Abraham (1962:iv) even
derives the name "*Hausa*" from the Arabic *al-lisan*,
"the language," although Skinner (1968) attempts a
derivation based on historical circumstances involving the Songhai Empire. The term "*Ur*-Hausa" was
suggested by A. H. M. Kirk-Greene (1967:86).
2. The best study in English of Muhammed and the
origins of Islam is Watt's work *Muhammed at
Medina* (1953) and its companion volume *Muhammed at Mecca* (1956). Brief surveys of Islam may be
found in Guillame (1956), Cragg (1969), and Gibb
(1975). Islam in West Africa is treated in Trimingham (1959, 1962).

teachings of Muhammed." According to the Koran, these revelations were given by God to the Prophet through the angel Gabriel, who laid them upon Muhammed's heart "for a guidance and good tidings to the believers" (Sura II, 90ff.). These revelations were recited by Muhammed and eventually were written down to form the Koran (in Hausa, *Alkur'ani*), the holy book viewed by Muslims as a direct manifestation of God among men, mediated through the person of Muhammed.[3]

The fundamental doctrine of the Islamic religion is that there is only one God, Allah, and that Muhammed is the Prophet of God by whom this revelation and its attendant duties are made known.[4] The recitation of this creed in Arabic is the prelude to becoming a Muslim, for by adhering to it one acknowledges the supremacy of God, the validity of the revelation of the Koran to Muhammed, and acceptance of that teaching as the foundation for one's life. The Koran exhorts this belief and practice most emphatically:

> O believers, believe in God and His Messenger
> and the Book He has sent down on His Messenger
> and the Book which He sent down before.[5]
> Whoso disbelieves in God and His angels
> and His Books, and His Messengers,
> and the Last Day, has surely gone astray
>   into far error.
> (Sura IV, 135ff.)

The Islamic doctrine of God is uncompromising. There is but one God, Allah, and He is supreme, the Creator and Ruler of the universe.

> God
> there is no god but He, the
> Living, the Everlasting.

3. Muhammed is seen as being the last prophet (Hausa, *annabi*), the capstone of the relevations given to the Old Testament prophets and to the Prophet Jesus (who is given respect and status in Islamic theology as a forerunner of Muhammed, but who is often deprecated in practice by Muslims hostile to Christianity).
4. This dogma is treated at great length in Wensinck (1932).
5. This refers to the previous revelations in the religious writings of the Christians and Jews which are seen as superceded by the teachings of Muhammed.

Slumber seizes Him not, neither sleep;
>   to Him belongs
all that is in the heavens and the earth.
Who is there that shall intercede with Him
>   save by His leave?
He knows what lies before them
>   and what is after them
and they comprehend not anything of His knowledge
>   save such as He wills.
His throne comprises the heavens and earth;
>   the preserving of them oppresses Him not;
He is the All-high, the All-glorious.
(Sura II, 256ff.)

The universe is seen as the creation of God, ordained by Him and run by His will. Watt has written (1969:33): "The regularity in nature is imposed on it by God's will, thought of as analogous to a human will." God Himself is seen as the active force in sending the rains, the crops, the harvest, in ordering the seasons and the forces of nature. One popular nature study book in Hausaland is even called *Ikon Allah*, "the power of God"—a manifestation of this belief (East and Imam 1949).

God's control goes beyond the realm of natural phenomena, however; it also extends to the affairs of men. Man's will is completely subordinate to God's will, so much that man cannot do or will anything unless God wills it too (Watt 1970:150).

>   That is the
bounty of God; He gives it unto
whomsoever He will; and God is of
>   bounty abounding.
No affliction befalls in the earth
or in yourselves, but it is in a
Book, before We create it; that is
>   easy for God.
(Koran, LVII, 22)

Even death, as life, comes from God alone:

God gives you life, then makes you die,
then He shall gather you to the Day
of Resurrection, wherein is no doubt.
(Koran, XLX, 26)

It is not given to any soul to die, save by the
leave of God, at an appointed time.
(Koran, III, 139)

Islam, in Arabic, means literally "submission" or "surrender," used in the sense of "submission to the will of God." A *Muslim*, therefore, is one who submits to the will of God and does His commandments. In Hausa this divine will is *nufin Allah*, "the desires of God," and *tuba* is the verb by which one indicates submission, surrender, or repentance. A person vanquished in a fight or a child being beaten will kneel and say *na tuba*, "I give up," while crossing his arms over his chest in an attitude of vulnerable submission. The word is also used for a pagan who converts to Islam. Of him it will be said *ya tuba ya ri'ka salla*, "He has 'surrendered' [his pagan ways] and has taken up Islamic prayers." This notion of surrender leads directly to the Hausa concept of *rabo*, "fate" or "destiny," and explains why the expression in *Allah ya yarda*, "if God agrees" is so common as a qualifying phrase when the Hausa discuss future plans or expectations.

The verb *raba* meaning "to divide" or "to portion out" is the root from which *rabo* is formed. In its broadest sense *rabo* refers to someone's lot in life, that which the world has dealt him. It is used to describe the share one gets in the division of things, as in *raban gado* the "portion of an inheritance" that a man receives from the estate of a kinsman. It is the "portion of life" given to a man by God, and when one says *rabansa ya 'kare*, "his share is finished," it is a euphemism for "he died." All that happens to a man comes from God: *Kowa ka gani da abu, Allah ne ya ba shi*, "Whoever you see with something, it has been given him by God." The fates of men are part of God's structuring of the universe: *Abin da mutum zai samu, da wanda zai same shi tun ran halitta*, "What a man gets, and what 'gets him' has been determined since creation day." The justice of this fate should not be questioned, for God is all-knowing, all-powerful; hence the proverb quoted at the beginning of this chapter: *Allah shi ke da rabo, da mutum ya ke da rabo ba zai ba wani ba*, "God shares out to all, did man apportion he would not give to anybody." There is a divine justice in the world, inscrutable though it may sometimes be. It should not be surprising that one of the greatest of Hausa virtues is *ha'kuri,* "patience."

A man's lot in life may be of several kinds: trouble (*wahala*) and misfortune (*masifa*), reasonable comfort (*daidaici*), or prosperity (*arziki*). Within this world (*duniya*) there are gradations of fortune and position in society: *Duniya matakin soro, wani na gaba da wani,* "The world is a flight of stairs, one ahead of another." For the Muslim, however, the end of this life means a passage into the next world (*lahira*). One of the strongest beliefs of Islam is the existence of the Day of Judgment and a just retribution in the life after death. The wicked, the unjust, the unbelievers (*kafirai*) will be thrown into a fiery hell (called *jahannama* in Hausa) with seven gates (Koran, XV, 44) guarded by angels (Koran, XL, 49–52), from which there is no escape for those "who have purchased the present life at the price of the world to come" (Koran, II, 81). The unbelievers will be like kindling for the fires of hell (Koran, LXXII, 15). The Koran contains fearfully explicit passages on this subject of eternal damnation:

> Leave Me to those who cry lies,
> those prosperous ones, and respite them a little,
> for with Us there are fetters, and a furnace, and
> food that chokes, and a painful chastisement,
> upon the day when the earth and the mountains shall
> quake
> and the mountains become a slipping head of sand.
> (Sura LXXIII, 12–14)

> Woe unto every backbiter, slanderer
> who has gathered riches and counted them over
> thinking his riches have made him immortal!
> No indeed; he shall be thrust into the Crusher;
> and what shall teach thee what is the Crusher?
> > The Fire of God kindled
> > roaring over the hearts
> > covered down upon them
> > in columns outstretched
> (Sura CIV)

for the insolent awaits
an ill resort,
Jahannama, wherein they are roasted—
an evil cradling!
All this; so let them taste it—boiling
water and pus,
and other torments of the like kind
coupled together.
(Sura xxxviii, 55–58)

For the believer, however, who has submitted to the designs of God and truly has tried to live according to the counsel of the Koran, God is merciful, compassionate. God has created paradise, *aljanna*, for the true Muslim, a garden of delights where the faithful will dwell forever (Koran, XLII, 68–73) separated from the unbelievers, whom they will see burning in hell (Koran, VII, 44). The gardens of paradise will pass all human comprehension, everything desired will be had and no one will want for anything:

And those that believe, and do deeds of righteousness,
them We shall admit to gardens underneath
which rivers flow, therein dwelling forever and ever;
therein for them shall be spouses purified,
and We shall admit them to a shelter
of plenteous shade.
(Koran, iv, 60ff.)

This is the similitude of Paradise
which the godfearing have been promised:
therein are rivers of water unstaling,
rivers of milk unchanging in flavour,
and rivers of wine—a delight
to the drinkers,
rivers, too, of honey purified;
and therein for them is every fruit,
and forgiveness from their Lord—
Are they as he who dwells forever
in the Fire, such as are given to

drink boiling water, that tears their
    bowels asunder?
(Sura XLVII, 15ff.)

    As for the unbelievers,
for them garments of fire shall be cut,
and there shall be poured over their heads
    boiling water
whereby whatsoever is in their bellies
and their skins shall be melted; for them await
    hooked iron rods;
as often as they desire in their anguish
to come forth from it, they shall be restored
into it, and: Taste the chastisement
    of the burning!
God shall surely admit those who believe
and do righteous deeds into gardens
underneath which rivers flow; therein
they shall be adorned with bracelets of gold
and with pearls, and their apparel there
    shall be of silk;
and they shall be guided unto goodly speech
and they shall be guided unto the path
    of the All-laudable.
(Sura XXII, 20ff.)[6]

6. Popular visions of *aljanna* are often couched in crudely sensual or materialistic terms, almost as if the bounds of morality had been lifted in the next world. I recall vividly one discussion with a village youth who was concerned about the fact that I was not a Muslim. He went to great lengths to describe paradise to me, a place where rivers ran with milk, beer, and honey. He said a man could wear 100,000 suits of clothing at once, but still feel light and comfortable. He said a man could have 7,000 wives, and a huge bed big enough for all of them at once! Moreover, all traveling was done by airplane—even on the bed—and all you had to do was desire to go there, and you would be taken wherever you wished, to any wife you wanted. All of these wives would be surpassingly beautiful, with shining hair and breasts the size of water pots. It would be impossible to fall in any direction without landing on these breasts and being embraced by your wives. Not only that, but a man would always be potent, able to enjoy the benefits of all these heavenly women. He thought it was such a terrific bargain that a man would have to be crazy not to become a Muslim.

To gain the promises of paradise and escape the damnation of hell, a man or woman must uphold the five "pillars of the faith." He must declare his belief in the oneness of God and the prophethood of Muhammed as the Messenger of God as revealed by the Koran. He must perform the five required sets of prayers each day. He must keep the fast during the month of Ramadan—the month during which the Koran was revealed to Muhammed. He must attempt to make a pilgrimage to Mecca at least once in his lifetime if it lies within his abilities. And finally, he must give alms to the poor and support the work of the *mallamai*, the religious teachers and scholars. Adherence to these five things includes one among the *jama'a*, the community of believers. Since Hausa society is a Muslim society, the term *jama'a* is used to mean "everybody," irrespective of his religiosity or devotion. If one is born a Hausa he is considered a Muslim unless he apostasizes—something that is exceedingly rare; but irrespective of one's diligence in living up to the demands of Islam, these institutions pervade the whole of Hausa life, setting the strictures of morality and view of the world that tie them to the wider "house of Islam."

There are two types of prayer in Islam: obligatory ritual prayer (*salla* or *salla ta farilla*) and voluntary personal prayer (*addu'a*). The form of the *salla* prayers is rigorously set forth by Islamic custom and varies little in Muslim cultures throughout the world. They must be performed five times per day and their performance is the surest sign of one's being a Muslim. The *salla* is the most obvious external manifestation of a man's allegiance to Islam; in fact, the Hausa query as to a person's religious status is not "Are you a Muslim?" (*Kai musulmi ne?*) but rather *kana salla?*, "Do you perform the *salla?*"—the espousal of Islam and the performance of the *salla* are identical concepts in the Hausa mind.

The manner in which the ritual prayers are performed is carefully prescribed. Each time a man performs the *salla* he must be in the proper state of purity (*tsarki*), which is assured by ritual washing (*alwala*). To undertake the washing a man pours a little water out into his hand from a clay pot or one of the plastic teakettles sold widely in northern Nigeria for this purpose. The right hand is washed three times, then the left. The mouth is washed out three times, then the nose and nostrils a similar number of times, followed by the same washing of the face and eyes. Then the right arm is washed three times, followed by the left three times. The head is washed from front to back and then back to front. The right ear is washed, then the left, and the process is ended by washing the right foot three times, and then the left foot three times. The washing completed, he now is ready to perform the prayers. Each of the five *salloli* is broken up into a sequence of repeated movements, each grouping of sequences being known as a *raka'a*. The number of *raka'u* required at each performance of the *salla* varies with the time of day. More may be performed than are required as an act of greater piety; but whatever the number, the sequence of acts is the same.[7]

To perform a *raka'a* the believer faces Mecca, raises his hands palms upward to shoulder level[8] and says *Allahu akbar*, "God is great." He then recites the prayers that go with the bowings, beginning with the *Fatiha*, the opening chapter of the Koran:

> Praise belongs to God, the Lord of all Being,
> the All-merciful, the All-compassionate,
> > the Master of the Day of Doom.
> Thee only we serve; to Thee alone we pray for succour
> > Guide us in the straight path,
> the path of those whom Thou has blessed,
> not of those against whom Thou art wrathful,
> > nor of those who are astray.

Other verses may follow; then the believer bows toward Mecca from the waist, his hands on his knees, says another formula, and rises to an upright position with the exclamation *Allahu akbar*. He then sinks to his knees, his legs curled under him off to the right side, and prostrates himself, touching his hands, forehead, nose, and face to the ground. He then raises up on his knees and repeats the prostration, thus completing the prayers of one *raka'a*. He will then perform the additional prayers necessary to complete a particular *salla* and will finish the last *raka'a* by reciting the credo: "there is no God but God, and Muhammed

7. Brief accounts of these procedures may be found in Guillame (1956:66–69) and Gibb (1975:42–43). A much more complete description, with illustrations of the positions, can be found in Edwin W. Lane's remarkable classic *The Manners and Customs of the Modern Egyptians* (Lane 1860:71–91).

8. This is one difference between the Hausa and most of the Islamic world. The more usual way is to touch the earlobes with the thumbs, palms outward.

Table 1   Obligatory ritual prayers (*salloli*)

Hausa name of prayer	Time of prayer	Number of raka'u
Asuba	Dawn	2
Azahar	After midday (2:00–3:00 P.M.)	4
La'asar	Late afternoon (4:00–5:00 P.M.)	4
Magariba	Sunset	3
Lisha	At night (8:00–9:00 P.M.)	4

is his Prophet." He will end by running through the thirty-three beads of the Muslim rosary (*cazbi*) to finish his devotions. The names of the prayers, the times of their performance, and the number of obligatory *raka'u* necessary at each performance are shown in table 1.[9]

The prayers may be performed individually or in groups. Women invariably perform the *salla* alone, excluded from the view of others, inside their own compounds. Although the dawn prayer is done individually, men prefer to pray in groups if possible.[10] Usually they will attend regular *salla* groups in their neighborhood. These groups meet at the same place at each *salla*—a prayer circle constructed in front of a man's house, or at a personal mosque (which may be quite large) that a man has built next to the entry-hut of his compound. The man who has built the structure in question will probably act as the *limam*, or prayer leader, for the group.

Each Friday afternoon, however, the men of the village and the surrounding countryside gather at the communal mosque to perform the two o'clock *salla* of *azahar*. Old women may be present as well but they will sit outside, away from the men.[11] The Friday mosque (*masallacin juma'a*) is one of the most prized buildings in the community. Built with the contributions of the faithful, it is usually large, spacious, and well built, a roof of sheet metal standing out sharply in a village where the roofs typically are of thatch or mud. When it is

9. See Taylor and Webb (1932:94–101), Madauci et al. (1968:29–32), and also Gibb (1975:42–43).
10. "In Maliki law, the dominant rite throughout the central and western Sudan, even the daily prayers are twenty-seven times better if said in congregation" (Fisher 1977:326).
11. In strict Maliki Islamic law women are prohibited from attending the Friday mosque unless they are past menopause (Ruxton 1916:24).

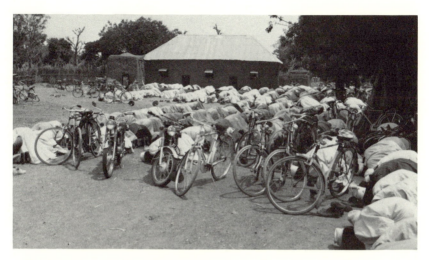

7. *Friday prayers at the village mosque.*

time for the prayers on Friday afternoon the mosque will be filled to
overflowing; the interior will be jammed full and men will crowd outside on either side and behind the mosque, facing Mecca. The *limam*
will mount a platform facing Mecca in front of the crowd and begin
the call to worship. Each *raka'a* of the *salla* will be performed collectively in a choreography of devotion which cannot but impress the
observer. The prayers finished, the crowd will disperse in short order,
a jumble of gowns and bicycles going their separate ways.

The prayer leader of the Friday mosque, who is known as the
limamin juma'a, "the Friday *limam*," *limamin masallaci,* "the limam
of the mosque," or simply just as the *limam,* is regarded as the religious
leader of the entire community, but he is not a priest since the individual stands alone before God without any intercessors in Islam. The
limam is, rather, the officiant who leads communal prayer and guides
the people in solemnizing the various rites of marriage, naming, burial,
and so forth. His position is one of immense prestige, second only to
the village headman. He should be a scholar (*mallam*) of authority and
learning, and, in practical terms, should also be quite wealthy, for the
job is not without its financial requirements. The *limam* is selected by
the consensus (and the politicking) of the acknowledged Koranic
scholars of the community with the consent of the village headman,

who formally invests him with the turban of office. In villages where
the population is too large for one *limam* to handle all of the duties
incumbent upon him, there will be a senior *limam* to lead the Friday
prayers and a subordinate *limam* (perhaps more than one) to divide the
other duties with him.

The *limam* and the *mallamai* are also responsible for running the
Koranic schools, where children attempt to memorize the Koran and
are instructed formally in their religious duties. These schools are held
all over the village, particularly during the dry season when agricultural activities are minimal. They meet in an entryway of the Koranic
scholar's house, in front under a tree outside, or in a special room built
for the purpose of instruction. The number of children in attendance
at any one school is quite varied. There may be anywhere from one or
two students under the tutelege of a relatively minor teacher to twenty,
thirty, or more studying with a scholar of high local reputation such
as the *limam*. These students may be boys and girls from the village
sent to do their lessons at the home of a neighbor, or older boys sent
from far away as *almajarai*—"boarding scholars" living with a *mallam*
in order to study the Koran, work in the teacher's fields, and imbibe
his wisdom.

The subject matter of these schools is roughly of two kinds: rudimentary and advanced. The basic Koranic education is *karatu*, "reading," which entails memorization of Koranic verses, learning to read
and write Arabic, and an understanding of the rudiments of the religion. Advanced education is *ilimi*, "wisdom," and corresponds to more
complicated theological study undertaken after the basics have been
mastered. Only a few pass beyond the first stage, though it may safely
be said that the typical adult Hausa is somewhat literate in Arabic.
Only the devout make an effort to gain a theological grounding and
qualify as Koranic teachers themselves. To gain a sophisticated Islamic
education one must leave the village and travel to a city such as Kano,
Katsina, or Zaria to study with the renowned teachers there.

The Koran is the heart of the religion of Islam. It consists of the
uncreated Word of God, transmitted to the Prophet Muhammed by the
angel Gabriel. It was recited in Arabic by the Prophet as a guidance for
believers and is, for the Muslim, the epitome of absolute truth and
holiness. As such it forms the foundation (along with the *hadisi*, or

traditions of the Prophet) for all Islamic law.[12] The frequently encountered Hausa exclamation *Alkur'ani!* may be translated "God's
truth!" with little loss of meaning. The Koran itself states:

> surely it is
> a Book sublime;
> falsehood comes not to it from before it
> nor from behind it; a sending down from
> One All-wise, All-laudable.
> (Sura xli, 41ff.)

Since the Koran was revealed in Arabic, its essence is Arabic; it is held
to be untranslatable and, hence, every Muslim must study the Koran
in the original Arabic.[13]

Koranic education begins with the pupil being given a few verses to
memorize, gradually building up his knowledge of Arabic.[14] When he
begins making progress the teacher takes a wooden slate (*allo*) and
writes simple verses on it, teaching the child how to read them. The
child memorizes these verses, learning to read (though not necessarily
understand) Arabic, and gradually is given the task of copying out for
himself what the teacher has written. These verses will be written out
over and over again, memorized, checked with the teacher, and then
washed off the slate. Then the process will begin again. Whenever one
passes a Koranic school, be it during the day in the shade of a tree or
at night by the flickering light of large bonfires, the soprano droning
of small boys and girls struggling to master the Koran can be heard.
The object of this pious education is to memorize by heart all 6,200-odd
verses of the Koran. This is an enormous undertaking for anyone, let

12. The basics of Islamic law are explained in Schacht (1950, 1964) and Coulson
(1964). Of the four schools of law in orthodox Sunni Islam—Hanafi, Maliki, Shafi,
and Hanbali—Maliki law predominates in West Africa. The standard work in English on Maliki law is Ruxton (1916).
13. One might say the point is that if God speaks Arabic, you can take the trouble to learn His language. In point of fact, this means that many Hausa Muslims
know very little of what the Koran actually says and means, even though they can
read the Arabic words. A Hausa version of the Koran is in preparation by some
of the Koranic scholars of Kano.
14. See the description of a Koranic school in Taylor and Webb (1932:46–59) and
also that in Madauci et al. (1968:41–46).

alone a child in his formative years. Few manage to accomplish it; most attend a Koranic school for a few months or a few years, enough to gain minimal literacy in Arabic and a store of the most important verses. The philosophy behind this education is that by memorization and repetition of the text a man will gradually enter into the wisdom of the Koran (Watt 1969:165).

Through the Koranic school the child is socialized to accept that there is a divine authority to which men must submit, the idea that success is attained by imitating a fixed traditional pattern, and the belief that adherence to established order and authority ultimately brings success. These ideas exert a profound influence on Hausa society.

Religious liturgies and formulas, and their memorization and re-iteration play an important role throughout a Hausa Muslim's life. The most important of these, of course, is the continuous repetition of the *salla* prayers and the liturgical phrases that accompany them. But there is also a spontaneity beyond the prescribed rites that gives vitality to the religious life of the Hausa. Besides the formal *salla*, Islam recognizes another kind of prayer, the informal supplication or devotional prayer known as *addu'a*. *Salla* prayers have a fixed Arabic form, but the *addu'a* may be in any language—it may be a voluntary ejaculation of the credo, a repetition of a Koranic verse or chapter such as the *Fatiha*, or simply a plea to God (*ro'kon Allah*) in a time of anguish or stress such as a death or illness. *Addu'a* may be said as part of the ceremony of naming or marriage, or informally in the course of every-day life. Religious expressions and exhortations are very much a part of the daily experience, and pious phrases readily fall from Hausa lips: *Allah Sarki!* "God is king!" *La ilaha illallahu!* "There is no God but God [Allah]!" *Alhamdullilahi!* "God be praised!" *Wallahi, tallahi!* "By God! By God!" Even the expressions for "please" are couched in religious terms: *Don Allah, don Annabi,* "For God, for the Prophet."

This spontaneous side of religion finds constructive outlets in activities such as *wa'azi,* "instructive preaching." It is common for devout men to meet in public places to lecture to the community, particularly the young. At night in the dry season by the glow of a kerosene lamp one man will read out a passage in Arabic from the Koran. The preacher will then attempt to translate the passage into Hausa and make exhortations to good conduct and proper belief and behavior, based on the passage that has been read. The lector then continues, reading another passage which again is expounded by the preacher, long into the night. Similarly, men may gather at the home of a pious member of the community to chant or sing passages from books such as the *Ishirimiya,* a popular collection of Muslim religious songs. People will gather around and listen, making offerings of coins on mats in front of the singers. Exceptionally intellectual types may join a *tarika,* a Sufi brotherhood, in which they contemplate the mystic teachings of their order. In general, however, such Sufi groups are confined to the large cities and metropolitan areas, where they can flourish in the more learned and cosmopolitan environment necessary for the appreciation of theological subtleties.[15]

Even so, religious duties are taken seriously in the village community. As the proverb says, *Ko 'daka da gabas sai da a ki yin salla,* "Every room 'faces east' unless you spurn prayers." The most arduous require-ment of the religious year is the fast of Ramadan, in Hausa *azumi.*[16] The Muslim month of Ramadan is, according to the Koran, the month in which the revelations of God to Muhammed began:

> the month of Ramadan, wherein the Koran
> was sent down to be a guidance
> to the people, and as clear signs
> of the Guidance and the Salvation
> So let those of you, who are present
> at the month, fast it.
> (Sura II, 185ff.)

The beginning of the fast is determined in Hausaland by the sighting of the new moon, which marks the beginning of the month. This infor-mation is announced from Sokoto throughout Hausaland by Radio-Television Kaduna to mark the start of the requirements of abstinence.

15. The most important Sufi order in Hausaland is the Tijaniyya. There were a few people in the village in which I lived who claimed to have some knowledge of the Tijaniyya and to follow their teachings. In broad terms, however, they were unim-portant as a group and were regarded by many with some suspicion. As several people put it to me, *ba Muhammidiyya ba ne,* "It's not the teachings of Muham-med." For an excellent study of Hausa Sufism and its importance in the city of Kano see Paden (1973). On Sufism in general see Arberry (1950) and Trimingham (1971).

16. On the fast in Islam see von Grunebaum (1976:51–65). On Hausa observance of the fast see Taylor and Webb (1932:114–30) and Madauci et al. (1968:32–36).

Believers are required to fast from sunrise to sunset throughout the entire month—a requirement that will last until the new moon is sighted at the start of the following month. This means total abstinence from food, water, tobacco, and sexual intercourse during the daylight hours for the entire month. Since the Islamic calendar year is based upon a lunar, not a solar, cycle, this means that over a period of time the fast may fall during any season. For the fast to come in the agricultural season, when work in the fields cannot be avoided, is a burden of no small proportions. Men must hoe and sweat in the hot sun with no prospect of relief until nightfall. Arduous as this may seem, it is adhered to scrupulously (at least in public). It is not uncommon to see a man lying down in the shade, completely worn out, and hear him say *"Wayyo. Hankalina ya kwanta. Azumi ya kama ni."* "God. My brain is asleep. Ramadan has caught me." Hard work, hot sun, and no food or drink can be quickly exhausting. Because of its rigors, the sick, the aged, children, nursing mothers, and pregnant women are excused from the fast—although in theory the lost days should be made good by fasting at other times throughout the year (Koran II, 18off.; Ruxton 1916:55–57). People not excused by religious law from the fast may be suspected of eating secretly behind closed doors. To paraphrase a proverb slightly, *An ce da arne "Azumi da wuya"; ya ce, "Kun kula da ita ne."* "One says to the pagan, 'Fasting is difficult.' He says, 'You're the ones who worry about it.' "[17]

For the devout, however, the fast can be an experience of heightened religious awareness in which Islam takes on a new and deeper meaning, and in which his commitment is strengthened. Early in the morning, before sunrise, a crier stalks the village streets calling out *Ku zo lafiya! Ku zo lafiya!* "Arise well! Arise well!" ensuring that the village is up before sunrise so they will have time to prepare and eat their food before the interdicting rays of the sun appear. Every morning during Ramadan groups of men meet in the mosque to recite the Koran and read commentaries (*tabsiri*) upon it. Men will enter, listen for a while, and present a few coins to the lectors. Some will stay until the reading stops at midday. In the course of the thirty days of the fast the entire Koran will be read out for the edification of the listeners.

17. The actual proverb is *An ce da arne salla da wuya, ya ce kun kula da ita na,* "One says to the pagan, 'Doing the *salla* is difficult'; he says, 'You're the ones who worry about it'."

During the fast the days are spent as leisurely as possible, often in contemplation or Koranic study, men counting the hours until *lokacin shan ruwa*," the time for water-drinking." With temperatures well over one hundred degrees in the dry season, not to touch liquids can be agonizing. When the sun falls below the horizon the Islamic community tucks into their meals with immense gladness and relief before retiring for the night in preparation for another day of fasting.

As the end of Ramadan approaches, excitement mounts in the village. The end of the fast marks one of the two major festivals of the religious year in Hausaland.[18] This is *Id-el-Fitr*, known in Hausa as *'Karamar Sallah*, "the Lesser Festival." The other major festival (or *idi* in Hausa) is *Babbar Sallah*, "the Greater Festival," (*Id-el-Kabir*, the Islamic Festival of the Sacrifice), performed on the tenth of the Muslim month of Zulhaji, the month of the pilgrimage. The *Sallah* is a time of rejoicing, of giving and receiving presents, of eating and enjoyment. At *Sallah* people get new clothes, and youths send presents to woo their sweethearts. Although the Lesser *Sallah* is not as important theologically, the fact that it comes at the end of the hardships of Ramadan makes it more important socially than the Greater Festival which follows later in the year.

The *Sallah* is the largest communal display of religious solidarity in Islamic Hausaland. The fundamental principle of Islamic government is the unity of the religious and the political community. The community of believers (*jama'a*) forms a single legal and social body, deriving its values and political structure ultimately from the Prophet and his teachings. At *Sallah* this ideological principle is emphasized heavily, for if the structure of the community is descended ultimately from the Prophet (and hence from God), it follows that whoever occupies the apex of the social and political structure in a Muslim society is very much an authority ordained by God. In the traditional order of things this position is held by the *sarki* of each emirate, under the nominal suzereignty of the sultan of Sokoto. Therefore, at *Sallah* there is a marshaling of the faithful, who troop to the capital of the kingdom in which they live to pay their homage to the emir and to reaffirm their

18. On Hausa festivals see Taylor and Webb (1932:114–30) and Madauci et al. (1968:36–41). Throughout this work I have designated the prescribed prayers as *salla* and the Greater and Lesser Festivals as *Sallah* in order to avoid confusion, although in Hausa the same word (*salla*) is used to refer to both.

commitment to the Islamic values on which their society is based. In Katsina this show of support is particularly impressive.

Village headmen do not spend *Sallah* in their villages. They must accompany their district chief to Katsina for the ceremonies there, affirming their support both for him and for the emir. A day or two before the end of the fast all the village headmen and their retinues meet at the district headquarters to prepare for the journey northward. Horses are loaded into lorries, bags and baggage are sorted out, and finally the procession sets off, accompanied by much drumming and blowing of horns. By lorry it takes only a few hours to make the trip, so by midday the party has reached Katsina and unloads, the headmen scattering to various compounds in the city, the district head going to his own house. The arrival in Katsina of all the village headmen and the district chiefs makes it an event of major importance. The approaching end of the fast and the arrival of so many dignitaries adds to the atmosphere of expectation.

Ramadan ends at sunrise on the morning of the first day of the month of Shawwal. The rising of the sun also lifts the burden of the fast, and there is something special about this first meal of the new month. The food is eaten with delight and relief, and no doubt helps instill a sense of gratitude in the fasting Hausa. Finally sated, the community begins to drift toward the communal prayer ground (*masallacin idi*) outside the city, each district chief and his retinue of subordinate village heads and followers traveling together. All the officials of the emirate will be there, dressed in the most opulent clothes they possess. Even the townspeople and the country bumpkins in from the rural areas will have new clothes, for this is one time of the year when extravagance is the order of the day. Everyone in the city who can be there attends the communal prayers performed at this time. Led by the chief *limam* and the emir, the enormous crowd of Muslim believers at their prayers presents a spectacle of enormous power and religious solidarity that is difficult to convey, a power that is obviously very important in contributing to the feeling of living in a divinely ordered system which is characteristic of so much Hausa thought.

Once the communal prayers have been performed an enormous procession forms, each district chief and his retinue occupying a place in sequence within it. The procession winds its way around the old city walls of Katsina and through the streets, amidst the cheers and applause of the masses of Hausa spectators jammed on the roadsides and lining all the rooftops. At points along the route prominent individuals emerge from the crowds and address the dignitaries, who stop their progress in the procession to receive the blessings and engage in *addu'a* before moving on. As the parties pass along the route each noble is recognized and greeted by cries of his title: *Galadima! Makama! Makama! Sarkin Fawa!* The shrill ululations of the women break through the noise of the crowd. Drummers and trumpeters accompany each dignitary, engaging in their own little processions and displays of musical virtuosity. Noble after noble passes by with his followers: hordes of dancers in green with feathers, mounted horsemen clad in orange, troops of turbaned swordsmen in flowing robes, and finally, bringing up the rear, the emir of Katsina himself, clad in brilliant white, riding a dark horse and protected from the mounting heat of the sun by a richly ornamented red-and-yellow parasol carried by an attendant, and followed by his guard of mounted spearmen, drummers on camels, and ceremonial cavalry.

The procession ends in the central parade ground near the prison and the emir's palace, where a huge reviewing stand has been set up. The emir enters the parade ground and mounts to the reviewing stand, where from his position of command he receives the *jafi*—a succession of massed cavalry charges by the chiefs from each district with their subordinate village headmen and retainers, who pull their mounts up short and salute in front of the stand. When the last district has paid homage in this fashion the district chiefs and other dignitaries attend a brief reception for the emir inside the palace grounds before dispersing. This procession and the massed cavalry charges are repeated again on the following day, after which the delegations from the districts begin to pack up and return home.

Besides keeping the fast during Ramadan, a Muslim is obliged to carry out a pilgrimage (*hajj*) to the holy city of Mecca at some time during his life.[19] Pilgrimage to Mecca was a pre-Islamic ritual, claimed by Muhammed to have been initiated by the patriarch Abraham, and enjoined on all true Muslims:

---

19. A general description of the pilgrimage may be found in von Grunebaum (1976:15–49). The best account, however, is Sir Richard Burton's *Personal Narrative of a Pilgrimage to Al-Madinah and Meccah* (1893).

Say: "God has spoken the truth; therefore follow
the creed of Abraham, a man of pure faith
 and no idolater."
The first House established for the people
was that at Mekka, a place holy, and a guidance
 to all beings.
Therein are clear signs—the station of Abraham,
and whoso enters it is in security.
It is the duty of all men towards God to come
to the House a pilgrim, if he is able to
 make his way there.
As for the Unbelievers, God is All-sufficient
 nor needs any being.
(Koran, III, 90ff.)

The obligatory pilgrimage (*hajj*) is performed during the month of Zulhaji, the twelfth and last month of the Muslim calendar. A lesser pilgrimage, or "visitation," (*umra*) may be made at any time as an act of piety, but does not by itself fulfil the obligation of making the *hajj* (Ruxton 1916:61). Each year a few wealthy men from the village sign on with the Northern Pilgrims' Board to make the flight to Mecca. Pilgrimage takes two weeks, leaving from Kano aboard chartered aircraft. As such, it no longer holds the same prestige it had earlier in this century or before, when a man needed months or even years to make the hazardous Sahara crossing.[20] At that time a primary motivation was learning (*ilimi*) and a man spent long days in study with all the great *mallamai* he encountered, gathering religious wisdom as he made the trip. Upon his return—if he managed to return, and many did not—he was regarded as a true doctor of the law, a theological authority and figure of respect who would occupy a place of high standing in the community. There is still a great deal of prestige attached to being an *alhaji*, "one who has made the pilgrimage." Rather than a sobriquet of pious learning, however, *alhaji* increasingly has the connotation of "one who is wealthy enough to travel to Mecca," and it is used as a form of polite address to people in positions of power and authority much the way *mallam* has come to mean "mister" in Hausa in addition to refer-

20. On the pilgrimage to Mecca by West Africans see particularly Works (1976) and Birks (1978).

ring to Islamic scholars. Nonetheless, the pilgrimage and the prestige
of the title that goes with it is open (at least in theory) to all believers,
and is not dependent upon previous status or rank of birth. As such
it is a golden hope to which all aspire.[21]

Numerous regulations surround the *hajj* to ensure that it is performed according to the correct ritual specifications.[22] These matters
obviously are of great concern to the pilgrim; but in realistic terms
only a small number of the total Muslim community ever manage to
make the journey to the holy places. This was a difficulty Muhammed
foresaw, and those unable to make the pilgrimage because of age,
penury, sickness, or other circumstances are given alternative forms of
purification, especially sacrifice:

> Fulfil the Pilgrimage and the Visitation
> unto God; but if you are prevented,
> then such offering as may be feasible.
> (Koran, II, 192)

The ritual of sacrifice is the basis of the Festival of the Sacrifice
(Arabic, *Id-el-Kabir*), the *Babbar Sallah* or Greater Festival of Hausaland. On the tenth day of Zulhaji, while the pilgrims carry out their
sacrifices in the Arabian city of Mina, the entire Muslim world joins
them in a worldwide ritual of blood sacrifice, which is for many Hausa
villagers the highlight of the festival celebrations.

The *Sallah* festival in the village is much like that in Katsina, although on a much more modest scale. While the village headman, the
district chief, and the occasional rural tourist depart for the celebrations
and processions in the capital, the people of the village ready themselves for their own celebration. The first thing done in the morning
is the preparation of the *tuwon Sallah*, the festival *tuwo*—the finest of
the year. Carefully made, covered with the best sauce, and topped with
meat—chicken, duck, or even beef (for several cattle are slaughtered

21. The cost of the pilgrimage was reckoned at roughly ₦1,000 in 1976, or about
the same cost as two oxen and a metal plow. When I asked my friends which they
would rather have—the oxen and plow or the title of *alhaji*—they responded almost uniformly that they would rather have the former—and then earn enough in
short order to make the pilgrimage as well!
22. An outline of regulations concerning the pilgrimage may be found in Ruxton
(1916:61–64).

by village butchers before *Sallah,* a practice unheard of at any other time of the year due to the enormous expense and the slim chance of selling all the meat)—this is a gourmet's delight. *Tuwon girma miyarsa nama,* "The *tuwo* of authority has meat sauce," says the proverb. There is also plenty of it: *Tuwon Sallah maganin mai-hadama,* "Festival *tuwo* is the medicine for a greedy man"—he can eat until he's stuffed.

The meal eaten, at mid-morning the villagers begin moving through the fields surrounding the town, dressed in their best clothes, to the *masallacin idi,* the festival prayer ground, located under a tree in one of the cotton fields. People gather under the shade of a large locust-bean tree, and bicycles are parked everywhere in the fields and along the paths, with perhaps a lorry or two drawn up nearby. Led by the *limam* of the village mosque, the communal prayers are said and then a great procession forms back to the village: hordes of brightly clad men, women, and children, riding bicycles, donkeys, and motorcycles, girls clapping, chanting, and singing together move through the main street down past the headman's compound toward the village mosque, breaking into the side streets and returning home, stopping to greet friends and exchange presents.

When the communal activities are over it is time for the individual compound heads to make their sacrifices, to kill the *ragon Sallah,* the festival ram. If a household head is not wealthy enough to afford the extravagance of a ram, then a lesser animal, a chicken perhaps, will do—and the very poor are excused altogether. The slaughter of animals is ritually prescribed in Islamic law. In Maliki law, "slaughtering is an operation which must be performed by a Believer in full possession of his faculties. It consists in severing the wind-pipe and the two jugular veins in one operation without removing the knife, the cut being directed from the front and not from the side of the neck." (Ruxton 1916:65). A hole is dug to receive the blood of the animal, whose neck is then forced to the ground while its throat is cut. Properly, the wielder of the knife should say *Bismillah!* "In the name of God" as he draws the blade across. The animal is held until it has bled to death, and then is carted away to be skinned and butchered.

Butchering follows the established Hausa pattern. One of the hind legs of the ram is slit open and the fascia is separated by poking a stick up underneath the skin. With his mouth the butcher then inflates the animal, bloating the carcass and drawing the skin taut. Following this, the chest and belly are slit open and the animal is then skinned, the hide coming away easily due to the internal pressure of inflation. The viscera are then removed and the edible remnants washed and hung up on a stake to be divided into portions for cooking later on. *Sallah* and the days following are always days of exceptionally fine eating.

The remainder of the festival day is passed in many ways. Perhaps the most common is *yawon Sallah*, "taking a *Sallah* stroll" to circumambulate the village, greeting friends and catching up on the latest gossip. One Hausa proverb states *Zumunta a 'kafa ta ke*, "Amicable relations lie in the feet," meaning that the maintenance of good feeling depends on frequent visits. *Sallah* is an excellent time to take care of these obligations. Everyone is relaxing and no work is being done (except, perhaps, by a few tailors who are behind on their holiday orders). The round of greeting is continuous, everyone is dressed up in new clothes, and there is as much vanity as friendliness involved in going by to greet one's friends. Everywhere the phrase *Barka da Sallah* is heard—"May the *Sallah* bring you blessings!" The recipient of such a greeting is expected to return the favor with a coin or kolanut— especially if he has been greeted flirtatiously by an attractive young girl dressed in her finest clothes. In the evening *Sallah* presents an admirable occasion for dancing, and drummers will be found around the village making music for the girls to dance by. Elsewhere in the countryside or in the village (particularly in the compounds of prostitutes) *bori*[23]—the dances of spirit possession—will be staged, adding to the festival atmosphere in a peculiarly non-Islamic way.

Besides the major festivals which form the core of Islamic celebrations in Hausaland, there are a number of minor religious holidays during the year. On the tenth day of the first month of the year, Almuharram, there is the minor *Sallar cika shekara*, "festival of completing the year" or *Sallar cika ciki*, "festival of filling the belly," when devout Koranic students "open the Book" (*bu'de takarda*) in an effort to divine the portents for the coming year, and others content themselves with eating to satiety in hopes of encouraging good fortune and prosperity in the coming seasons. The second month, Safar, is devoid of

23. *Bori* and the spirits are discussed in some detail in the next chapter.

celebrations, but the festival of *Mauludi*—the birthday of the Prophet—falls in Rabi'i Lawwal, the third month. This is marked by minor prayers at the village mosque. Three months follow with no religious holidays: Rabi'i Lahir, Jimada Lawwal, and Jimada Lahir. The seventh month (Rajab) contains the day of *azumin tsofaffi*, the "old people's fast," designated as a day of atonement for those aged Muslims who were unable to keep the fast of Ramadan the previous year. In the following month of Sha'aban there is a day called *sallar tsofaffi*, the "*Sallah* of the old ones," a day of prayer in commemoration of deceased parents and grandparents. The ninth month is Ramadan, the month of the great fast—the most important month in the Muslim calendar. It ends on the first day of Shawwal, when the Lesser Festival begins. The eleventh month (Zulaidu) has no celebration, but leads into the month of the pilgrimage, Zulhaji, and the Festival of the Sacrifice, *Babbar Sallah*.

The structrue of Hausa religious life centers around these yearly festivals and the observance of the five daily times of prayer. Passage through the crises of life is mediated by simple Islamic ceremonies, as described in chapter 2. Adherence to the five pillars of the faith of Islam—declaration of belief in one God (*Allah*) and the Prophethood of Muhammed, prayer, fasting, pilgrimage, and almsgiving—assures one of a place in the *jama'a*, the company of believers, and guarantees salvation from the wrath of God on the Day of Judgment. As the village headman put it, "You will hold the next world in the palm of your hand." These five duties stamp one as a Muslim, but even so there are obvious gradations of personal worth and varieties of moral excellence found throughout the community. Merely being a Muslim is not enough. To reach the pinnacle of moral and religious veneration a man must meet standards other than the mere outward performance of required duties. There are many people who would be accepted as "Muslims" in a Hausa village, but not regarded as men of moral excellence. To understand fully the Hausa moral order it is necessary to examine their concepts of moral virtue in some detail, to delineate the Hausa values that make a person a *mutumin kirki*, a "man of excellence" or a "good man."[24]

24. An invaluable treatment of this subject is that of A. H. M. Kirk-Greene (1974), a work which has greatly influenced the discussion that follows below. Much of this same material has also been treated by Barkow (1974).

■ The Components of Virtue

The moral attributes of a man lie in his *hali*: his character, temperament, or disposition. A man's *hali* is the aspect he presents to the world, the general tenor of his being. *Hali*, therefore, is something possessed by everyone, but it is not the same for all: *Hali, kowa da irin nasa,* "Character, everyone has his own kind," as the proverb says. While a man's mood or state of mind may change with circumstances, his basic character remains and manifests itself over the course of time. One proverb declares *Sai an da'de a kan san hali,* "Only by waiting is character known." Character is the fundamental determinant of what a man is, the ultimate, overriding value of a man: *Kan da hali muni kyau ne, in ba hali ba, kyau muni ne,* "If accompanied by [fine] character wrong becomes good; if there is no character, good becomes wrong." *Kirki,* "moral excellence," is the finest expression of a man's *hali*; its opposite is *mugunta,* "badness" or evil—a word that also means "pus." *Mugun hali,* "vile character" is disruptive, a moral sickness that destroys a man's worth as surely as a sickness destroys his body; and the most damning comment of all upon a man is to say *ba ya da hali,* "He has no character at all."

The foundation upon which the character of a good Hausa man is erected is *tsoron Allah,* "fear of God." The Biblical injunction that the fear of the Lord is the beginning of wisdom (Proverbs I:7) is equally applicable to Hausa notions of virtue. *Imani,* "maintaining the faith in Islam and living by Islamic precepts" is the groundwork that underlies all manifestations of moral excellence. Strict adherence to the faith and its ritual observances are prerequisites for any sort of moral stature. To be a *mutumin kirki* a man must first manifest *ibada,* service to God. Those foreigners who have won the approbation of the Hausa as good men are always adherents of other religions, who likewise manifest such a devotion to God; the concept of a "good atheist" is a contradiction in terms for the Hausa villager. *Wanda bai gode Allah ba, ya gode wa azabarsa,* "He who does not thank God will be thanking his time of anguish."

One of the primary requirements for moral excellence is *gaskiya,* "truth." The Hausa concept of *gaskiya* goes beyond the English notion of mere truth or honesty. It implies a fundamental orientation toward the world that transcends the ebb and flow of daily living. *'Karya ta shekara 'karya, gaskiya tana matsayinta,* "A lie is a lie even after a year, but truth has its abiding place." A *mutumin gaskiya,* a "man of truth," is more than an honest man. He is a man who is open and forthright, one who has clearly seen the proper structure of the world and cleaves faithfully to it.[25] He perceives rightness and acts upon it. His actions are characterized by *adalci,* "fairness and justice." His speech is truthful and appropriate (*daidai*), confined to the requirements of the situation, and not extending beyond them. His maxim is *Kowa ya yi 'karya ta dame shi,* "Lies will recoil on those who bear them." He is no boaster or busybody, knowing that *'Daurarriyar magana wadda ta fi sukam mashi ciwo,* "A libel hurts more than the thrust of a spear," and *Yawan magana ita kan kawo 'karya,* "A plenitude of talk always brings forth lies." The truthful man deals rightly with everyone and extends an even hand to all. The outcome of *gaskiya* is, therefore, *amana,* "trust." One can loan him a farm without fear, give him credit, or leave land or money in his care while making a journey, secure in the knowledge that all will be well when one returns. He is dependable, reliable, a constant (as is truth) upon which one can count.

In addition to these attributes, the good man among the Hausa must possess *ha'kuri,* "patience." Indeed, this is one of the most widely invoked of all Hausa virtues. The angry or impatient man is told *yi ha'kuri,* "Be patient. Calm down." Islam exhorts submission to the will of God, and so the Hausa exhort each other to be patient, enduring, steadfast, forbearing. *Duka 'daya ba shi kada 'kato,* "One blow will not knock a strong man down." Through patience all obstacles may be overcome. *Wanda ya yi ha'kuri ga masifa sai shi zama kama ba a yi ba,* "He who bears misfortune patiently remains as though it had never been." *Kome ka yi ha'kuri da shi ka ga bayansa,* "By bearing troubles patiently one soon sees the end of them." Each man's lot in life (*rabo*) is determined by God in His omniscience. Resignation to the will of God and acceptance of whatever befalls one leads to peace in this world and blessings in the next. *Kowa ya yi ha'kuri shi ka samun riba,* declares the proverb: "The patient man makes the profit." No better summary of the importance placed by the Hausa on this virtue of stoic

25. The name of the most prominent Hausa language newspaper is, appropriately, *Gaskiya ta fi kwabo,* "Truth is worth more than a penny."

fortitude called *ha'kuri* can be found than the simple proverb *Ha'kuri maganin duniya*, "Patience is the world's medicine."

God-fearing, truthful, trustworthy, patient—these are all characteristics of the *mutumin kirki*; but even these are not sufficient by themselves. A good man must also be characterized by *aminci*, "friendliness." *Son mutane*, "love of people" or "humankindness" should characterize his relations with others. As one proverb declares, *Mai-da'din kai ya fito daga Allah*, "A man with a pleasant personality comes from God." This friendliness should manifest itself in another primary Hausa virtue, *karamci*, "liberality." The good man shares what he has with others and is attentive to their needs.

In large part these virtues of generosity are an expression of the Islamic duty of charitable almsgiving, one of the five basic obligations of the faith. Two forms of charity are enjoined upon Muslims: in Hausa, *zakka* and *sadaka*. The *zakka* is a tithe on the harvest, paid formerly to the rulers of the Hausa emirates in the pre-British days as part of the general system of taxation (see Orr 1911:155), but now a voluntary yearly contribution given to the *limam* and the Koranic *mallamai* to support them in their religious duties and to aid in other charitable endeavors. *Sadaka* refers to personal charitable contributions made to beggars, the indigent, the feeble, or other needy persons. Demanded as a religious obligation for the alleviation of suffering, charitable offerings and personal intervention form virtually the only social services in Hausaland. An ailing relative, the leper who crawls through the streets of the village, a madwoman who lives half-naked in the market—the only solace these people have is individual charity. If they are not taken into someone's home (usually that of a relative) or supported by what they can beg, they have little hope and must eke out an existence as best they can. The moral imperative to engage in charitable acts is vividly expressed in one somber proverb: *In an 'ki maraya da rigar buzu, wata rara an gan shi da ta 'karfe*, "If you spurn an orphan clad in skins, one day you will meet him clad in armor."

The stricture to be generous makes itself felt throughout all levels of Hausa society and colors all social relationships. Small coins or foodstuffs are often given as *sadaka* to beggars or small children; but the practice does not end there. The Hausa custom of *goro* is a proper and necessary part of all personal encounters of any significance and dovetails fully with the Islamic demand for charitable giving. Strictly speaking, *goro* refers to the kolanut, the seed of the *Cola acuminata*, ubiquitously traded and eaten throughout Hausaland for centuries.[26] High in caffeine, it is one of the few stimulants permitted to Muslims, and is highly valued both for its flavor and for its effects. It holds a place very similar in Hausa culture to that occupied by a cup of coffee in the United States or a cup of tea in Britain. Old men so toothless they cannot chew anything solid will still take kolanuts, making a small grater (*magogi*) out of a piece of tin or the lid of a can by which they can shred the nut into fine pieces and savor the flavor without the burden of mastication. When two friends meet one will offer the other a kolanut as an act of friendship. If one man comes to visit another, he will bring kolanuts as a present of greeting, or a few coins as a substitute— coins which in this case are likewise called *goro*, "kola."

What is the purpose of all this? The institution of *goro* in Hausa society is but one manifestation of the impulses that spring from the Islamic precepts of charity and the values attached to generosity. It is but one link in a chain of prestations[27] which binds much of Hausa social activity together into a coherent social whole. The belief is very strong among the Hausa (as among all Muslims) that God is the ultimate source of all blessings and well-being. The Koran makes this point very clearly:

> Your wealth and your children are
> only a trial; and with God is
>   a mighty wage.
> So fear God as far as you are able,
> and give ear, and obey, and expend
> well for yourselves. And whosoever
> is guarded against the avarice
> of his own soul, those—they are
>   the prosperers.
> If you lend to God a good loan, He
> will multiply it for you, and will

26. On the kola trade in Hausaland see Lovejoy (1971).
27. The term "prestation" is Mauss's and refers to "any thing or series of things given freely or obligatorily as a gift or in exchange; and includes services, entertainments, etc., as well as material things" (Mauss 1954:xi).

forgive you. God is All-thankful,
  All-clement.
Knower He of the Unseen and the Visible,
  the All-mighty, the All-wise.
(Sura LXIV, 15–18)[28]

The prosperity of men is here depicted as a test of man's stewardship
of the blessings tendered to him by God. Those who hoard greedily
what they have been given ultimately will not prosper. Only those who
treat men as generously as God has treated them will benefit. A prosperous man (*mai-arziki*) is so because God has favored him. He is therefore obliged to give to others—through *zakka* and *sadaka*—as a means
of returning to the service of God the things which have passed his
way. In this sense the alms given to the poor or the tithes given to the
Koranic scholars complete a circle of exchange from God to man and
back to God.

In the general realm of human relations a man who gives a gift places
himself in a position of superiority to the man who receives from his
hand, putting the latter under an obligation to respond with gratitude
and with like generosity at a future time. Mauss has written of this
situation in his perceptive study of gifts and exchange (1954:72): "Between vassals and chiefs, between vassals and their henchmen, the hierarchy is established by means of these gifts. To give is to show one's
superiority, to show that one is something more and higher, that one is
magister. To accept without returning or repaying more is to face sub-
ordination, to become a client and subservient, to become *minister*."
One Hausa proverb is practically a translation of these thoughts: *A ba
mu a fi mu an 'hana mu daidai a mu a ke*, "Who gives to us is our superior, who refuses us is our equal." In giving a gift one gives more than
the gift; the giver gives part of himself as well. Giving a gift, even a
small one like a kolanut, is an indication of a greater willingness to give,
a sign of a superior moral generosity. *Wanda ya ba ka barin goro, in ya
san guda ya ba ka*, "He who gives you half a kolanut would give you a
whole one if he could."

Such generosity should evoke a similar response in others. *Yar da
alheri baya ka 'dauke shi a gaba*, "Throw favor behind and you will pick

28. The importance of this passage was suggested by the comments of Mauss
(1954:75–76).

it up in front"—hence the continual exchange and counterexchange that goes on throughout Hausa life. A man feels humble respect and "shame" in the presence of his parents-in-law because *sun ba ka mata*, "they have given you a wife." You give coins to a praise-singer who extols you because he has placed you under an obligation by giving you praise—and to refuse may result in diminishment of your status and a "change of tune" from adulation to obscene abuse. Similarly, on one of the festival days when a girl or young boy says *"Barka da Sallah,"* the recipient of the blessings is obliged to respond in material fashion with a coin or kolanut or face a diminishment of status and a minor stain upon the excellence of his character. A generous man will give *taimako* "aid" or "assistance" or *gudummawa* "help" to his needy friends— such as those who have suffered a personal disaster or fire in their home—thus indicating his generosity and raising himself higher on the moral plane. When a friend has been instrumental in completing a sale he should receive *la'ada*, a "commission" as repayment for his generous help, also indicating that the seller is a man of equal good character. At a *bi'ki*, or feast, on the occasion of a marriage or birth, those invited come and *yi bi'ki*, "make contributions toward the feast," giving presents of money, food, and other items to help defray the costs—all these items being listed and called out by a crier to the crowd and duly entered (if someone literate is present) in a book. The recipient is then under an obligation to assist the others in their own times of similar need or face diminishment of his own status. Even the institution of *adashi*—a kind of rotating credit association in which each member contributes a sum each week or month to a general fund, which is used by all the participants in turn—has manifestations of this concept inherent in it.

On days of sorrow, when there is a death in a family, friends will come and leave gifts of coins or kolanuts as *gaisuwa*, "greeting," thereby establishing a common bond with the grieving family and showing sympathy. Greeting and gift giving go hand in hand; one is the giving of one's time and respect, the other is the giving of material goods and is a manifestation of moral correctness, superiority, generosity. The elaborate rituals of greeting and the constant exchange of verbal blessings so characteristic of Muslim piety are all manifestations of this total system of prestations by which generosity enhances one's position and respect. In confronting a social superior one always brings a small gift, thereby placing a little of oneself before him as a token of respect and an effort to win his favor. *Toshi*, the money of persuasion and courtship, is a similar kind of institution, and *ku'din aure*—the marriage money—is a kind of partial compensation given to the bride's family for their trust and reciprocal gift of a wife to the other family. Special friendships are marked by gift giving, the material exchange being an outer indication of the deeper personal interchange that goes on. A man's "big friend" (*babban aboki*) aids with the marriage arrangements, the courtship, and the expenses that may occur. A girl's "best friend" (*'kawa*) is her similar confidante; their personal interchanges are marked by the giving of small gifts. Special relationships may exist between older and younger men or women (sometimes even between men and women), called the *wan rana* and the *'kanen rana* ("elder brother of the day" and "younger brother of the day") and the *'kanwar rana* and *'yar rana* ("younger sister of the day" and "elder sister of the day"), similarly cemented by gifts. These people have a privileged place in the wedding arrangements. A youth's relationship with his *budurwa* ("special girlfriend," though not necessarily a fiancée), is likewise reinforced by small tokens and presents. Longstanding liaisons between otherwise respectable citizens and village prostitutes may have a similar character. The importance of patronage and clientship in traditional Hausa politics should not be underestimated, and the distinction between mutual help, the repayment of obligations, and outright corruption is often a fine one.

The good man, therefore, is a generous man. The more generous and giving of himself and his possessions, the more merit he obtains in the eyes of his fellows and in the sight of God. Generosity marks all his actions and relationships; it clearly establishes his moral ascendancy. For some, of course, hard-pressed as they are by their economic circumstances, munificence is hard to practice; but for a prosperous man to be niggling and stingy is a gaping flaw in his character. It breaks the proper and commended circle of moral relationships. A *tsogo*, "skinflint," or a *bahili*, "miser," is disdained. The proverb says *Bahili ya fi kowa rowa*, "A miser exceeds everyone in greed"—for he has but does not give, only seeks to accumulate more. To be a miser is to be selfish, to look only after one's own interests to the exclusion of others, narrowing the moral community down to one individual and thus diminishing the well-being of the community and undermining its ideal state. Taken to extreme conceptualizations, the miser becomes the user of *wone*, a charm designed to assure his own success at the expense of others—such as taking the milk from a neighbor's cow and transferring it by means of occult power to his own. In the ultimate image of selfish iniquity the miser becomes the owner of a *dodo*, an evil troll-like spirit which guarantees wealth and prosperity to its owner, but at the price of taking the life of a kinsman or friend. Selfish greed here reigns supreme, the very antithesis of solidarity and well-being.

Generosity, truthfulness, patience, trustworthiness, attention to religious duty, friendliness—these all characterize the *mutumin kirki*; but one other virtue is necessary to set the others in their proper places. This virtue is *hankali*, which may be translated loosely as "common sense." It is not the same as *wayo*, "cleverness," or *dabara*, "guile"—both of which are respected (particularly in traders), but which are not necessarily (or even commonly) characteristics of a good man. *Hankali* lies much closer to *sani*, "knowledge," particularly knowledge of the proper and just order of affairs, human relationships, and one's place in the general structure of the world. Without this ability to gauge the proper order of the world a man is lost. *Rashin sani ya fi 'dare duhu*, "Lack of knowledge is darker than night"; or, more poignantly: *Rashin sani ya sa makaho ya taka sarki*, "Lack of knowledge caused the blind man to tread on the chief." A man who cannot evaluate relationships or ascertain the ways in which the world runs is permanently crippled: *Jahilci cuta wadda ba ta da magani*, "Ignorance is a sickness for which there is no medicine."

Hankali, then, is "sensibleness," level-headedness, prudence, the ability to make good judgments. It is the foundation for proper action: *Amfanin hankali aiki da shi*, "The purpose of sense is to *use* it." A man with sense will know his duties and take care of them. If a man possesses *hankali* he will, as a result, possess other related virtues: *kunya* or "modesty," *ladabi* or "good manners," and *mutunci* "treating others with courtesy and respect." He will manifest propriety in all his actions, knowing the proper bounds of behavior and the correct response in any situation. He will greet those he meets politely, giving no offense in any way. He will exhibit modesty and respect in the presence of his social superiors, when dealing with his in-laws, or when addressing prominent men.

To be said to lack sober judgment—to be without *hankali*—is a great condemnation. If one says *ba shi da hankali*, "He has no sense," it is almost equivalent to saying *shi mahaukaci ne*, "He is crazy." *Hauka*, "madness," is diametrically opposed to *hankali*. Madmen (*mahaukata*)—those pitiful, naked creatures one sees squatting by the roadsides or wandering in the empty marketplaces—are beyond the limits of human society. They have no ability to gauge correct behavior or move in the ways of civilized men. The destruction of their sensibilities has rendered them effectively nonhuman. Only with *hankali* is orderly social life possible. The Hausa proverb is truly apropos: *Zama da mutanen hankali shi ke raya zuciya*, "Living with sensible men keeps the heart alive."

The acme of all virtues, present when the others have reached their fulfillment, is *hikima*, "wisdom." By diligently cultivating all the other virtues the good man strives ultimately to obtain the capstone of them all. The route to this wisdom is through *ilimi*, "knowledge," but especially knowledge of religion and theology. This religious knowledge must be internalized. It must be lived, felt, and experienced, not just "known." Of this "knowledge" (in Hausa *ilimi*, from the Arabic *'ilm*) Watt has written (1969:62):

> This distinctive meaning of "knowledge" in Arabic may provisionally be indicated by the English word "wisdom." It is wisdom in respect of the general conduct of human life. Further, it is looked upon as something which only very few persons possess in an eminent degree, persons who may be spoken of as "sages" or "men of wisdom." Men other than this select few attain a measure of wisdom only in so far as they are able to enter into the thoughts of the sages. The ordinary man or woman can add nothing to the human race's store of wisdom, but only the sage. Thus, study, learning and the acquiring of knowledge come to be identified with the process of memorizing the words of the sages. Presumably the idea in this is that, if one memorizes the exact words in which wisdom is expressed, one will be able to meditate on these words continually; when some event happens to a man he will remember an appropriate saying; and so in general one will "enter into" the wisdom of the sages.

This wisdom is, therefore a received corpus of perceptions about the world, a closed system of tradition extending back to the Prophet, the mastery of which leads to enlightenment. The authoritative values are essentially fixed; one must merely strive to master them. In his quest for wisdom, then, the good man comes full circle. The foundation on which the *mutumin kirki* stands is *tsoron Allah*, "the fear of God." His aspiration—*hikima*, "wisdom"—is obtained finally from the study of the Word of God as sent down in the Koran and interpreted by the sages. The moral community begins and ends with Islam.

■ Islam and the Social Order

The prototype of moral excellence and *hikima* was the charismatic Fulani cleric Shehu Usman 'Dan Fodio, who early in the nineteenth century started a holy *jihad* against the "unbelieving" Hausa kingdoms and eventually toppled them to build in their place a Muslim empire centered in the city of Sokoto.[29] As the founder of the new social and political order and as the real establisher of Islam in Hausaland, Shehu Usman 'Dan Fodio came to be regarded as a culture hero of near mythical proportions. His descendant, the late Sardauna of Sokoto, Alhaji Sir Ahmadu Bello, described him as a man of utmost piety, an Islamic combination of John Wesley and Oliver Cromwell (Bello 1962:10). During his lifetime Shehu 'Dan Fodio was accorded great honor as a religious teacher and Koranic scholar noted for his unswerving devotion to religious duty. As a Sufi mystic he had seen a vision of God arming him with a "sword of truth" to carry out his holy war to establish an Islam devoid of heresy and pagan accretions. He based his life on imitation of the Prophet Muhammed and, because he established Islam in Hausaland much as Muhammed founded it in Arabia, Shehu Usman was often accorded a similar position in the minds of his followers.

During his lifetime he was seen by many as the *Mahdi*, the last great Muslim "renewer" before the end of the world, or at least as a forerunner of that messiah. The hairs of his head were venerated by his followers as holy relics (Clapperton 1829:206). It was said that he knew the secret name of God, something which, seen within the framework of Muslim theology, would have given him almost unfathomable power. Stories spread concerning his unnatural powers, his superhuman abili-

---

29. The establishment of Islam and the *jihad* of Usman 'Dan Fodio are considered in more detail in chapter 4.

ties, his miracles.[30] He was said to converse with the spirits, to know their ways and how to control them—even to have been a descendant of them himself (G. Nicolas 1975:612–17). The *bori* adepts, devotees of the cults of spirit possession, paled before his powers. He was said to be able to divine the sex of cattle before their birth and was able to converse with animals, who calmed in his presence. After his death his tomb became a shrine for pilgrims and on one occasion he was reported to have risen from the dead.

The tale is told how, when he was still a wandering preacher, he foiled a plot by Yunfa, king of Gobir, to assassinate him (Last 1967a: 13; Hiskett 1973a:70–71; Skinner (1977b:1–2). Fearing 'Dan Fodio's growing influence and power, Yunfa summoned him to court for an interview, in reality plotting to kill him. He prepared a large pit in the floor of his royal audience chamber and lined the bottom with spears. This chasm was then covered with a large woven mat to mask it from 'Dan Fodio when he appeared for the audience. When he seated himself on the mat he would fall into the pit, impale himself on the spears, and be killed as the courtiers stoned him to death from above. On the appointed day of the interview, however, Shehu Usman walked onto the mat, sat down, and conversed with the king until the interview was over, at which time he got up and walked away unhurt. Furious at the failure of his plot, Yunfa removed the mat to discover to his amazement that the pit had been miraculously filled in with sand.

Shehu Usman 'Dan Fodio was also said to possess powers of levitation, the ability to traverse great distances instantly, and powers of omniscience. He knew what was happening in his domains hundreds of miles away, even as the events were taking place. One popular folktale, called "The Shehu and the Caravan Leader," offers dramatic evidence of these powers (Johnston 1966:124–25; Skinner 1977b:9–12).

There once was a caravan leader who was returning to Hausaland from Asante with a hundred thousand kolanuts. When he reached the banks of the Niger River it was necessary for him to ferry his load across. All went well until he himself was being carried across the river. A terrible storm blew up, threatening to capsize the canoe and kill all the passengers. In his fright the caravan captain called out, "Oh Shehu

30. On the miracles of Shehu Usman 'Dan Fodio see Last (1967b), Hiskett (1971, 1973a:150–52), and Skinner (1977b:1–12).

'Dan Fodio! Come and save us!" No sooner had these words left the man's mouth than the figure of a man appeared at the bow of the canoe, righted it against the storm, and saved the party. The caravan leader vowed to give Shehu 'Dan Fodio ten baskets full of kolanuts in thankfulness when he finally arrived in Sokoto.

While this was happening on the distant banks of the Niger, the Shehu was teaching some of his followers in Sokoto. Suddenly, he arose and went into his room. Upon returning shortly thereafter, his gown was seen to be dripping wet. His disciples asked him what had happened and he replied cryptically, "In twenty days you shall know what has transpired." When that time had passed the kola trader arrived and told the tale of his adventure, presenting the Shehu with only five baskets of kolanuts in thankfulness, slyly seeking to minimize his promised gift. The Shehu immediately asked him what had happened to the other five baskets he had promised. Had not his vow been to present him with ten full baskets as alms? Abashed and ashamed at the discovery of his secret deceit, the caravan master returned with five additional baskets and begged for forgiveness. Shehu 'Dan Fodio promptly forgave him and sent him on his way to Kano with assurances that no misfortunes would befall him on the way. The trader set forth, arrived in Kano without incident, and made a fortune from the sale of his goods.

Shehu 'Dan Fodio acknowledged his preeminent position in the Islamic community by taking several important Arabic titles: *Amir al-mu'minin* or "commander of the faithful," (translated into Hausa as *Sarkin Musulmi*, "chief of the Muslims"), *Imam* or "congregational leader," and *Khalifa* or "caliph."[31] In Arabic this latter word is especially important, as it means "successor," in the sense of successor to the Prophet Muhammed as the leader of the community of believers (cf., Levy 1957:277). Shehu 'Dan Fodio, who was a learned scholar, consciously set out to establish an Islamic government based on received principles of Muslim political organization. He set forth his basic assumption of government in a work with the Arabic title *Kitab al-farq bayn wilayat ahl al-islam wa bayn wilayat ahl al-kafor*, "The book of the difference between the governments of the Muslims and the governments of the unbelievers." Of the ideas embodied in it Hiskett has written (1960:578–79):

31. See Last (1967a:46). On the significance of the titles in Islamic thought see Watt (1968:32–35).

It is clear that Shehu conceived the Fulani empire as a microcosm of the ideal Islamic polity of the 'Abbasid jurists, evolved retrospectively to justify the political realities of the day. Yet this largely theoretical structure reflected a clear political image and a defined objective. The Shehu recognized the significance of the imamate as a concept of unifying the divided kingdoms of Hausaland, and in consequence was able to propound a theory of government which succeeded, for a time, in realizing most of his aim.

In classical Islamic thought the religious community and the political structure are coterminous.[32] There is no such thing as a separation of religious and secular authority. Islamic law is ultimately religious law, derived from God through the Koran and the traditions about the Prophet Muhammed. Established by Shehu and consolidated by his son, Muhammed Bello, the Fulani Empire was thus buttressed by Islamic values that proclaimed its legitimacy as the true community of Islam descending ultimately from Muhammed. Hausa social organization therefore was idealized as a pyramid with Allah at the apex and the peasant community at the bottom. God had decreed the Islamic community to be the proper order of human society and had delegated the authority to lead it to Muhammed. Muhammed's cloak fell upon his successors, who functioned as "substitutes" for him in leading this community. The Fulani conquerors claimed that the powers of these successor-substitutes resided in the sultan of Sokoto, who delegated powers to the emirs he appointed under him. They in their turn supervised district chiefs and their emissaries and confirmed village headmen, who then organized hamlets and wards in their own small territories. At the lowest level the *mai-gida* ("household head") exercised proper authority over his compound and the members of his family. Rather than being overturned by the British colonial rulers, these political arrangements were confirmed and strengthened, giving the community of Islam a yet firmer hold on Hausa society.[33] Authority in Hausa thought thus flows from God down through the social structure.[34]

32. A good summary of Islamic political thought is Watt (1968).
33. A complaint voiced by many Christian missionaries in the era of British rule. See, for example, Miller (1936).
34. This idea is developed by D. Dry (1952). The pitfall faced by Islamic rulers is, however, that they are also placed under the obligation to use their power according to Muslim principles of justice. Failure to do this can result in the proclama-

This view of the social order has important implications for the way the Hausa view the world. The *jama'a* of Islam, as a moral, political, and religious community ordained by God, has an aura of correctness and permanence about it. It is static, the institutionalization of God's wisdom. The Islamic social order itself is sanctioned by God as the organization of the community of salvation in this world. The Hausa notion of *rabo*, "fate" or "one's lot in life"—determined by God— tends to freeze ambition and initiative, leading to a passive acceptance of the existing social situation. *Hankali*, "common sense," carries with it the implication that one should recognize one's place in the world and dutifully take care of the obligations that arise from it. The Hausa view of *ha'kuri*, "patience," exhorts an acceptance of things as they are, and the correlative virtue of generosity, *karamci*, declares that those in power should dispense favors to those who are loyal, patient, and supportive of them. The administration of power should be benign. Its benefits should trickle down through the social structure to one's supporters even as the blessings of God trickle down through His established community. As one Hausa proverb puts it: *Wanda bai ci arzikin wani ba, sai ya mutu matsiyaci*, "One who does not share another's prosperity will die in poverty." The ideal of the successful Hausa man appears to be the officeholder who faithfully supports his superiors and rewards his followers.[35] The structure of the social order is thus fundamentally right in the eyes of its members. As an Islamic community it is ordained by God. Its primary stricture is that those in power should uphold Islamic values and strive to be "good men" themselves.

The distillation of Hausa feeling about the moral order lies in their word *lafiya*. Usually this word is translated as "health," for it often has implications pertaining to the proper state of the body; but a more accurate translation would render it as "peace" or "well-being." It is the ideal state of affairs with everything running smoothly, each com-

---

tion of a holy war against them, as was so often the case after the introduction of Islam in West African history. The responses of dissent in Islamic Hausaland have been treated briefly by Last (1970b).

35. LeVine's (1966:36) study is a fascinating comparison of the values of achievement and success in Ibo, Yoruba, and Hausa cultures as manifested in the dreams and essays of Nigerian schoolboys. Clientship and patronage in Hausa society are dealt with in M. G. Smith (1964b).

ponent of existence in its ordered, assigned, and rightful place. When a friend asks about the state of the village, if all is well he will be told that it is *lafiya*, peaceful and undisturbed. When a man sets out on a journey, his friends offer their blessings for the trip by saying *ka sauka lafiya*, "May you descend safely at the end of your journey." When things are going smoothly in one's compound, the family is *lafiya*, all healthy, content. *Lafiya* is safety, security, order—all the things a Hausa finds in the Islamic foundations of his society and the prescribed duties of his religion.

Conversely, those things which are disruptive and unsettling injure *lafiya*. When fortune strikes a savage blow at the harvest and people fear for the coming year, the *lafiya* of the village has been disrupted. When sickness or disease invades a body, its *lafiya* is overturned. When the moral failures of children or relatives bring hurt and consternation the *lafiya* of a man's household, his peace of mind, is injured. The path to *lafiya* lies in the guidance of Islam and the pursuit of the values that make one a *mutumin kirki*. Moral excellence and *lafiya* are intimately intertwined. Without *lafiya* nothing much in this world has any value: *Zama lafiya ya fi zama sarki*, "Obtaining peace is better than becoming chief." In the next chapter we shall see how *lafiya*, the peaceful ordering of life and its concomitant interconnection with Islam, is threatened with disruption by forces originating outside the moral community and how evil is seen symbolically as an assault on the *jama'a* of Islam and its values.

IV

Antitheses of Islam: The Forces of Moral Disorder

Gaba da maye, ba a san 'karewa tata ba.

(Quarreling with a witch —no one knows how it will end.)

HAUSA PROVERB

In rural Muslim Hausa society, centered on its villages, periodic markets, and mosques, the moral order is delimited essentially by Islamic values and duties as described in the preceding chapter; but it is not a sophisticated religion, that is found there. It is rather the simple "little tradition" of an Islamicized, rural peasantry that looks for true learning to the "great tradition" of the religion nurtured by scholars in the large cities.[1] The implantation of Islam provided an institution that could unify and strengthen, and eventually spread, Hausa culture and civilization, but this was not always the case. Islam finally

1. The terminology is derived from Redfield (1953: 228). He later elaborated the concept (Redfield 1960:41–42):

> How shall we begin to take mental hold of this compound culture that deserves a special word, "civilization"? Let us begin with a recognition, long present in discussions of civilization of the difference between a great tradition and a little tradition. (This pair of phrases is here chosen from among other, including "high culture" and "low culture," "folk and classic cultures" or "popular and learned traditions." I shall also use "hierarchic and lay culture.") In a civilization there is a great tradition of the reflective few, and there is a little tradition of the largely unreflective many. The great tradition is cultivated in schools or temples; the little tradition works itself out and keeps itself going in the lives of the unlettered in their village communities. The tradition of the philosopher, theologian, and literary man is a tradition consciously cultivated and handed down; that of the little people is for the most part taken for granted and not submitted to much scrutiny or considered refinement and improvement.

These notions are discussed for the Islamic world in particular in von Grunebaum (1967).

took root in the nineteenth century—upon a pagan foundation that still exerts strong influences throughout much of rural Hausa life. These influences represent forces of moral disorder which are seen as standing in antithetical contrast to the moral community of the Islamic order that forms the boundaries of the village community. To understand these forces, now largely subdued but still lurking in the background, as potential threats epitomizing the forces of evil that threaten the Muslim community, it is necessary to know something of how Islam was first established in Hausaland and was then reforged and reformed in the Fulani *jihad* of the early nineteenth century as the final triumph over these forces of darkness.

■ The Islamic Conquest of Hausaland

The most important influence on early West African history was probably the trans-Saharan caravan trade.[2] Although the Sahara Desert is sometimes seen as a vast, impenetrable barrier separating the Mediterranean littoral from the black countries to the south, it is less an impenetrable barrier than an ocean of sand, whose obstacles could be navigated with appropriate skill and courage to bring great financial rewards. The caravans were the fleets that sailed over this ocean of sand to the centers of trade on either side, and the Arabic word *sahel*, which was used to describe the more favorable lands directly south of the Sahara reflects this, for it means "shore," and was used of those places where the caravans could harbor in safety following their hazardous journey across the desert.

The trans-Saharan trade has existed since prehistoric times and for most of its history was based upon a desire for African gold, brought up from the south and exchanged for salt from the north.[3] Combined

2. The trans-Saharan trade in classical antiquity is discussed by R. C. C. Law (1967). A brief survey of the trans-Saharan trade is given in Hopkins (1973:79–87). A more complete treatment is found in Bovill (1970). See also Boahen (1962) and Newbury (1966).

3. Until the discovery of the mineral riches of the Americas, the African Sudan was the most important source of gold for Europe and the Mediterranean world (Levtzion 1976:141). The availability of gold in the African interior was counterbalanced by a lack of salt. The sixteenth-century traveler and geographer Leo Africanus, for example, writing of his visit to the trading center of Timbuctu, stated "Corne, cattle, milke and butter this region yieldeth in great abundance;

with these staples of trade were luxury items from the Mediterranean shore and slaves captured in bloody, predatory wars in the African interior and sold to masters in the central Sudan and along the Mediterranean coast.[4]

There were numerous trade routes across the Sahara throughout West African history, and as trade flourished and then declined, so did a succession of empires based upon control of this trade: Ghana, Mali, Songhay, Kanem-Bornu. Most of these empires were unstable coalitions of rival factions held together only by a strong leader whose authority was buttressed by semidivine status in the traditional pagan religions of each area. Trimingham has captured the flavor of these states thus (1962:35):

> Empires were spheres of influence, defined not by territorial or boundary lines but by social strata, independent families, free castes, or servile groups of fixed status as royal serfs. The ruler was not interested in dominating territory as such, but in relationships with social groups upon whom he could draw to provide levies in time of war, servants for his court, and cultivators to keep his granaries full. He held the allegiance of village groups or *civitates* who recognized his spiritual authority by paying tribute, for the collection of which he appointed agents to live in provincial villages. He possessed his "royal domains" as did all noble clans and high officials, but the principle behind these was lineal, not territorial.

Continuous trade with the Arabs in the north gradually brought Islamic ideas to the south. The Muslim influences were limited at first to the more sophisticated urban centers where traders and travelers congregated. In general the Arab rulers of the north were not interested in conquest as much as they were in keeping the trade routes open, and

---

but salt is very scarce heere; for it is brought hither by land from Teghaza, which is five hundred miles distant. When I my selfe was here, I saw one camel's loade of salt sold for eighty ducates" (L. Africanus 1896:824).

4. Discussion of the trans-Saharan slave trade has been neglected in favor of the better known trans-Atlantic slave trade; but in fact the Saharan trade antedated the Atlantic by over 1500 years and may have carried more slaves at its height than did the more famous Atlantic slaving routes (see Hopkins 1973:82–83; and also Fisher and Fisher 1970).

along these trade routes came scholars, learned divines, and religious teachers, who established themselves at the courts of pagan rulers where their knowledge of Arabic script, law, theology, and divination made them influential. Gradually, some of these pagan rulers became Muslims themselves, but in general the depth of penetration of Islam was superficial and the mass of common people continued in their traditional ways—a fact of which their rulers were not uncognizant.

From time to time, however, there was direct military conflict between the Arab north and the fragmented kingdoms in the African interior. The most important of these wars, for our purposes, was that which resulted in the collapse of the Songhay Empire in 1591, which ultimately led to the closure of the Taghaza salt mines, the destruction of the principal western routes of the trans-Saharan caravan trade, and the diversion of this trade to a new set of routes farther east which led right into the heart of Hausaland. The consequences of this were profound.

When they first appeared the Hausa kingdoms seem to have been based around fortified towns that were swollen by immigration from the countryside. The fortified capital (*birni*) was a haven to which peasants could flee from the towns and hamlets in times of trouble, and also served as a focal market for the hinterland.[5] As these small, territorially based Hausa chiefdoms expanded and grew more prosperous they were gradually brought into the wider circle of West African trading relationships. The most important result of these contacts over the long run was the penetration of Islam into Hausaland. According to the *Kano Chronicle*, the principal source for the early

5. This version of the early history of Hausaland has been advanced by Abdullahi Smith (1970) and has been the view that has generally found its way into the textbooks (Hunwick 1976; A. Smith 1976; Fisher 1977). It marks an advance over other, earlier theories advanced by such people as Palmer (1928 III:132–38), M. G. Smith (1964a), Hallam (1966), and Johnston (1967:4–6), who described the formation of the Hausa states as the cultural impress of sophisticated immigrants upon a backward, more primitive, indigenous population. Abdullahi Smith's thesis has the intellectual appeal (as well, perhaps, as the disadvantage) of describing a process whereby the sophisticated hierarchy of the recent Hausa states could have been built up from below in a series of stages. Recently, Fuglestad (1978) and Sutton (1979) have made criticisms of this theory as being too simple, and have proposed modifications to allow for a more complex process influenced by outside forces to a greater degree.

history of the Hausa kingdoms, these first contacts were made during the reign of Sarki Yaji of Kano (1349–1385), when the Wangarawa came from Mali, bringing the Muslim religion.[6] Yaji was said to have observed the five times of daily prayer, appointed a *limam* to oversee the rituals, slaughtered cattle in the prescribed ritual forms, and built a mosque at the site of the sacred tree of Kano.

The religious practices of these pagan Hausa states appear to have centered around the veneration of trees and sacred places associated with spirits, with the ruler acting as a sort of high priest for the performance of the ritual offices.[7] The coming of Islam posed a potential threat to these traditional beliefs but, as in the case of the other states of the central and western Sudan, the Hausa kingdoms adopted Islam only as an adjunct to general court procedures and rituals.[8] Rarely did Islamic practices extend to the mass of the population and in times of crisis traditional beliefs often reasserted themselves, pushing Islam aside (Palmer 1928, III:107–8).

Gradually, however, both the volume of trade and the influence of Muslim beliefs grew in importance. By the end of the fifteenth century Islam was an important social force to reckon with and the ruler of Kano, Muhammed Rumfa (1463–1499), began the celebration of Islamic festivals on a wide scale and introduced the practice of wife seclusion (Palmer 1928, III:112). He also became a patron of scholarship and for his efforts was rewarded with the composition of a famous treatise in his honor, *The Obligations of Princes*, composed by 'Abd

6. Palmer (1928 III:104). On the role of the Wangarawa in the central Sudan see especially Lovejoy (1978b).

7. Palmer (1928 III: 97–98). As will be seen below, these practices are very similar to those found today among the pagan Maguzawa Hausa. See Greenberg (1946) and Gilliland (1971).

8. All northern Sudan states, except the Mossi, adopted Islam as the imperial cult. This strengthened commercial links with North Africa, facilitated the introduction of new elements of material culture, and above all brought a written language and clerical class. But its adoption did not lead to either confessional or cultural homogeneity and had no effect upon the cults of the lineage groups. It introduced new elements into the elaborate ceremonials that manifest the authority of the ruler, such as the formal corteges with which he proceeded to the *jami'* or *musalla* for Friday or festival prayer, but its adoption did not affect the mythic basis of the chief's authority, caused no breach between him and the community, and he never thought of imposing it upon his subjects (Trimingham 1962:37).

al-Karim al-Maghili, a famous Muslim lawyer and divine who urged the waging of a holy war (*jihad*) against all pagans to spread the message of Islam (al-Maghili 1932; Hiskett 1962; Trimingham 1962:133).

The overall picture that one obtains of Hausaland in the centuries before the Fulani conquest, therefore, is of a number of small, but growing principalities gradually being drawn into a wider circle of relationships. The *Kano Chronicle* suggests the growth of a number of petty kingdoms constantly at war with each other, reporting wars involving Katsina, Kano, Zazzau (Zaria), Gobir, Kwararafa, the Beriberi, and others, occasional civil wars, and intermittent peace—threats that were never really allayed until the consolidation of Hausaland under the Sokoto Empire in the nineteenth century.

The internal politics of the Hausa kingdoms showed tensions as well. The *Kano Chronicle* lists many ostensibly Muslim rulers, but always interspersed with oppressors and pagan revivalists. Muslim practices were twisted and perverted: one king, for example, appears to have offered sacrifices of cattle to the Koran (Palmer 1928, III:116, 127)—truly an abomination in Muslim eyes—and other kings introduced oppressive programs of taxation in violation of the Muslim spirit of justice. To one particularly heavy-handed chief, Kumbari (1731–1743), his advisers reportedly said, "*Sarki*, if you do not let this *Jizia* (taxation) alone, there will be no one left in the town but yourself and your servants" (Palmer 1928, III:124).[9]

9. The Arabic word *djizya* technically refers to a poll tax levied by Muslim rulers on non-Muslim subjects (see Becker 1961). In Hausa practice everybody seems to have been taxed and the taxes then named according to whether the person was pagan or Muslim. For example, Murray Last writes regarding the tax structure of the early Sokoto Caliphate: "Classically the Sa'i was the collector of zakat. In Sokoto the Sa'i was responsible for taxing the Fulani cattle, and the tax, popularly known by its Hausa name jangali, was officially referred to as zakat, if the Fulani were Muslims, or jizya if they were pagans" (1967a:51).

Meek noted (1925, I:296) that it was not clear how far the introduction of Islam affected taxation in the earliest times among the Hausa, or what taxes were collected by local chiefs on their own account and what taxes were for tribute imposed by a foreign power. This seems to be the case in the instance described in the quotation from the *Kano Chronicle* cited in the text. The rest of the quotation is as follows:

> The thirty-eighth Sarki was Mohamma Kumbari, the son of Sharefa and Luki. He was a liberal Sarki but quick to anger. His counsellors liked him but the

The Hausa kingdoms of this time present us with a picture of numerous petty states of varying strengths, intermittently at war with one another for the sake of plunder and the glorification of their rulers, and buttressed by a syncretistic religion stemming from a mixture of traditional pagan religions of the area and an uneven blending of Islamic elements. Into this amalgam another element was added that eventually was to prove an explosive catalyst: the Fulani.

A pastoral people of puzzling origins and obscure ethnological relations to the rest of Africa,[10] the Fulani first appeared in Hausaland in the reign of Sarkin Kano Yakubu (1452–1463). According to the *Kano Chronicle:* "In Yakubu's time the Fulani came to Hausaland from Mali, bringing with them books on Divinity and Etymology" (Palmer 1928, III: 111). Over time they came to form a significant minority of the population in the Hausa kingdoms and their herds of cattle soon became a source of revenue which the Hausa rulers eyed covetously and began taxing greedily. The cattle tax (*jangali*), first levied by Sarkin Kano Kutumbi (1623–1648) (Palmer 1928, III:119), was an inevitable point of friction between their Hausa overlords (whom they contemp-

---

common people hated him. In his time there was fierce war between Kano and Gobir. . . .

Mohamma Kumbari was active in collecting *Jizia* from the Kasua Kurmi so that the market was nearly killed. The next year he collected *Jizia* in Kano and *made even the mallams pay* [my emphasis]. There was so much disturbance that the Arabs left town and went back to Katsina, and most of the poorer people in town fled to the country.

Turaki Kuka Tunku said to Kumbari, "Sarki, if you do not let this *Jizia* alone, there will be no one left in the town but yourself and your servants." The Sarki listened to him. (Palmer 1928, III:124)

The picture that thus emerges is one of a nominally Muslim ruler using any excuse possible to collect taxes, imposing *djizya* (Hausa *jiziya*), a tax technically on non-Muslims, on everybody, even attempting to make Koranic scholars ("mallams") pay. The taxation was so intolerable that the teachers and Arab traders fled the city and went to Katsina, along with a substantial exodus of the poorer segments of the population. Kumbari would therefore appear to fit well into the picture of a nominally Muslim ruler using Islamic law in accord with his own notions rather than in a strictly legal and proper manner. The traditional Hausa tax structure was complex and the reader is referred to Hill (1972: 323–25) and Lord Lugard's *Political Memoranda*, especially number 5 on taxation, for more details.

10. On the Fulani see St. Croix (1945), Hopen (1958), Stenning (1957, 1959), Van Raay (1975), Azarya (1976, 1978), and (Riesman 1977).

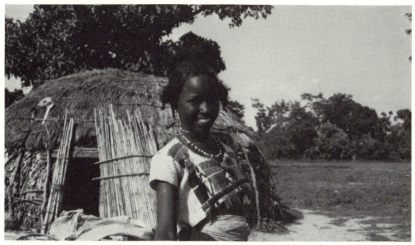

8. A Fulani girl in her family's wet-season cattle camp.

tuously referred to as *Ha'be*) and the proud, independent Fulani people, who hold that "cattle surpass everything, they are even greater than one's father and mother" (Hopen 1958:26).

The Fulani were not all nomadic pastoralists. Many took part in a kind of transhumance, based from semipermanent camps and supplemented by agriculture. Others were *Fulanin gida*, "settled Fulani," who lived in the towns and built permanent houses of mud-brick and clay. As might be gathered from the quotation from the *Kano Chronicle* cited above, they were Muslims. While the pastoral Fulani were often only nominally Islamic, living close to the traditional beliefs of their ancestors in the course of their wanderings, their more settled brothers were devout, ascetic Muslims with formidable reputations as Koranic scholars and preachers.

On December 15, 1754, in the village of Maratta, a son was born to a devout Muslim scholar named Muhammed Fodio, who named the boy Usman. As he grew up, Usman 'Dan Fodio became an exemplary scholar and eventually he traveled as far north as Agades to study with an unbending Tuareg *mallam* named Jibril b. Umar, who taught that "disobedience to the Shari'a, the Islamic legal and social ordinances, was a sin sufficient to invalidate a man's Islam and turn him into an unbeliever, destined for eternal punishment in hell fire" (Hiskett

1973a:40). Jibril's radical teachings were unorthodox, but in his demands for strict observance of the law, his revivalistic agitation for
purity in Islam, and his demands for *jihad*—be it an internal war of the
spirit or an ultimate military crusade against the unbelievers—he was
following a longstanding and potent tradition in Sudanic Islam. The
thoughts of Usman 'Dan Fodio traveled similar paths.[11]

Usman early developed a reputation as a powerful teacher and
preacher, receiving license to preach at the young age of twenty. He
soon developed a substantial following in the Hausa kingdom of Gobir
where he lived, and as he traveled about he became more and more
aware of the syncretism between Islam and the traditional pagan beliefs of the country. In his preaching he devoted himself to the presentation of a purified Islam, unsullied by unorthodox local accretions. His
success was impressive and he built up a large number of devoted
followers.

'Dan Fodio was also a mystic, a devotee of the Sufi order of the
Qadiriyya, and as such he always preferred to be known by the title of
"*shaik*," or in Hausa *shehu*, as befitted his position. In 1794 his beliefs
were strengthened by a vision in which he saw God give to Muhammed,
the cohorts of the Prophet, and Abd al-Qadri (the founder of the Sufi
Qadiriyya order) a "sword of truth." This impressive group of holy
men strapped the sword to Usman 'Dan Fodio's side and told him to
carry on a *jihad* against the Ha'be rulers and their misguided supporters
(Hiskett 1973a:63–69). 'Dan Fodio's preaching of reform and revival
was further enhanced by the widespread Islamic belief that God will
send a renewer at the beginning of each century to strengthen the community of believers, and his followers had no doubt as to who God's
chosen instrument was (Hiskett 1973a:121–25).

Examining the Hausa kingdoms—in particular the Kingdom of Gobir
in which he lived—Shehu 'Dan Fodio saw many evils. In a later work,

11. The best general study of the life of Usman 'Dan Fodio is by Hiskett (1973a).
His early life is treated in El-Masri (1963). See also Balogun (1975). The theological background is described in a number of works, among them Palmer (1913–15),
Hiskett (1957, 1962, 1973b), Last and Al-Hajj (1965), Bivar and Hiskett (1962), and
Willis (1967). The account of the Fulani Caliphate which follows is based on several sources: Arnett (1922), Waldeman (1965), M. G. Smith (1966), Johnston
(1967), Last (1967a), and Adeleye (1971). The techniques of Hausa-Fulani warfare
are discussed in Smaldone (1977).

called *Kitab al-Farq*, he detailed the corruptions of the Hausa kings as he saw them (Hiskett 1960). His major complaint was that although the Hausa kings professed to be Muslims, their governments were based upon the whims of the rulers and pagan traditions, rather than on the rule of the Shari'a. In his eyes such governments had no legal standing. They were corrupt. Kings were chosen by hereditary rule, without the consultations and elections demanded by Islamic tradition. The rulers were arbitrary, killing or exiling whom they chose, violating men's honor, expropriating their wealth, imposing unjust taxes unrecognized by the Islamic codes, such as *ku'din 'kasa* (land tax), and *ku'din salla* (festival money). Additionally, they demanded and received bribes (*gaisuwa*). They ignored precepts to live righteously and in moderation and ate whatever they liked, married whom they wished with no regard for Islamic marriage regulations, kept houses full of concubines and prostitutes in violation of Islamic rules, and lived in sumptuous palaces contrary to Shehu Usman's personal ascetic beliefs. The Hausa kings, he said, usurped alms, raked off a percentage of market sales, and adorned themselves with non-Islamic titles taken from pagan courts. In his view they were no better than unbelievers. The Islam they practiced was so adulterated as to be unrecognizable.[12]

Much of what Shehu 'Dan Fodio preached was undoubtedly true, but demanding that the Hausa kings base their rule strictly on the Shari'a was revolutionary. It meant that they must overthrow the entire system of government that has grown up around traditional practice with the support of their non-Muslim subjects. A community based solely on the Shari'a would have as its ruler the *iman*, the "congregational leader" or "head of the community of believers." Since this was the very position held by Shehu 'Dan Fodio, it appeared to the king of Gobir that these clerics were setting up a government to challenge his own and were drawing supporters to the banner of Islam under the pretext of religious revival to effect just such a revolution and change of rulers. Conflict was becoming inevitable.

It was not long before open hostilities broke out. On February 21,

12. The state of Islam in these kingdoms before the Sokoto Caliphate reminds one of the Hausa proverb, *Son 'doya da man ja*, "The love of a yam for palm oil," that is, exceedingly superficial, not going beneath the surface to the heart of the matter—in this case only a superficial covering of Islam over the "yam" of paganism.

1804, Usman 'Dan Fodio and his followers were forced to flee the Kingdom of Gobir into the western desert in a *hijira* that soon assumed for the Fulani Muslim community the same importance that Muhammed's flight to Medina had for the first Muslims. His followers swore allegiance to him, and Shehu Usman 'Dan Fodio became the *Imam*, "leader of the community," and *Amir al-Mu'minin*, "commander of the faithful." The Sokoto Caliphate had been born.

War was soon declared and as 'Dan Fodio's message spread, the Fulani tribesmen in other Hausa kingdoms joined the revolt. One by one the Hausa kingdoms toppled as the Fulani warriors and their allies swept across the savannah. By 1810 the Fulani armies and their followers had consolidated the kingdoms of Gobir, Zamfara, and Kebbi; brought about the collapse of the Hausa dynasties in Kano, Katsina, and Zaria and replaced them with Fulani rulers; forged new emirates out of pagan lands in Adamawa and Bauci; overrun the ancient kingdom of Daura; and had received homage from the emir of Air and Adar in the north. The southern kingdom of Yauri submitted and its ruler was allowed to retain his position. Numerous smaller states had been created or absorbed on the fringes of the larger ones. When 'Dan Fodio's son, Muhammed Bello, built the capital city of the empire at Sokoto in 1810, his father and his followers controlled an enormous amount of territory in the West African savannah. Under the rule of Muhammed Bello this territory was to increase to include the emirate of Ilorin, which was carved out of a portion of the old Oyo Yoruba Empire, and the emirate of Nupe, brought into the Sokoto Caliphate through Fulani intervention in the civil strife resulting from internal Nupe factionalism.

Usman 'Dan Fodio himself took only a minimal part in the generalship of the military campaigns, entrusting most of the leadership in the field to his brother Abdullahi and to his son, Muhammed Bello. As the Fulani-Muslim revolts spread in the Ha'be kingdoms and their leaders pledged allegiance to him, 'Dan Fodio gave them standards and delegated his authority to them as his emirs for the furtherance of the *jihad*.

In 1809, with complete victory at hand, Shehu 'Dan Fodio retired from active service and administration to Sifawa to devote himself once again to the study and teaching that had always been his primary interest. He remained there until 1815, when he moved to Sabon Gari on the outskirts of the new capital city of Sokoto, which had been con-

structed five years earlier by Muhammed Bello. On April 20, 1817,
Shehu Usman 'Dan Fodio died in Sokoto. His son Muhammed Bello
was elected to succeed him as ruler of the empire.

Shehu and his successors established a form of government that
maintained much of the structure of the old Ha'be kings, but at least
outwardly was based on traditional Muslim concepts of administration.[13] Acknowledged as the formal ideology of the ruling hierarchy
and carrying with it substantial political and social advantages under
the new regime, Islam made tremendous progress in establishing itself
at the local level.[14] The fact that the British, after their conquest of
Hausaland at the turn of this century, left the Hausa-Fulani structure
of administration and government essentially intact and were loath to
let Christian missionaries operate in the northern regions, gave the
process of Islamization a further boost which has continued to the
present day.[15]

It is not the object here to trace the subsequent history of the Sokoto
Empire, detailing how corruption, political intrigue, and maladminis-
tration often brought about marked deviations from the Islamic ideal
and finally political collapse under the onslaught of British imperial
power—that task has been admirably done by Johnston, Last, Adeleye,
and others[16]—but the importance of the Fulani *jihad*, the achievements
of Shehu 'Dan Fodio, and the enduring consequences of the establishment of the caliphate merit some elaboration. Above all it established

13. See particularly Last (1967a), Adeleye (1971:38–51), Hiskett (1960, 1973:134–59),
and Abubakar (1974) on the administration and legal structure of the caliphate.
Detailed studies of the political structure of Zaria and Daura, respectively, are by
M. G. Smith (1960, 1978). The emirates of Gombe, Katagum, and Hadejia are
treated by Low (1972), and Kano is treated by Fika (1978). On the Nupe see Nadel
(1942, 1954). On Adamawa see Abubakar (1977).

14. It is essential to note that it was only with the jihads of the eighteenth and
nineteenth centuries that extensive Islamization of the Sudan can be said to have
begun (Awe 1965:70).

15. See, for example, Schacht (1957), Last (1970b), and Hiskett (1973b) for the
progress of Islam in northern Nigeria. The importance of Islam in contemporary
politics in the north is detailed in Means (1965), Dudley (1968), Whittaker (1970),
and Paden (1973). The progress of Islam among the pagan tribes of the north and
the importance of governmental power as a force in promoting it is considered in
Gilliland (1971, especially pp. 253–78).

16. Johnston (1967), Last (1967a), Adeleye (1971). The fall of the Fulani Sultanate
is detailed in Orr (1911), Muffett (1964), and Dusgate (1985). See also Fika (1978).

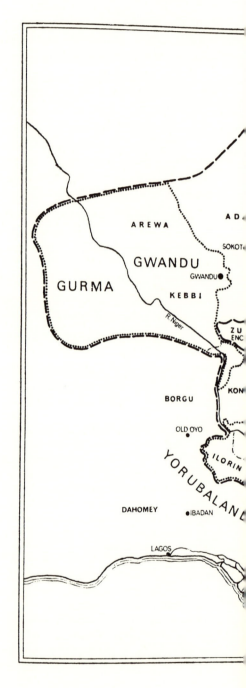

Figure 4   The Fulani Empires of Sokoto and Gwandu at their greatest extent.

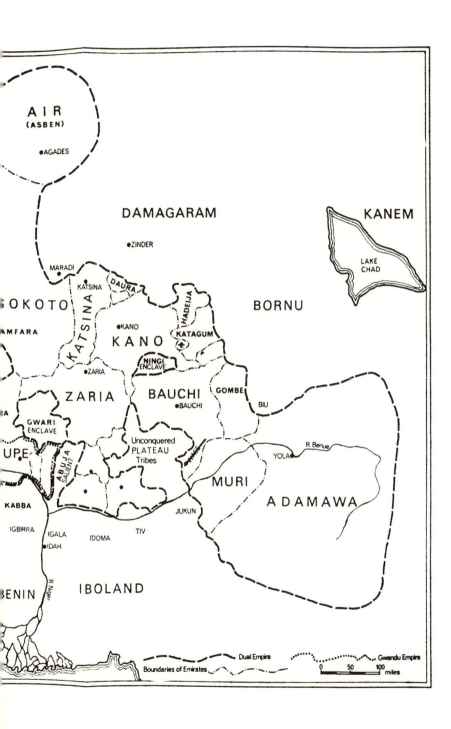

AIR
(ASBEN)

•AGADES

DAMAGARAM

•ZINDER

KANEM

MARADI

LAKE
CHAD

OKOTO

KATSINA

DAURA

BORNU

KATSINA

•KANO

HADEIJA

KANO

KATAGUM

MFARA

•ZARIA

NINGI
ENCLAVE

ZARIA

BAUCHI

GOMBE

GWARI
ENCLAVE

•BAUCHI

BIU

UPE

ABUJA
SALIENT

Unconquered
PLATEAU
Tribes

YOLA

R.Benue

MURI

ADAMAWA

KABBA

IGBIRRA

IGALA

IDOMA

TIV

JUKUN

•IDAH

BENIN

R. Niger

IBOLAND

Dual Empire

Gwandu Empire

Boundaries of Emirates

0   50   100
miles

an Islamic basis for Hausa society by ending the fragmentary, feuding Ha'be kingdoms and giving them a central focus in and a common allegiance to the ruler in Sokoto. It established Islamic Shari'a law as the ideal basis for society, and as a result of the political unification and consolidation of power in the hands of a reforming and dedicated group of Muslim rulers, gave enormous impetus to the Islamization of Hausa society. Whereas the Ha'be had tolerated traditional religious practices and had been in easy harness with pagan rituals and ceremonies, now the hierarchy of society was Muslim, and dedicated (at least in theory) to the establishment of Islam as the only basis for justice.

The achievements of the Fulani warriors, as they themselves saw them, were recorded by Muhammed Bello, son and successor to Usman 'Dan Fodio, in his work *Infaku'l Maisuri*:

> now in our times these countries have become Moslem, for God has taken away their corrupt practices and left what is good by the blessing of Shehu who is God's gift to this land, for he has enriched it with many blessings, he has given it a surpassing glory. Those who have been fortunate and found salvation have been profited by his call. For they heard him and obeyed, those that were stubborn in heart and found not salvation, yet he saved them and they obeyed him by force. He removed all grounds for contention and error and there are none remaining. God laid open these countries to him. He established justice among them and set up a ruler in each land to rule it in the right way. Prayer became constant, *zakka* was given, strife was put down, the disobedient were punished, extortioners brought to justice, the roads made safe and the faith made secure in the world. In truth Shehu became the expounder of the Law to the Moslem chiefs and settled the disputes of the people. He was firm in purifying the faith, God takes pleasure in his servants even to the end of time. (Arnett 1922: 124–25)

It may be doubted whether the just administration of the state and the devotion of the people to Islam were quite as spectacular as Muhammed Bello reports,[17] but there is no question that the Islamic ideal

17. See, for example, the comments of Spencer Trimingham (1962:200–207, 219) and M. G. Smith (1964b).

was established and that Shehu Usman 'Dan Fodio became the per-
sonification of that ideal. He became a culture hero who brought Islamic
order out of unbelieving chaos. He established *Dar-al-Islam*—"the
house of Islam"—in Hausaland, waging his holy war against the forces
of darkness and evil, overthrowing *Dar-al-Harb*—"the house of the
unbelievers," the enemies of Islam against whom perpetual war is man-
dated by the Prophet Muhammed.[18]

These two spheres, *Dar-al-Islam* and *Dar-al-Harb*, encompass the
world. One is a member of either one or the other. The sphere of Islam,
the *jama'a*, or society of believers, is the community of salvation, both
in this world and in the next. To be a *kafiri*, an unbeliever, is thus to be
outside the moral order. Worse still is to be a *ridadde*, an apostate, one
who has been within the fold but has abandoned it to work actively
against it, joining forces with the Devil himself. Small wonder, then,
that Muslims are urged to undertake holy war (*jihad*) against the unbelievers, to convert them or crush them, and are enjoined by law to
execute apostates and blasphemers, even if in the contemporary world
of practical affairs such things are never done.[19]

18. See Watt (1968:14–19) for a further explanation of *jihad*.
19. "The charge of infidelity is . . . the most terrible accusation a Muslim can
make against a fellow man. The Shehu even went so far as to state its grim corol-
lary: that such renegade Muslims must be slain and buried, without washing or
prayer, in unhallowed graves" (Hiskett 1973a:108).

In Maliki law apostasy, which is "to be received into the faith of the Unbelievers," is punishable by death. The apostate is, however, allowed three days in which
to recant. If he fails to do so, he should be executed on the evening of the third
day, irrespective of sex, status, or social position. Blasphemy is unrecantable. See
Ruxton (1916:325–26, 328).

In strict legal terms there is not a man alive—Muslim or otherwise—who could
not be condemned to death for apostasy or blasphemy. According to Ruxton (1916:
325–26): "The crime of apostasy may consist in saying words in contradiction of
the principles of Islam, or by giving forth opinions implying renunciation of those
principles. . . . Any act which implies outrage to or renunciation of the faith of
Islam is held to establish the crime of apostasy. Thus, a Muslim is guilty of apostasy who: throws a copy of the Koran, or even a single letter of it, into the dirt;
who wears any part of the dress of an Infidel; or who practises witchcraft."

Executions for apostasy are extremely rare in the Islamic world. It was Ruxton's
belief in 1916 that the last such execution had taken place in the Ottoman Empire
in 1844. Such things are unheard of in modern Hausaland, but the fact that such
legal strictures exist gives an indication of the depth of feeling such matters can
touch upon in Islamic communities.

Thus, it should be seen that the moral order of Islam, the sphere of justice, truth, and righteousness described in the last chapter and personified for the devout Hausa or Fulani Muslim by Shehu 'Dan Fodio, was established only after centuries of intermingling of Islam and paganism and was brought to pass finally only after prolonged and bloody warfare against the pagan Ha'be kings. It should come as no surprise, therefore, that paganism and the beliefs and practices associated with it should be seen as malevolent, satanic forces, subdued for the present but ready to raise themselves as threats to the *lafiya* of the community.

■ The Dark Underside of the World:
Paganism, Witchcraft, and Sorcery

Within the immediate environment of a Muslim Hausa village the most striking contrast to the *jama'a* of Islam is the paganism found in the surrounding countryside. In southern Katsina, the focus of this study, these pagans are the Maguzawa Hausa, a subculture in the wider Hausa civilization generally considered to be the scattered descendants of the original Hausa stock, especially the pagan Hausa rulers of Dala Hill described in the *Kano Chronicle* (Krusius 1915:279; Palmer 1928, III:97–99; Greenberg 1946:vii; Gilliland 1971). The general Hausa term for pagans is *arna* (sing. *arne*), a term the Maguzawa feel is pejorative, though certainly less so than *kafirai*, "unbelievers," one of the most derogatory words in the Muslim vocabulary. The term *Maguzawa* (sing. *Bamaguje*) is said to be related to *majusi*, the Arabic word for "magician" or "Zoroastrian" (Robinson 1925, I:282; Greenberg 1946: 13, n.7; Trimingham 1959:39). Maguzawa is the term these pagan people themselves prefer. Although conquered by the Fulani in the *jihad* of Usman 'Dan Fodio, the Maguzawa were not forced to convert, but remained as tribute-paying farmers and have been politically subordinate to their Muslim overlords ever since (Trimingham 1962:200).

Unlike their Muslim cousins, the Maguzawa do not live in towns or villages but prefer rather to settle in large, kin-based settlements among their farms in the bush. Their aversion to the crowding and strangeness of the Muslim villages is proverbial: *Ana zaman 'karya, in ji Bamaguje*, " 'They can't really live there!' said the pagan Maguzawa man [when he saw the village]."[20] These large settlements are composed of a father, who serves as the compound head (*maigida*), his married sons, and their children. It is much more common for Maguzawa brothers to remain together in the compound after their father has died than for brothers in the villages, and as a result Maguzawa compounds may have a hundred or more people living in them. Greenberg has used the term "patrilineal sib" to describe the local groupings of these patrilineal groups and has discussed the wider relationships of these sibs in terms of "clanship," even though there is no native Hausa word that can be translated accurately as such (Greenberg 1946:22, 1947; Barkow 1973:65–66). These wider clan relations are found in common group names, common praise songs (*kirari*), common "totems" or mutually held food avoidances (*kan gida*), and common patterns of scarification—but aside from the acknowledgment among them that some sort of common relationship exists, these clans have no political, economic, or religious significance and the "members" of these groups never gather or act together as a unit. In terms of their impact on the daily life of the Maguzawa they are completely otiose (Krusius 1915: 297; Greenberg 1946:25–26; Barkow 1973:63–64). Politically, there is a *sarkin arna*, or "chief of the pagans," a *sarkin noma*, or "chief of the farmers," and a *sarkin dawa* or "chief of the bush" (important in hunting) in each community, although these titles are mainly honorary. The real power lies with the village headman of the Muslim village in whose village area the Maguzawa live.

The economic foundation of Maguzawa life is farming. Living fairly secluded lives away from the villages, often quite deep in the bush, they are cut off from the mainstream of village commercial activities (Greenberg 1946:19; Barkow 1973: 68–69). Trading, by and

20. This attitude toward the towns may carry over as part of the Maguzawa ethos, even under the impact of conversion to Islam. One Maguzawa man of my acquaintance who had become a Muslim years before and had even made the pilgrimage to Mecca proudly boasted to me that he had never spent one night in the village in all his life—even though he owned a substantial compound there which he rented out. He had many friends in the village and was frequently present at the market, but even under the foulest possible conditions of weather he would slog his way several miles through the bush to avoid spending the night in town—even if he had to leave his motorcycle in the village because of the condition of the paths.

large, is foreign to them as an economic livelihood. The proverbs say
Cinikin arna noma, "The 'commerce' of pagans is farming"; and *Ana zaman 'karya wai Bamaguje ya zo gari ya iske ba masussuka,* " 'They can't really live here!' as the Maguzawa man said when he found the town had no threshing floors." Farming arrangements are similar to those among the Muslim Hausa, but the *gandu* arrangement whereby each compound head directs the cultivation of the family farms by his sons and brothers and controls the distribution of grain after the harvest appears much stronger, in keeping with the stronger cohesiveness of the Maguzawa family unit. Men and boys also have their own personal plots to farm, as do the women of the household—who also participate extensively in farm labor, in marked contrast to their secluded Muslim counterparts. Indeed, the importance of women in Maguzawa agriculture is great; they supply a large portion of the produce that supports the compound.[21] Hunting plays an important role in Maguzawa life as well, but is diminishing as the countryside increasingly is domesticated and land brought under cultivation.

In an article comparing Muslim Hausa villagers with the pagan Maguzawa Hausa, Jerome Barkow (1973) lists what he considers to be the major differences between them. The Maguzawa live in rural, isolated homesteads, which are less solidly constructed and less enclosed than the mud-brick compounds of the village. Maguzawa family structure is strongly centered on a close-knit patrilineal group which practices marital exogamy with respect to other, neighboring groups, in contrast to the less cohesive kin structure of the Muslim village. In addition, the Maguzawa economic pattern is less diversified and more heavily centered on agriculture, with stronger *gandu* organizations than those found in the village.[22] Maguzawa women participate fully and significantly in the agricultural pursuits of their families, while the secluded Hausa women of the Muslim village are left free to pursue their own crafts and trades. The Maguzawa ethos is more open and permissive, with frequent group beer drinking (forbidden to Muslims by Koranic injunction), less emphasis on feminine modesty (Maguzawa

21. Barkow reports (1973:67–68) that Maguzawa men often say "our women feed us" when discussing their role in the economic life of the settlement.

22. Among the Maguzawa it is considered shameful for a son to leave the compound while his father is alive. While some villagers agreed this might be somewhat shameful, they felt it was a frequent occurrence (Barkow 1973:66).

women are not secluded and habitually go about bare-breasted), greater scope for adolescent sex play, and a generally wider range of emotional spontaneity and display. Without question, however, the major dividing difference between the two groups is religion.

The essence of Maguzawa religion is the veneration of and sacrifice to various spirits, called *iskoki* in Hausa. This word is actually the plural form of *iska*, meaning "wind" or "air," and serves as an indication of the nature of the spirits. They are invisible, ethereal beings, innumerable in number, present everywhere. Similarly, they are sometimes referred to as *inuwa* or "shade"—dim reflections of another world capable of interacting with men for good or evil. The Maguzawa have been in contact with Islam long enough to have accepted the notion of Allah as supreme high God, controlling and ruling the universe, but in the terms of practical Maguzawa religion, Allah is unimportant and is ignored.[23] Many of these spirits have known names, characteristics, and powers. Many of them are directly responsible for the onset of illness which, in the Maguzawa view, must be alleviated by supplication, sacrifice, and medicines derived from plants and trees associated with the places that the spirits frequent. It is through the manipulation of these powers that the Maguzawa attempt to control their world and mitigate the misfortunes that befall them—an intercourse abhorrent to their Muslim village neighbors.

Although anyone may sacrifice to a spirit individually, the most important rituals are performed on behalf of a compound by the compound head. Each *maigida* performs these ceremonies when he sees fit, and they are usually performed during the hot season before the onset of the rains, to assure bountiful crops during the agricultural portion of the cycle of the seasons. Family groups may sacrifice to the same spirit or different spirits; the larger bonds of kin relationship play no role in Maguzawa religion. There are no corporate ceremonies beyond those undertaken by a compound and its members.

Sacrifices to the spirits are undertaken at trees in the bush associated with them, at special "spirit poles" (*jiguma*) or trees planted in front of

23. "It must be understood that the concept of Allah as the Supreme Being is only elicited by direct questioning. Ordinarily the Maguzawa pay no attention to Allah, and His name is only heard in the oaths and common expressions involving God's name which these folk share with their Moslem neighbours, but which, unlike them, they use less frequently" (Greenberg 1946:27).

the compound, or in places kept secret by the members of the settlement. Often, items associated with that spirit, objects symbolic of his
or her particular nature, will be taken along and placed at the sacrificial
site. Then a goat or appropriately marked fowl (for the type of sacrifice
also varies according to the characteristics of the particular spirits) is
led to the site, its throat slit, and the blood is allowed to pour out on
the ground and over the sacred objects while the officiating priest
makes his invocations and requests. The blood of the sacrificial animal
is given to the spirit to drink, and the body of the animal is cooked
and eaten by the participants in the ceremony. Not infrequently, such
sacrifices are referred to as "alms" (*sadaka*) for the spirits, borrowing
the Islamic term (M. F. Smith 1954:227).

Sacrifices may be made to the spirits by individuals for their own
purposes as well as on behalf of the group. Since the spirits are seen
as frequent causes of illness, those afflicted by a particular spirit will
offer sacrifices in order to restore their own health. In cases of spirit
possession related to severe illness or mental disorder, mere sacrifice
may not be enough. The individual may have to become one of the
'*yam bori* ("children of the cult of spirit possession") through an
elaborate ritual known as *girka*. After this experience these individuals
develop a special relationship with their "familiar spirits," who then
reveal to them medicine appropriate for the treatment of disease and
aid them in the healing of illness.[24]

Sacrifice by the compound or settlement head and the rituals of spirit
possession (*bori*) are two aspects of Maguzawa religion that give the
worship of the spirits both a communal and an individual aspect, a
complementarity that aids in ordering life on a collective as well as a
personal level.

For the Muslim Hausa the worship of the spirits and sacrifice to
them are *tsafi*, "pagan ritualism," and as such are viewed as religious
abominations, participation in which marks one as an unbeliever and
puts him outside the community of salvation. The Muslim community,
however, does not deny the reality of these spirits, nor does it deny
their powers to work evil. Besides the words *iskoki* and *inuwa*, mentioned above as words for "spirits," there are two others in Hausa, both

24. *Bori* is discussed in more detail later in this chapter. Medical aspects of *bori*
are dealt with in the two chapters that follow.

of which carry (for the Muslim Hausa) approximately the same meanings: *aljannu* and *iblisai*.

Aljannu is a word derived from the Arabic *djinn*, and the existence of these spirits, originally the pagan gods and spirits of pre-Islamic Arabia, are recognized specifically by orthodox Islam (MacDonald and Masse 1965:546–47): "Djinn, according to Muslim conceptions, are bodies (*adjsam*) composed of vapour or flame, intelligent, imperceptible to our senses, capable of appearing under different forms and of carrying out heavy labours. They were created of smokeless flame (Koran LV:14) while mankind and the angels, the other two classes of intelligent beings, were created out of clay and light." Furthermore, "In official Islam the existence of the djinn was completely accepted, as it is to this day, and the full consequences implied by their existence were worked out. Their legal status in all respects was discussed and fixed, and the possible relations between them and mankind, especially in questions of marriage and property were examined." (MacDonald and Masse 1965:547) The reality of the spirits is therefore not seriously questioned.[25]

Some of these spirits heard and submitted to the teachings of Muhammed, and thus were saved.

> And when We turned to thee a company of jinn
> giving ear to the Koran; and when they were
> in its presence they said, "Be silent!"
> Then, when it was finished, they turned back
>   to their people, warning.
> They said, "Our people, we have heard a Book
> that was sent down from Moses, confirming
> what was before it, guiding to the truth and
>   to a straight path.
> O our people, answer God's summoner, and
> believe in Him, and He will forgive you
> some of your sins, and protect you from a
>   painful chastisement.

25. Some of my Muslim informants did deny that spirits existed, maintaining that God is the only controlling power. These people usually seemed anxious to avoid any possible hint that they were involved with spirit worship, and under closer questioning admitted that spirits did exist, but that they wanted nothing to do with such *tsafi*, being good Muslims.

> Whosoever answers not God's summoner, and
> cannot frustrate God in the earth, and he
> has no protectors apart from Him; those are
>   in manifest error.
> (Koran XLVI, 28–31)

These "believing djinn" in Hausa are the *iskoki masu salla*, the "pray-ing spirits" or the *farin iskoki*, "white spirits." Their counterparts are the *iskoki mara salla*, "spirits who do not pray" or *ba'kin iskoki*, the "black spirits" or "spirits of evil."[26]

In respect to these *iskoki*, however, a word more in keeping with the Muslim Hausa viewpoint is *iblisai*, "demons" or "devils." The singular form, *iblis*, like *aljani* and its plural form *aljannu*, comes into Hausa from Arabic and is related as well to the Latin *diabolus* or "devil" (Robinson 1925, I:161; Tritton 1934; Bargery 1934:492; Abraham 1962:394). The chief of these demonic *iblisai* is *Shaitan* (Satan), and devout Muslims may identify this Koranic figure with the *Sarkin Aljannu* or "chief of the spirits" venerated in pagan Hausa religion and the cult of *bori*. The spirits—the *iskoki, aljannu, bori,* or *iblisai*— are the demons whom infidels and unbelievers obey while disobeying God. They are the powers that oppose God's will, corrupting the hearts of men away from the true religion of Muhammed.[27] Pious village Muslims have no doubts that Maguzawa religion is dominated by wor-ship of the unbelieving black *iskoki* and involves the veneration of the powers of evil.

Related in Muslim minds to pagan religion (*tsafi*) is witchcraft, *maita*. For many villagers the two terms are synonymous. The witch (m. *maye*, f. *maya*) is a person possessed of the power to capture and eat the soul (*kurwa*) of an individual, resulting in that person's sick-ness and death. The *kurwa* of a man is an ethereal, spirit-like thing intimately related to, but different from, his life or life force, *rai*. It is very much like one of the *iskoki*.[28] While the *rai* resides in the body of

26. The classification and organization of spirits in this manner is rather diffuse and not rigidly formalized. The significance of these evil spirits is discussed in more detail in the next chapter.
27. As for Shaitan, Tritton writes (1934:286): " 'Every proud and rebellious one among *djinn*, men, and animals' is the meaning given in the dictionaries."
28. See Krusius (1915:290–92), Greenberg (1946:59), and also chapter 5 of this book.

a man, his spirit is free to travel about, often dissociating itself from the body out of wanderlust or curiosity. Dreams, for example, are thought to be the mental images seen by the *kurwa* on its nocturnal travels. Irrespective of its location, however, the *kurwa* maintains a metaphysical link with the body and with the *rai*. Should the spirit be captured, killed, or "eaten," that person's *rai* will suffer. He will sicken, progressively weaken, and die.

Maita (witchcraft) is an actual physical substance present within the body of the witch. Often it is described as *kankara*, "flint" or "ice" residing in the belly of the witch. It can affect men, women, or children and may be inherited from the mother or the father. It can also be obtained by purchase, for it is said to be vomited up by the witch, who will then sell a portion of it to someone who wants to become a witch himself. This person then swallows it, and through this act of ingestion obtains the powers of witchcraft for himself. This witchcraft substance is said to come in all shapes, sizes, and colors: black, red, yellow, blue, striped—a rainbow assortment of evil.[29]

A better translation of *maye* than "witch" would be the more cumbersome "eater of souls," for this is the nature and main activity of the witch. Although it is invisible to the normal human eye, the witch has the ability to see the *kurwa* of a man as it ambles around the village or the countryside, and to waylay it, capture it, and eat it. The witch's own *kurwa* is especially adept at catching the souls of others and sets out (mostly at night) on these hunts. It may even transform itself into other shapes, appearing as a wild animal.[30] The witch will

29. While there may be much joking about witchcraft there is also a real underlying fear of it. One Maguzawa man, a pagan, lived in the village and did odd jobs as a day laborer. He was widely regarded as a witch, and on several occasions I tried to make arrangements with him to have him show me his witchcraft substance. I reported to some of my Muslim neighbors that this fellow was going to give me some of his witchcraft, and they immediately expressed strong concern that I not eat any of it—for I would then be captured and myself transformed into a witch. Unfortunately, before I could make final arrangements with the witch and pay him the money he requested, he converted to Islam, at which time his witchcraft "became inoperative," *ya kwanta* (literally, "it lay down").
30. There is some controversy as to whether all animals have a *kurwa*, or only humans. A number of informants told me that all animals have them, and that all animals also have their own witches which prey on these souls. One informant told me that you should never let a witch pick up your chickens in the market to

then take the soul to his compound for safekeeping until he desires to eat it, at which time he will cut it (*yanke*, the same verb as is used in describing the ceremonial slaughter of an animal) and gorge himself on his victim's soul.[31] The victim will then find himself prostrated, vomiting blood or bleeding from the nose, as he weakens toward death. There is a parallel here with pagan ritual, for even as the pagans will sacrifice the life and blood of a chicken or goat to the spirits, here the pagans in their role as witches will sacrifice the life of a human victim. It is easy to see how the two notions flow together in Muslim Hausa thought.

Apart from the power of the witch there is another way of catching and killing someone's soul. In this case an individual enters into a relationship with an evil spirit called a *dodo*. The *dodo* is a bush spirit of enormous powers, which figures prominently in Hausa folklore,[32] and like an evil genie can be made to do the bidding of a human master. The *dodani* (pl.) reside in the bush away from human habitation, but if one seeks diligently enough they can be found. By using convincing words and the right sacrifices one can persuade a *dodo* to come and live in his compound. Usually, the spirit is given a large pot or granary in

---

feel their weight, for he would eat their souls while he held them and give them back to you dead!

A being similar to the witch is the *kambultu*, or "were-hyena." These individuals are said to have the inherited power to transform themselves (*riki'da*) into hyenas. This they do predominantly at night and kill other peoples' sheep or cattle for a feast. Another favorite pastime is to transform themselves into hyenas on the road or path, frighten people into dropping their loads, and then change back to men to make off with the loot. One man of my acquaintance confided in me that he had had an affair with a female *kambultu*, who suddenly transformed herself into a hyena in the midst of their amours and made out through the door, scaring him nearly to death. Several healers told me that they had given these people medicine to cure them of this unwanted affliction.

31. All appetites have limits, however, and the witch is no exception. It is said that when a witch has eaten 1,000 souls his hunger will be satisfied and his witchcraft will no longer be effective. This belief has also been reported by Last (1970) and Darrah and Froude (n.d.:6).

32. See, for example, the tales in Johnston (1966) entitled "The Girl, Her Young Brother and the Ogre," "Auta and the Ogre," and "The Husband, the Wife, and the Ogre." Tremearne (1913) gives two such folktales involving the *dodo*, and Skinner (1977a) present another large selection of such stories.

which to live and thereafter acts as a protector for its master.[33] The *dodo* will kill thieves who enter the compound and will guarantee successful farming and the accumulation of great wealth for its owner.[34] The one condition that must be fulfilled in this Faust-like pact, however, is that the *dodo* must be fed regularly on the souls of the other members of the compound—wives, sons, mothers, daughters, brothers, or on the souls of friends and neighbors. The lives of these people are sacrificed for gain to the *dodo* owner.[35] The *dodo*, therefore, is a symbol of boundless personal greed. Involvement with such an ogre for personal gain involves the destruction of all ties that bind an individual to family, friends, and community, and ultimately, as he runs out of available sacrifices, the owner himself.[36]

There remains one last form of evil power, aside from spirit worship, witchcraft, and the *dodo*, that threatens the moral order. This is sorcery, *sammu*, and although it is linked in the minds of many Hausa villagers with paganism, it is not exclusively so. *Sammu* is a poison which works on its intended victim through occult means rather than by immediate physical ones. It may be contrasted with *dafi*, substances known to be poisonous on ingestion or injection such as the seeds of the *kwankwani* plant (*Strophanthus sarmentosus*), which are used in making arrow poisons. The cause-and-effect relationship of this latter kind of poison is obvious—attack by a snake and death from the resulting bite are easily linked—but such is not the case with *sammu*.

33. I was told that an alternative way to obtain a *dodo* was to find somebody who already had one (no doubt a dangerous business in itself) and to make arrangements with him to buy some of the *dodo's* offspring—described as being small and furry, like kittens—to raise in one's own compound, much as one might buy fowl or livestock to raise.
34. The fact that village Maguzawa perceive the Maguzawa as excellent and successful farmers no doubt helps to heighten suspicion of their way of life for reasons similar to this.
35. Greenberg (1946:47) reports that Maguzawa who make sacrifices to individual spirits take pains to insure that these are done outside of their compounds to avoid imputations that they have struck up a relationship with a *dodo*.
36. The concept of the *dodo* thus lends itself to allegorical use in moral exhortations such as the proverb that runs *Munafunci dodo ne; wanda ya yi shi, shi ya kan ci*, "Slanderous backbiting is a *dodo*; he who engages in it is eaten up himself."

Those who know the secret of preparing these sorcery poisons may use them to destroy their enemies by driving them mad, blinding them, turning them into lepers, causing dissension to engulf their compounds, destroying their crops, withering their limbs and crippling them, stealing their wives, or killing them outright.

While it is usually a physical substance, *sammu* does not necessarily have to be ingested by the victim, it only needs to come in contact with his personal sphere of existence. It may be placed in his footprint on a path, poured out in the grass where he has urinated, mingled with a strip of his clothing, tossed over the wall of his compound in the dead of night, or brought into his immediate world by some other means. The desired effects will then follow insidiously to their conclusion.[37]

The ability to use *sammu* comes when one obtains the proper knowledge of the occult. This knowledge is obtained only from a pagan priest who knows the ways of *tsafi*: a *boka* (herbalist), a member of the cult of spirit possession ('*yam bori*) or, paradoxically, from a "big Koranic scholar" (*babban mallam*)—people whose knowledge transcends the sphere of everyday affairs and reaches into those realms where the average villager is a stranger. A pagan sacrifice by definition lies beyond the moral community of Islam, and because the *boka* and the *bori* devotee both deal extensively with spirits, they are seen as suspect, living on the border of paganism. Similarly, those scholars immersed in the depths of Koranic study—especially if they are members of a sufi *tarika*—may be suspected of wandering from the narrowly defined path of *Muhammadiyya*, "the ways of the Prophet."

All these forces—witchcraft, sorcery, spirit worship, and the *dodo*—come from areas either clearly beyond the community of Islam or from the liminal areas that touch upon pagan practices or knowledge unknown in everyday life. At the level of the rural Hausa village this is an important part of the conceptual structure of the world. The village community (*gari*) is identical with the *jama'a*, the congregation of Islamic believers. To use the term *jama'a* within the village is not to say "the community of Muslims," but simply "everybody." With its

---

37. *Sammu* may be looked upon as a negative kind of *magani* (medicine). The main purpose of *magani* is to restore the balance of *lafiya*, to correct and restore proper order and health. *Sammu*, on the other hand, is disruptive, and aims at maximizing disorder, destroying balance, and bringing illness and death. These concepts are described in more detail in following chapters.

Koranic teachers, public observations of prayer, and mosque the village is inextricably identified with Islam. Islam, the domestic world of the family, and the cultivated fields are *gari*, "the village." It is the place of life. In stark contrast to this is the wild, uncultivated bush (*daji*) surrounding the village, with its lack of habitations, wild animals, uncontrolled forces, and malevolent spirits; and the pagan Maguzawa with their blood sacrifices, witchcraft, and sorcery. When a person dies he is removed from the village, taken outside its precincts and buried. Outside the village is the place of death. The polarity between the civilized village community of Islam and the uncertain, wild domain of the bush is a basic component of Hausa thought, and is mirrored succinctly in the proverb *Alheri gida, mugunta daji*, "Kindliness at home, evil in the bush." Indeed, one Hausa synonym for "goodness," "worth," or "value" is *nagari*, literally "of the village"; its antithesis is *na daji*, "of the bush."

If these concepts are ordered schematically, the polarity becomes clearer:

Nagari	*Na Daji*
Village	Bush
Islam	Paganism, witchcraft, sorcery
Mosque	Sacrificial sites for spirits
Order	Disorder
The known	The unknown
Open	Hidden
Life	Death

These two spheres are extremely important in shaping Hausa thought and symbolism. As will be seen later, they have an additional focus in Hausa beliefs about health and illness.

■ Women: Wives, Lovers, and Prostitutes

If the forces of evil and disorder listed above lie outside the village community, there is one powerful disrupting force present at the very center of domestic life. This discordant element is women.

Islam is a religion dominated by men and although it guarantees certain rights to women it nonetheless proclaims the supremacy of the male. The Koran declares of women that "their men have a degree above them" (Sura II, 228ff.), and later it is written:

> Men are the managers of the affairs of women
> for that God has preferred in bounty
> one of them over another, and for that
> they have expended of their property.
> Righteous women are therefore obedient,
> guarding the secret for God's guarding.[38]
> And those you fear may be rebellious
> admonish; banish them to their couches,
> and beat them. If they then obey you,
> look not for any way against them; God is
>   All-high, All great.
> (Sura IV, 34ff.)

The inferiority of women does not, however, preclude their ultimate reward in the next life. Paradise is open to the God-fearing, obedient, and faithful among them even as it is to men:

> Men and women who have surrendered,
> believing men and believing women,
> obedient men and obedient women,
> truthful men and truthful women,
> enduring men and enduring women,
> humble men and humble women,
> men and women who give in charity,
> men who fast and women who fast,
> men and women who guard their private parts,
> men and women who remember God oft—
> for them God has prepared forgiveness
>   and a mighty wage.
> (Sura XXXIII, 35ff.)

Although women are not excluded from the rewards of ultimate salvation, the expectations for them are less. The descriptions of paradise in the Koran have a distinctly male-oriented tone and less stringent religious obligations are placed upon women in light of their lesser capabilities (see Barkow 1972:321). They do not attend the communal prayers at the village mosque unless they are both old and exceptionally

38. That is, "guarding themselves and their husband's property, in return for God's guarding them" (Watt 1967:64).

devout. As children they receive less Koranic schooling than their brothers. Less attention is given to ensuring their devout compliance with the times of daily prayer and the obligations during the fast at Ramadan. In classical Islamic law a woman who commits apostasy is not executed but rather is forced to recant through beatings and imprisonment (Schacht 1964:126). Similarly, in classical Islamic law the blood money paid in compensation for the murder of a woman is only one-half that paid for the death of a man (Schacht 1964:126). In matters of inheritance and in the giving of evidence, she is counted as only half a man: one man and two women would be required to testify in case another male witness could not be found (Schacht 1964:126). The unreliability of women is echoed in the Hausa proverb, *Bin shawara mata, ita ka sa "da na sani!"*, "Following the advice of women leads to 'If only I had known!' " (i.e., regret).

In marriage the woman's rights are protected by specific Koranic safeguards (Sura II, especially 220ff.), but she is not an equal partner with the man. She is the ward of her husband, who has invested his money in her through marriage payments to her family for the use of her reproductive powers. The Koran puts it bluntly (Sura II, 223ff.): "Your women are a tillage for you; so come unto your tillage as you wish, and forward for your souls."[39] Indeed, Hausa men state quite frankly that the usefulness (*amfani*) of women is children, which they regard as the profit (*riba*) derived from their outlay of marriage money. If a divorce takes place before a child has been born, ideally the marriage money should be refunded to the husband. If a child has been born, the child remains with the father and the woman returns to her own father's compound.

The virtues to which a woman should aspire are, not surprisingly, virtues related to accepting this secondary position in society. The general background for moral excellence in women is much the same as it is for men: women should fear God, be diligent in religious obligations, be honest, patient, generous, and so on; but above all a woman should exhibit the virtue of *kunya*, "modesty," "shame," or "respectful submission." She should acknowledge men as her superiors and do their bidding without complaining. Women should greet men by kneel-

---

39. The phrase "forward for your souls" is often interpreted as uttering a pious phrase before intercourse. See Cohen (1969:58).

ing on the ground, and should go about in quiet modesty with their heads covered and eyes downcast. As the proverb succinctly puts it: *Matar na tuba ba ta rasa miji*, "A submissive woman will not lack for a husband."

The Islamic custom of *purdah*, or wife seclusion, known in Hausa as *auren kulle* ("locked-in marriage") is based on Koranic injunction and nurtures the virtues of shame and obedience desired in women:

> And say to believing women, that they
> cast down their eyes and guard their private
> parts, and reveal not their adornment
> save such as is outward; and let them cast
> their veils over their bosoms, and not reveal
> their adornment save to their husbands,
> or their fathers, or their husbands' fathers,
> or their sons, or their husbands' sons,
> or their brothers, or their brothers' sons,
> or their sisters' sons, or their women,
> or what their right hands own,[40] or such men
> as attend them, not having sexual desire,[41]
> or children who have not yet attained knowledge
> of women's private parts; nor let them stamp
> their feet, so that their hidden ornament
> may be known. And turn all together
> to God, O you believers: haply so
> you will prosper.
> (Sura xxiv, 31ff.)

Ideally, all married women should be kept thus in *purdah*, secluded within the confines of the household with the other wives and female relatives. As the proverb puts it, *Kakkyawar 'kwarya tana ragaya da faifanta a rufe*, "The best calabash stays hung up at home with its lid fastened on." Not only is this domestic policy sanctioned by Islamic ideals, but it gives added prestige to the compound by indicating that

40. That is, slaves (Watt 1967:164).
41. That is, old men and possibly eunuchs (Watt 1967:164).

the head of the household is wealthy enough to maintain such an arrangement (Cohen 1969:59–61; Hill 1972:22–24, 279; Barkow 1973: 322–23).[42]

42. Verses such as these quoted above delineate the virtues of modesty, shame, and obedience expected of Muslim women, values which certainly undergird the system of wife seclusion in Islam. The social origin of this custom probably lies within the practices of the Quryash tribe of Arabia of which Muhammed was a member. Several passages of Sura XXXIII of the Koran contain exhortations by Muhammed to his wives urging modest comportment and veiling and give concomitant instructions on proper behavior to his companions regarding women:

> Wives of the Prophet, you are not as other
> women. If you are Godfearing, be not
> abject in your speech, so that he in whose
> heart is sickness may be lustful, but speak
> > honourable words.
> Remain in your houses; and display not
> your finery, as did the pagans of old.
> And perform the prayer, and pay the alms,
> and obey God and His Messenger.
> People of the House, God only desires
> to put away from you abomination
> > and to cleanse you. (Sura XXXIII, 33ff.)

> O believers, enter not the houses of
> the Prophet, except leave is given you
> for a meal, without watching for its hour.
> But when you are invited, then enter; and
> when you have had the meal, disperse,
> neither lingering for idle talk
> that is hurtful to the Prophet; and he
> is ashamed before you; but God is not
> ashamed before the truth. And when you
> ask his wives for any object, ask them
> from behind a curtain; that is cleaner
> for your hearts and theirs. (Sura XXXIII, 53 ff.)

Reuben Levy, writing on the custom of wife seclusion among Muslim people in general noted: "On the whole, the exceptions that can be enumerated to the general practice of the veiling and seclusion of women are comparatively few, and the practice is entirely in keeping with the supremacy of the male over the female postulated by the Koran. But the vagueness of its provisions placed great authority in the hands of the Muslim doctors of law, who frequently interpreted them as

Of course, total seclusion of women is impossible. Women are allowed to visit friends and relatives, provided they first obtain the permission of their husbands. These visits—aside from such special occasions as a marriage or naming ceremony—usually take place at night, and it is interesting to note that women are released from their compounds to go abroad in the world under the cover of darkness at the same time that witches and evil spirits are thought to be most active.[43] Women may also undertake extended trips to other parts of the country for the purpose of visiting relatives but (ideally) should be accompanied by a chaperon or guardian under such circumstances.

In Hausa society, therefore, women are forced to function as a subculture separate from the men. Their mental and moral inferiority is recognized in the legal provisions which equate them with half-men, and the social conventions of greeting in which they must kneel in the presence of men. These categories of rank are further delineated by the fact that women suffer from recurrent impurity in the course of their menstrual cycles. By their biological nature they are less pure than men. The Koran declares:

> They will question thee concerning
> the monthly course. Say: "It is hurt;
> so go apart from women during
> the monthly course, and do not approach them
> till they are clean. When they have cleansed
> themselves, then come unto them as God
> has commanded you." Truly, God loves

---

local customs demanded, particularly where no pertinent *hadith* existed" (1957: 129).

Wife seclusion in Hausaland is an Islamic phenomenon, as the freedom of women among the pagan Hausa readily attests, and has its roots within the larger traditions of Muslim culture. The firm foundation of this cultural practice within the mainstream of Islamic customs and attitudes toward women is well known, and Muslim Hausa attitudes toward women fit the general cultural pattern nicely. For a further discussion see Callaway (1984).

43. Christian Nigerians obtain great mirth from the fact that while Muslims jealously guard their women during the day, they give them license to wander the village streets at night at the time when sexual escapades are most likely to occur—a predicament which also weighs heavily on the minds of many Muslim husbands.

those who repent, and He loves those
  who cleanse themselves.
(Sura II, 223ff.)

Biologically there is no compelling reason to abstain from intercourse
during a woman's menstrual period, but in Hausa thought the menstrual blood is more than merely aesthetically displeasing, it is both
condemned by the religion and related to the pathophysiology of certain illnesses and bodily states. Leprosy and albinism, for example, are
both said to stem from sexual relations that take place during the
menstrual period and lead to the conception of a defective fetus. The
menstrual blood (*jinin haila*) may also be found as an ingredient, so it
is said, in sorcery poisons.

The polarity of the sexes is symbolized in other ways, as well. Men
and women do not eat together. Eating is an intimate act not to be
engaged in together by men and women who have proper modesty—
only prostitutes would eat from the same bowl as a man. The milk from
a mother's breast—another fluid unique to the woman—is likewise
charged with power. If a few drops of milk were to fall on the genitals
of a nursing baby boy he would likely become sterile or impotent as
an adult. In symbolic terms women are classified as cold (*sanyi*), while
men are hot (*zafi*). Hot, spicy foods (*yaji*) are therefore used by men as
aphrodisiacs to increase their own sexual heat, which is drained off
into the coldness of the woman. Indeed, this "coldness" in the woman
is a source of illness in men. While environmental cold (also *sanyi*) is
seen as a major cause of illness, penetrating the body and disrupting
its proper functioning, *sanyin mata* ("the coldness of women," as
apart from environmental cold, to which women are also subject), is
seen as the cause of *ciwon sanyi*, literally "the illness of cold" but actually the term used to describe the clinical symptoms of gonorrhea, a
disease rampant in northern Nigeria. Since gonorrhea produces a puru-
lent urethritis in males but usually does not do so in females— in
whom it is often entirely asymptomatic—the symbolic polarity of the
sexes fits in nicely with the natural course of the disease.

The untrustworthiness of women is manifested especially in their
sexual nature. Hausa Sufi poetry refers to the world as a profligate
woman, ready to snare the unwary (Hiskett 1975:80–87). Partly be-

cause women are seen as vehicles for reproduction, it is assumed by
men that they have a constant sexual appetite. In polygamous households in particular, maintaining the proper sexual diplomacy among
the several wives presents a challenge to the husband.[44] As has been
noted earlier, the Hausa word for co-wife, *kishiya,* stems from the word
for jealousy, *kishi,* and the combination of sexual frustration and wifely
rivalries represents a volatile mixture in many a Hausa household. Men
fear that their wives will seek a *kwarto,* a lover, to ease their frustrations and thus do injury to their husbands; but conversely, since the
sexual desires in women burn so constantly, a woman no longer married, a *bazawara,* is eagerly pursued by the men of the village as an
object of sexual attentions. In this there is an explicit double standard.
Most Hausa men see nothing wrong in fornication with an unmarried
woman (even if they are married themselves); the moral injury comes
in thus abusing another man by damaging his property. It is the nature
of women to seek sexual enjoyment and men feel they cannot be
blamed for occasionally taking advantage of this fact (Cohen 1969:56–
57; Barkow 1971: 70–72, 1972:323). The fact that women have this
nature, however, means that men must also be vigilant in protecting
what is rightfully theirs.

From the masculine point of view, then, Hausa women are a necessary evil that must be controlled. One proverb declares of women:
*Kurasa, dangin Shaidan! In ba ku, ba gida; in kun yi yawa, gida ya
'baci,* "Kurasa, kin of Satan! Without you there is no home; if you
are many the household is spoiled!" Women are seen as quarrelsome,
petty, simpleminded creatures whose only power comes from their
constant nagging.[45] The untrustworthiness of women is proverbial in
Hausa folklore: *Kissar mata gomiya tara da tara ce; guda 'daya ta
cikon 'darin Iblis bai san ta ba,* "The deceits of women are ninety-nine,
and even the Devil himself does not know the hundredth." The virtue
of *kunya* or "shame" is so highly valued in women in part because they
are seen generally as so lacking in it, especially when compared to men:
Abin da mace ta yi, ta ce "na ji kunya," in namiji ya yi shi, ya bar gari,

44. In this regard it is of interest to note that the two presents the king of Katsina
requested from Heinrich Barth were rockets for war and aphrodisiacs to increase
his conjugal vigor! (Barth 1859:142).
45. The proverb says *'Karfin mata sai yawan magana,* "The strength of women is
only their plenitude of speech."

"An act that makes a woman say 'I'm ashamed,' if done by a man would force him to leave town."

These characteristics of sexual fickleness and domestic treachery figure prominently in Hausa folktales. Women are seen as impossible to control and full of wanton sexual desires, and a common theme is the betrayal of a husband by a wife who shamelessly seeks a lover, as in the story of "The Vigilant Husband" (Tremearne 1914a:148).

There once was a husband so jealous of his wife that he followed her everywhere. If she had to urinate, he went with her and watched. If she had to move her bowels, he went and observed her. One day she challenged him and said, "Ha! My lover and I will have sex even while you watch me!" This he angrily denied, but she persisted in her declaration.

She got word to her lover to come to their house and hide under a pile of chaff near the threshing floor. This he did, covering himself completely in the chaff except for his penis, which he left exposed. When the sun had set and it was growing dark the woman said to her husband, "I need to urinate." Ever vigilant, he accompanied her outside. She went over to the pile of chaff and squatted down upon her lover's penis. Her husband said impatiently, "Make your water and get up," but she paid no attention to him as she was enjoying herself immensely. She cried out, "Oh! Oh! Come on! Come on and finish me off!" Her husband said angrily, "Who are you talking to?" She replied breathlessly, "Do you see anybody?" He said, "Make your water and get up. You are certainly taking a long time about it!" But she paid no attention to him and kept exclaiming, "Do it! Do it! Finish me off!" Her husband, now growing angry, demanded, "Are you talking to the spirits? Enough of this!" But she kept on enjoying herself.

Finally she was exhausted and got up, but while she was standing there arranging her clothes her lover let out a long sigh of contentment from under the chaff. Her husband heard it and cried out, "Oh no! Oh no! You have tricked me." She smiled at him and said, "Of course I have. I told you I would." The husband saw that he had no chance and resigned himself to his unhappy lot, while his wife and her lover continued their adulterous ways.[46]

46. Two other folktales can be cited as further examples of this set of themes.
   Once upon a time, two Koranic scholars had an argument on the deceits of women. The first one maintained that women's lechery was not inherent in their nature but was, rather, absorbed by girls from their mother's milk—a common

Such tales all center on the treachery of women and the impossibility of controlling them. In real life, however, there is a continuum of female behavior from the ideal submissive and obedient wife to the pro-

---

Hausa view as to how many characteristics (including some illnesses) are transmitted. The second *mallam* insisted that all women were deceitful and adulterous from birth, but the first scholar maintained his position. Then it happened that a girl was born in the town. The first scholar, eager to prove his point and defeat his friend, arranged to marry the baby girl and took her away from her mother. He raised her on goats' milk and eventually she grew into a beautiful young woman.

One day the chief of the town was telling his son about this longstanding argument. He said, "You know, there is a certain *mallam* in this town who has raised his wife from birth and claims she won't fornicate with anybody!" The chief's son thought, "We'll see about that!" and resolved to put her to the test. He draped his horse with all his finery and rode off to visit this reputedly chaste woman.

When he arrived at her compound he threw a bundle of twenty kolanuts over the wall to let her know there was a man outside who was interested in her. Some of these she ate and the rest she hid from her husband, lest he should question her about their origin. Three days later the youth returned, and again threw some kolanuts over the wall. She resolved to meet him and tied several of her body cloths together to form a rope. She threw one end over the top of the wall and climbed to the top. She saw the young man and told him to return in the morning when her husband went to the mosque to pray.

In the morning, before it was light, the *mallam* went to the mosque to perform the first ritual prayer. The chief's son came soon after and threw the woman another bundle of kolanuts. She climbed to the top of the wall and told him to bring his horse inside. The young man did so and tethered his horse in the center of the courtyard. Then he entered her hut and began to have sex with the eager young wife.

It so happened, however, that before they were finished the *mallam* returned from his prayers and saw the hoofprints of the horse leading into his compound. When he went inside he saw the horse tethered in the yard, richly caparisoned and shaking its fine head. The chief's son was afraid and felt they were lost. The young wife, however, said, "Don't despair. I have a hundred and one ways to take care of him! Let me show you." She tidied her body cloth and ran out into the yard.

"*Mallam!* Look behind you!," she cried. "The chief has sent you this fine horse as a present! You must not come back until you have gathered the other scholars and thanked him!"

Her husband was highly pleased at this and scurried out of the compound to gather his associates and go thank the chief. When he had left, the chief's son left the woman's hut, mounted his horse, and rode off. The young wife then got out her broom and swept out the courtyard, obliterating all the hoofprints and other traces of the horse.

miscuous, domineering prostitute. Moreover, the range of acceptable
behavior varies with a woman's age and marital status. Children, sexually immature girls (*berori*), and maturing, nubile maidens (*'yam*

Meanwhile, her husband and all the Koranic teachers in town had gathered before the chief. The husband gathered himself up and said, "While I was at the
mosque this morning you sent me a fine horse as a present. For this I am deeply
grateful and I thank you." The chief looked at him in amazement and said, "I
did no such thing!" The *mallam* insisted, saying, "You certainly did! You sent me
a very fine horse and he is tethered in the middle of my compound!" The chief was
adamant that he had not done such a thing and sent a party with the teacher to
his house to see the horse.

When they arrived there was no sign of a horse anywhere, not even a single hoof
mark. The man called out to his wife, "Where is the horse that I left this morning
in the middle of the yard!" His wife cried out, "*Wayyo!* My poor husband has
gone mad! Do you see any signs of a horse here?" The chief's servants grabbed
the teacher and prepared to subdue him before he became a raving madman.

The woman was then summoned to appear before the chief, who asked her to
explain what was going on. Was the *mallam* telling the truth or was he lying?
Under his close questioning she told him the whole story and said, "I did it because he once quarreled with his friend and said that women are not lustful by
nature. I wanted to prove to him that we are born full of cunning and that our
nature is deceit!" The poor scholar admitted his defeat and was released by the
chief, and his young wife continued to enjoy herself with whatever man she fan-
cied (Tremearne 1914:23–26).

A second, more somber tale relates the story of a hunter whose wife took a
warrior for her lover. Having become tired of her husband and eager to run off
with the warrior, she plotted to kill her spouse. One day when he was away she
went to his quiver and carefully removed all the tips from his arrows. Then she
carefully rearranged them so he would think nothing was amiss. She then ran off
to meet her lover.

In the meantime her husband returned and, finding that his wife had run away,
he picked up his bow and quiver and set off after her. He trailed her to her rendezvous and, outraged at what he witnessed, he challenged the warrior to battle
on the spot. As he readied his bow he discovered that his arrow had no tip. He
discarded it and reached for a new one, but to his horror he found that each shaft
was headless. By this time it was too late. The warrior, mounted on his horse with
his sword in his hand, was bearing down upon him. At the last minute, however,
the warrior suddenly wheeled his horse around, charged at the woman and cut off
her head.

Returning to the astonished hunter, the warrior proclaimed, "Friend, let us be
reconciled, for I have realized that if I had killed you now, some day she would
have done the same thing to me. Any man who gets mixed up with a woman will
certainly lose his life" (Johnston 1966:173–74; Skinner, 1969:229).

mata) have great freedom to go where they like, to talk and banter with the men and youths. As they reach maturity there is a great deal of flirting and discrete sex play (*tsarance*), which is regarded as a normal part of growing up. Old women no longer in their reproductive years regain much of the freedom they knew as girls, and may wander through the village freely, trading, visiting friends, and offering advice or criticism to the men they meet. So too, is it with sexually mature women who are between marriages, either having been divorced (which is very common), or widowed. These *zawarawa* also revert to the social behavior of young girls and have considerable latitude in their behavior with men. Since the natural state of a woman is assumed to be that of marriage and obedience to a husband, a *bazawara* is expected to remarry and leave the compound of her father. Mature, eligible women who persist in remaining single may come to be regarded as profligate women, *karuwai*.

The Hausa word *karuwa* is generally translated as "prostitute," but this simple translation gives a misleading impression of the meaning of the word. While it is generally applied to women, it may also be used to indicate any morally irresponsible person, male or female. Usually it refers to women, particularly women who are not under the authority of a man and who therefore do not conform to the expected subordinate role of women in Hausa society.[47] A *bazawara* who lives with her father but refuses to remarry and flaunts proper behavior may be referred to as a "prostitute," but generally the *karuwai* are women who live by themselves in their own compound in the town or village with a woman as compound head. Such a compound is known as a *gidan mata*, or

47. See M. G. Smith (1959:244–46). In this regard Barkow (1971:62, n.9) writes:

> *Karuwa* cannot be precisely rendered in English, and certainly not by "prostitute." The English verb "to prostitute" means to use something for a purpose of less worth than that for which it was intended. A prostitute, therefore, is a woman who demeans herself. In Hausa *karuwa* may be translated as "a profligate" (of either sex), a person extravagant and uncontrolled. The West traditionally views sexuality, especially female sexuality, as debasing: the Hausa view of sexuality, female sexuality in particular, is that it is strong and aggressive, dangerous unless controlled. So in the West the prostitute symbolizes sexual debasement; while among the Hausa the *karuwa* symbolizes dangerous, uncontrolled female sexuality. Wife seclusion, in turn, symbolizes control over that sexuality.

"house of women," and functions as a hotel for traveling strangers, a restaurant, tavern, gambling parlor, night club, salon, and whorehouse.

Although their compounds are not headed by men, ultimately the prostitutes are under male control. All the prostitutes in a village are responsible to the village headman, through the person of the *magajiya*, or "elder sister." The *magajiya* is the "chief of the prostitutes" and is one of their number selected by them to serve in this office. This is an official position, and the woman who is selected to hold it is invested with the title by the village headman. As with other official positions in Hausaland, performance of the social obligations attendant on the title often requires a substantial financial backing. Hence, the *magajiya* frequently is an older woman who has accumulated a certain amount of wealth through her trading enterprises. Similarly, the office may lie vacant for some time because no one wishes to take it up.[48]

The population of village prostitutes is changeable. Usually, there is a nucleus of women who have lived as *karuwai* together in the village for a long time; but if one keeps careful track of village activities, he will also notice a frequent turnover of women who live in the prostitutes' compounds for a few weeks or months and then move on to another location. The prostitutes' compounds may also have a male population. Many of these men are simply friends of the women who live there—musicians, praise-singers, village ne'er-do-wells who do odd jobs and run errands for the female compound head—but some of them are homosexuals who live with the prostitutes on a permanent basis. These men, called *'yan daudu*, dress in female clothes, adopt feminine mannerisms, and earn their livelihood by cooking and selling food commercially, especially snack foods such as fried eggs, fried potatoes, roast chicken, and the like.[49] Since the *gidan mata* serves as a

48. Such was the case in the village where I lived. The *magajiya* was an old woman who had held the title for many years. On her death, some three years before my arrival, no one was found willing to assume the office because of its expense. Instead, one woman was appointed *shugaba*, or "leader," of the prostitutes to take care of any political matters, but she did not have to face the ceremonial and economic burdens of the office.

49. A male homosexual is called a *'dan Daudu* in Hausa, after one of the *bori* spirits who represents a man dressing up as a woman. M. G. Smith (1954:262) has erroneously recorded this expression as *'dan dau'da* or "son of dirt," which does have a certain metaphorical flavor to it, considering the circumstances. A

hotel, there may be itinerant travelers or laborers renting rooms there as well.

The prostitutes' compounds conform to typical Hausa architectural styles. They possess an entry-hut which opens into a large courtyard with other huts or rooms facing the central area. They may be made of cornstalks and thatch or mud-brick. The various women who live there each have their own rooms in which they keep whatever material possessions they may have. By rural Hausa standards some of these rooms are quite elegant, with metal-frame beds, mattresses, pillows, mosquito-net canopies, and photographs on the walls. The rooms let to the transient population are generally bare by comparison.

A wide range of activities takes place in these *gidajen mata*. They are convenient places to buy candles, kolanuts, cigarettes, and similar items since many of the women are small market traders. (Since prostitutes are not confined to their compounds but are free to wander where they please, they may turn this to their economic advantage; on the other hand, their segregation from the main body of village women effectively precludes many profitable trading relationships within the local network of women. Only settled prostitutes can hope to accumulate much money.) The women prepare daily meals for themselves and also sell *tuwo* and snack foods to others. Although the consumption of alcohol is forbidden to Muslims, there is always a certain segment of society eager to drink, and there will be an enterprising prostitute who brews and sells beer, either the sweet, sugary *duma* or the more rustic *burkutu*. Very sophisticated establishments may even sell bottled Nigerian beer—the ever-popular Star and Double Crown in their dark green bottles. At night there is often drumming and music-making for entertainment, and dancing to the *kirari*—songs of the *bori* spirits. The women are always available to play cards with the men, host gambling matches, or just sit and chat.

Sexual favors are available as well. Such affairs may be quick, physical encounters for a few naira, or long-lasting liaisons between a village man and one of the women, who is then looked upon more as a mistress than the English word "prostitute" would indicate. Generally, if a patron is to obtain sexual considerations from one of these courtesans a

---

homosexual may also be called a *'dan lutsu*, meaning "son of Lot," after the Biblical and Koranic figure.

period of courtship and persuasion is necessary—it is by no means an impersonal financial transaction.[50] Men may even take wives from among these women, for their worldly experience and sophisticated ways give them an attraction not found in a normal village woman. However, the proverbial expression *Da auren karuwa gara kiwon zakara,* "It's better to keep a cock than to marry a whore," indicates a skepticism of such matches. Since nearly all these women have been married before and have left their husbands for the freedom and self-assertion of the life of a prostitute, there is reason to doubt that many of them would be content with the life of a secluded village wife. A man who marries one must possess great patience and a strong will if he is to exert any control (see Cohen 1969:54–64).

The style of living in the prostitutes' compounds is very free and open. Since prostitutes are, in a sense, "wives" to the whole male population, the normal constraints on relationships with unfamiliar men do not apply. Since they are by definition lacking in "shame," they may strike up joking relationships with almost anyone. Their relationships with men are marked by an easy familiarity lacking among their married, secluded counterparts.[51] They do not hesitate to eat with men, for example, whereas other women would not do so. They are open, direct, even blunt in their conversation with men, perfect examples of the proverb that says *Matar shige ba ta (da) daraja,* "A woman who accosts you has no honor."

50. Barkow (1971:62–63) in particular deals with this aspect of the sexual encounter.
51. A striking example of this behavior occurred just after my arrival in the village. I was sitting in the entry-hut of one of my neighbors talking with him when a woman of sexually mature years entered the hut selling *ganda,* a mixture of roasted meat scraps of generally poor quality. Instead of talking politely to the men from outside the entryway, she came right on inside and sat down with us, talking, laughing, and making jokes. She leaped right into the conversation and slapped one of the men on the back several times to emphasize her points. The conversation quickly turned to sex, and my neighbor pointed to the woman and made some unmistakable gestures indicating that she was a "good lay" for only three naira. At this point another man entered the hut and make a jokingly rude comment to her, at which time she jumped up, ran across the room, lifted up his shirt and grabbed him by the penis through his pants, and proceeded to shake him until he gave in and admitted his defeat. After considerable laughter she picked up her large enamel basin full of meat, put it on her head, and walked outside to continue her trading.

The fluidity of the relationships in these compounds makes them centers of disorder in a very real sense. The epithet of the prostitute is *Karuwa, tsumma ma'kunsar cuta,* "Prostitute, a piece of cloth in which disease is wrapped up." This not only refers to the spread of venereal diseases such as gonorrhea, but also indicates the disturbance of the moral order of the community which emanates from the prostitutes' way of life. Their compounds are places where the shiftless, unreliable, deviant population of rural Hausaland congregates. They are places where drunkenness, gambling, promiscuity, and dishonesty run rife. On market days, when the village is crowded and certain people are well into their cups, tempers often flare and fights erupt. The settled, ordered values esteemed by Islam find little place in the world of the prostitutes; in fact, *karuwanci* ("the ways of prostitutes") bears a striking resemblance in many of its aspects to paganism.

If one compares the behavior of prostitutes to that of pagan Maguzawa women, there are certain broad parallels between them that contrast distinctly with the behavior expected of a Muslim Hausa woman. Both pagan women and prostitutes sell beer. Maguzawa women bring their homemade brew into the village and sell it in the marketplace on market days, while prostitutes make and sell beer in their compounds throughout the week. There is a general feeling that pagan women are more sexually expressive than Muslim village women (Barkow 1971:62, n.9; 1972:324–27), and certainly prostitutes are uninhibited in this regard. Prostitutes eat with men and, in rural areas, go about barebreasted with little thought of the propriety of the matter. Maguzawa women habitually go about bare-breasted, and appear thus when they come to the village, while a Muslim woman would take great care to cover her entire body before going out. Like the village prostitutes, Maguzawa women are much more open and candid with men than are the secluded Muslim women. Maguzawa women work as the equals of men in the fields and shoulder a large part of the economic responsibility for the household themselves. Village prostitutes do not usually farm, but their economic independence helps engender a similar feeling of social independence in their relationships with men. But the most striking parallel between paganism and prostitution is the fact that the houses of the prostitutes are the centers for the devotees of *bori,* the Hausa cult of spirit possession which plays a very important part in the lives of pagan women. Since prostitutes have largely turned their backs on Islam, it is not surprising that they should turn to the spirits in its place. In this sense the compounds of prostitutes represent little islands of pagan spirit worship in an otherwise Muslim community, foci of religious as well as social disorder.

■ *Bori:* The Cult of the Spirits

The *iskoki*, or spirits, are ethereal, invisible beings whose presence can be felt even though they cannot be seen, like the wind (*iska*), whose plural form in Hausa (*iskoki*) means "spirits." As described earlier in this chapter, Muslim Hausa thought identifies these spirits with devils (*iblisai*) or with the Koranic *djinn* (in Hausa, *aljannu*). The *bori* are those spirits which cause spirit possession and they thus enter into a special relationship with the humans they afflict, particularly women. The *bori* cult is the social and religious institution that centers on inducing, maintaining, and regulating this intercourse between the spirit world and the members of the possession cult, called *'yam bori*, "the children of *bori*."

The pantheon of *bori* spirits is almost unlimited. Nearly every living entity may have a *bori* counterpart. There are elephant spirits and lion spirits, hyena, snake, and hedgehog spirits, to name but a few. There are noble spirits such as *Sarkin Aljannu*, "The chief of the djinn," and *'Dan Galadima*, to whom the others are subordinate. There are master spirits and slave spirits, like *Bawa and Bagobiri*, "the man from Gobir." There are Muslim spirits like *Mallam Alhaji*, and pagan spirits like *Arne*, the beer drinker. There are spirits of the town and spirits of the bush. A pantheon of ethnic spirits exists as well. Hausa and Fulani spirits predominate, but there are also Gwari spirits and even European spirits, who are said to fly airplanes, drive cars, and live in fine houses. There are water spirits like *Sarkin Rafi*, the "chief of the river," and *Gajimare*, the rainbow spirit. There are lepers, drummers, warriors, weavers, and hunters in the realm of the spirits. The spirits are also arranged in social hierarchies and kinship groups, having husbands, wives, and children—although many of these relationships are ill-defined and vary according to the informant one questions. In short, the

world of the *bori* is a pale, incorporeal reflection of the natural and social world in which the Hausa live.[52]

The organization of the *bori* cult is relatively loose and varies from
region to region throughout Hausaland. Within a given community
there may be someone regarded as the *Sarkin Bori* ("chief of the *bori*")
or *Sarauniyar Bori* ("queen of the *bori*"), a title that may represent an
actual invested position or may be merely an expression of local pre-
eminence in dancing, knowledge of spirits, and notoriety in the practice
of herbal medicine. Like as not, the head of the prostitutes (*magajiya*)
will play a role in organizing *bori* performances, for prostitutes' compounds are the setting for many of these dramaturgies. The prostitutes
within a given region have their own network of social relationships
along which much of the information pertaining to *bori* performances
is transmitted. In general, prostitutes are a highly mobile section of the
population, moving frequently from place to place. The more settled
members of the community of prostitutes provide stopping points for
their itinerant sisters and the constant shifting of prostitutes from one
location to another keeps one compound in contact with most of the
others within a given region.

At the village level the frequenters of *bori* will all be known to each
other, and word of an impending performance will travel along the
usual local networks of communication. For a performance held in connection with an important occasion, such as a wedding or a naming
ceremony, invitations will be sent out by special messenger to ensure
the participation of the more prominent *bori* personages within the
area. People may come from forty or fifty miles away in order to be
present at such an event.

Performances of *bori* vary considerably in style and content. Informal sessions are held frequently in the households of prostitutes. Here
men and women dance to the songs of the various spirits mainly for
amusement, with no serious attempt to induce possession. These ses-

52. The nature and characteristics of many of these spirits are described in the following chapter, "Illness and Its Causes." In addition, extensive lists of *bori* spirits
and information relevant to each may be found in the following works: Tremearne
(1912:254–57, 1913:530–40, 1914b:296–391, 1915), Palmer (1914), Greenberg (1946:
30–43), King (1966), J. M. Nicolas (1967:27–31, 1972:355–61), and Onwuejeogwu
(1969:293–303). The material in this last article derives in large part from the writings of Tremearne. The best overall discussion of *bori* is in Besmer (1983).

sions are roughly analogous to a show in a nightclub where musicians and dancers perform for the entertainment of the patrons. On the other hand, *bori* performances may be quite elaborate affairs involving a whole battery of musicians, singers, and devotees of the cult, culminating in the possession of several people simultaneously.[53] Such extravaganzas, which are held out in the street or in some comparable large, open public area, may involve a considerable financial outlay for food, body cloths, cigarettes, perfume, and sweets, which are disbursed by the hosts to the musicians, singers, dancers, and notable guests. At such events great formal displays of generosity center on the disbursement of these materials to their recipients, with concomitant ceremony surrounding the return donation of funds by the guests to help the host defer some of her or his expenses. Such return gifts are usually written down by a scribe appointed for the event. Yet again, an intimate *bori* performance may be held in a particular compound for a small, select group and staged primarily as a therapeutic encounter with a spirit or spirits for the benefit of a single individual. In this case the induction of possession in this person is the major purpose of the ceremony.

Music is an integral part of any *bori* performance. The dancers must have music to accompany their actions, but more important, the spirits require it. The *bori* spirits are not faceless entities but as remarked above have specific characteristics and personalities. Furthermore, each *bori* spirit has its own musical beat, its own epithet or *kirari*, and its own praise song (*wa'ka*).[54] When the spirits are summoned the musicians play the particular beat of the spirit, the vocalists (who may be the same as the musicians) sing the praise songs, and the dancers perform the movements unique to each spirit, often carrying the ritual objects identified with that spirit. The only requirements for a *bori* musician are that he must know the songs of the spirits in question. Music at a *bori* séance is a job to be performed, not a ritual office requiring special qualifications. This music is provided by a combination of five instruments: the large, single-stringed bow lute (*goge*) or its smaller version (*kukuma*), the large, resonant gourd drum ('*kwarya*), the gourd rattle (*caki* or *gora*), and the two-stringed plucked lute (*garaya*).[55]

53. See, for example, Besmer (1975).
54. Many of these are given in King's (1966) translation of "A Boorii Liturgy from Katsina." See also Besmer (1983).
55. These and other Hausa musical instruments are fully discussed in the compre-

At a *bori* performance the musicians generally sit at one end of an open space with the crowd of observers forming a circle or an oval within which the dancers can perform. At the other end of the space, surrounded by the crowd and facing the musicians, a line of dancers will form. These dancers are the "horses" that the spirits will "mount" and "ride" in the course of the possession. All the dancers, both male and female, dress as women, wearing a body cloth (*zane*) or blanket (*gwado*) during the dancing and possession—a further identification of *bori* with women and an expression of the marginality and femininity of the men who participate in these rites. The musicians begin to play the songs of the *bori*, usually starting with that of *Sarkin Ma'kada*, the "chief of the drummers," who prepares the dancing ground for the spirits. Then follow the songs of the other spirits played in varying order (see King 1966; Besmer 1975). As the musicians play, the dancers move out of the line toward them one at a time, dance in front of them for a few seconds, and then return to the end of the line of dancers, another moving out of the line to take the place of her predecessor, or perhaps to dance with her in front of the musicians, as in the dance of the spirit *Barahaza*. Usually, there is a piece of cloth or a shoe in front of the musicians, into which coins may be placed for their benefit. Each of the spirits in the progression has its own drumbeat and song, some faster, some slower. This part of the dance is mainly entertainment, a warm-up for the possession that will follow.

At some point in the proceedings, often preparatory to the induction of possession, the *faduwa*, or "fallings," will begin. The *faduwa* are the *bori* leaps, a striking characteristic of the dances. They are done by both male and female members of the cult, the most impressive usually (but not necessarily) being done by the men. There are several ways in which the *bori* falls are done, depending on the skill of the dancer. Usually, the dancer dances around to one spot and then stops briefly, with his or her legs spread apart. Stretching his arms out to the side and then quickly bringing them sweeping in, he bends over and drops his belly in, falling stiff-legged to the ground while slapping the taut body cloth between his legs with a resounding slap. There are many variations on this and some are very impressive indeed. A good dancer

hensive work of Ames and King (1971), *Glossary of Hausa Music and Its Social Contexts.*

may leap as high as four feet into the air, legs outstretched in front, landing flat on his buttocks while slapping the cloth hard, then flipping out straight back to slam his shoulders into the ground. This act may be completed by a full somersault into a seated position on the ground, slapping the ground, jumping up, and doing another fall. Describing these actions on paper does not do them justice, for if one were to apply an equal force to an off-center part of the body, serious damage could result. The proper performance of these falls marks off the true "child of *bori*" from the more casual participants, and these *'yam bori* are said by all to possess a medicine that strengthens their bodies and renders them impervious to the beating they take in these perfor-mances—medicines that also help them to control the spirits who possess them and to aid the suffering of others. This violent jarring of the body is most impressive, and members of the audience will run out and pay homage to the dancer (and the patron spirits) by placing coins on his forehead as he sits on the ground. These coins soon fall off into the dust and are collected and placed in the receptacle in front of the musicians, for distribution to the musicians and the devotees.

The actual onset of possession by one of the spirits comes under a variety of conditions. Sometimes it may happen spontaneously at the time of the falls, or under quieter circumstances when the dancers, anxious to induce possession, sit quietly on the ground in a circle con-centrating on the hypnotic rhythms of the throbbing music.[56] When the performance is done for the benefit of a single individual, the sup-plicant to the spirits may sit quietly on a mat, covered by a large, white cloth, while the spirits' songs are played. As the spirits come upon the individual, she will tremble and shake in succession as each new one comes to rest and then leaves, reacting violently when the main spirit of possession descends. Sometimes a combination of these pathways to the spirits will be seen.

Possession usually first manifests itself as a slight coughing, accom-panied perhaps by the twitching of an extremity. These build up into violent paroxysms of coughing and retching, with the expulsion of large quantities of mucus and saliva and increasingly marked spasms of the limbs, until the characteristics of the individual spirit take no-ticeable shape out of the amorphous movements: the clawing of the

56. See the discussion of possession and its relation to music in Erlmann (1982).

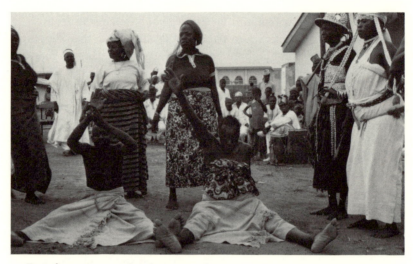

9. Bori *dancers preparing for possession.*

hands and bending of the limbs as *Kuturu,* the leper, comes; the groveling in the dirt on all fours, running and barking as *Kure,* the hyena, takes possession; or the wild striding and violent pratfalls, the pouring of dust on the head and the searching for water in the audience that characterizes the incarnation of *Sarkin Rafi,* the chief of the watercourse. Several spirits may enter and leave the same person in succession, passing in review for the devotees and the crowd. As the spirits leave at the end of the performance their departure is manifested as a series of sneezes (usually three) which indicates their passage out of the body.

Bori performances are great entertainment for those who watch them. The violent falls of the dancers are met with great approbation, and the antics of those possessed by the spirits are often greeted with gales of laughter. The music is loud and constant, and the crowd chatters and talks with one another. It is by no means a solemn, sacred ceremony done in hushed tones. A better sense of the nature of *bori* can be brought out by a description of one such performance that took place in front of a compound in a small hamlet as part of a wedding celebration at the home of the new bridegroom. A similar performance had taken place the previous day at the home of the bride.

We arrived in the village after dark, about 7:45 P.M., to find a typical wedding feast in progress. Lawai (a village friend) and I got some *tuwo* from the cooks and went inside the compound's entry-hut to eat. When we were finished we came outside to sit on the mats spread out on the ground around the kerosene mantle lamp lighted for the proceedings. Nothing much happened until about 9:30, when three men came out with the big, open-ended gourd drums. These instruments are held on the ground with the feet, one end slightly raised so as to let the sound escape, and beaten with wooden sticks. Accompanied by two lute players, the musicians started to play. After about half an hour a blind woman—she was suffering badly from *hakiya* (leucoma)—came out and began singing praise songs in a high, eerie, ululating voice. After a while one of our hosts, called 'Dan Maye ("son of a witch"), came out, clowned around, and did a few *bori* falls. Nobody started dancing until around 11:00 P.M.

The musicians were very good, laying down a loud, rapid, heavy beat, and a number of people began dancing, occasionally going into the much-applauded *bori* falls. Throughout these activities there were interruptions for the distribution of body cloths to important guests, and the receipt of money to aid with the finances of the event—all made much of by the *maro'ka* or praise-criers. Money was also pressed up against the dancers' foreheads when they performed the falls especially well. All in all, it was very good entertainment.

At about 2:00 A.M. the dancers decided it was time to get on with the process of possession. They formed a circle of four men and one woman (all dancers) around Yayi, the *Sarkin Bori,* and all removed their head-covers (including the woman). The drumming and strumming continued, loud and constant. Before too long the woman showed signs of possession. She started coughing, eventually quite violently. Large globs of saliva welled up to her lips. Her throat was distended, bulging out with the effort, and the saliva started to hang down her chin in a long, globular string. Before very long she started flopping on the ground, stiffened her arms upright, and squatted down in a hunched position while making sharp little barks. She was possessed with *Kure,* the hyena. 'Dan Maye came up behind her and squatted, then got a cloth and tied it around her waist. She ran off on all fours, yelping, barking, and howling, while he held the cloth at her back, as a hyena tamer might do when bringing his show through a village. He guided and restrained her. Eventually somebody came up with a stick of spitted roast meat and gave it to her. She carried it around in her mouth, but soon replaced it with a rubber sandal.

By this time one of the other dancers had started to show signs of possession. He didn't appear to cough, but did develop a violent, wild look in his eye, and began to gesticulate in the air with his hands, rather like making "shooing" motions. It looked to me as if he might be telling the spirits to go away. Suddenly he grew violent and began bouncing, falling, and flopping in the circle of seated dancers, several of whom moved away from him. He was being possessed by *Sarkin Rafi*, the chief of the watercourse and began to demonstrate the distinctive arm gestures, slapping and pounding his chest and doing the violent falls typical of this spirit.

While this was going on the woman who had been possessed by *Kure* had been led over to the side of the crowd and was sitting peacefully, watching the proceedings. She was quiet and subdued, but from her glazed eyes and expression it was obvious that she was still possessed. In the meantime, Yayi was possessed by *Kure* as well. At this point three people were possessed, two men and one woman. The other dancers who had been sitting in the circle got up and moved over to the edge of the crowd.

Kure now left Yayi and was replaced by *Bawa*, the slave. His arms were bound behind his back. While this was done somebody came out of the crowd with a large bowl of water and began pouring it over the head of *Sarkin Rafi*—the usual gesture of respect given to this spirit. At this juncture *Sarkin Rafi* became violent. Usually this spirit is vigorous and agitated, walking around stiff-legged at a rapid pace, and doing frequent *bori* falls. He did all these things, but then ran over to the edge of the crowd and tried to catch hold of a young boy (who was scared out of his wits). He pried the boy free from the crowd and carried him out into the center of the circle. 'Dan Maye and another man took the boy away and released him. When a motorcycle started up, at about 2:20 A.M., *Sarkin Rafi* ran away in the opposite direction as if scared by the noise.

Yayi was still possessed, sitting quietly in the circle formed by the crowd, saliva drooling from his lips. The woman was still sitting quietly at the edge of the crowd. *Sarkin Rafi* was spitting out prodigious amounts of saliva, half a mouthful at a time, again and again. It was running down his contorted face and chin and into the dust.

It was starting to get very late and the crowd began to disperse. 'Dan Maye and an assistant lined all three of the possessed dancers up in a row, one behind the other, facing the crowd: first the woman, then Yayi, then *Sarkin Rafi*. 'Dan Maye stood very closely behind *Sarkin Rafi* and began telling the spirit to leave. *Sarkin Rafi* was struggling— gurgling and beating his chest. Yayi, meanwhile, was whining in a high-pitched, howling voice, and the woman began sneezing. 'Dan Maye kept saying, *"Tafi gida. Tafi gida."* ("Go home. Go Home.") to the spirits. When the woman had sneezed three times, she got up and was led over to the side. At about 2:25 Yayi began sneezing. The spirits were leaving from the front of the line to the back. He regained control of himself and left the state of possession rather rapidly, but *Sarkin Rafi* wouldn't go away. He kept burbling and spitting, impervious to what was going on around him. Finally, he too began to sneeze. Yayi grabbed him and flung his arms up and down violently—a standard technique for helping the spirits leave those they have possessed in a *bori* séance. Finally, he gave out with his third sneeze and rolled over on the ground, slapping his chest. They lifted him up to his feet, but he remained bent over, crying softly and whimpering *"Cikina yana ciwo. Cikina yana ciwo."* ("My belly hurts. My belly hurts.") They began bouncing him up in the air a time or two, talking to him and admonishing him, but he clearly was affected by his spirit. Finally, he sat down, but didn't appear to be in very commendable shape. He was upset and perhaps physically ill, but unpossessed, at 2:30 A.M., when we began our journey home.

There is skepticism that possession is only feigned in many of these performances.[57] Hence the proverb says, *In bori gaskiya ne, a bar shi ya fa'da rijiya,* "If his *bori* is real, let him throw himself in a well," an allusion to the questing leaps for water seen in possession by *Sarkin Rafi,* which has caused some devotees in the past to jump into wells with imaginable consequences for their health. There is, however, a stronger reason for suspicion, especially among the devout male Islamic sector of the population, and that is the relationship of *bori* to paganism.

The vast majority of the important spirits found in the *bori* cults of

---

57. As, for example, the admonishments of Harris (1913:332–33) against "false *bori*" conducted in the barracks and by prostitutes for the purposes of arranging assignations.

Muslim Hausa communities are identical with those found in the spirit pantheon of the pagan Maguzawa Hausa. The conclusion strongly presents itself that sacrifice and spirit worship constitute the pre-Islamic religion of Hausaland, which still exists among the Maguzawa. Consequently, the *bori* rites appear to be a thinly veiled and partially modified paganism existing in an otherwise Muslim society.[58] For example, during the course of public performances of the possession dances alms are given to the spirits by placing coins on the forehead of the dancer, later to be divided among the devotees and the musicians—an Islamic substitution for the sacrifice of fowls which takes place in pagan religion. Devout Muslims regard *bori* as only one step removed from paganism; indeed the post-*jihad* Fulani rulers made little distinction between *bori* possession and pagan spirit worship (*tsafi*). *Bori* was prohibited and the performance of it was punishable by death; later, *bori* dancers were merely taxed—a good example of the state attempting to regulate an unpleasant social reality rather than suppress it entirely (Tremearne 1912:257; Meek 1925, I:298; King 1966:104). Since independence, formal harassment of this kind has largely disappeared. Indeed, *bori* rites have even been put to political use by Nigerian political parties in the cities (Cohen 1969:63–64; Onwuejeogwu 1969:291–92).

Nonetheless, there is a stigma attached to participating in *bori*. The numerous parallels between *bori* and pagan religion are well recognized by villagers. Devout Muslims fear the compromise of their ultimate salvation should they take part in it. One man, when asked if he would accompany me to a *bori* performance, replied: "No way. I have good sense [*hankali*]. *Bori* is a thing of [hell] fire." When asked what the use (*amfani*) of *bori* was he replied succinctly, "*sakarci*," that is, "worthless mischief."

The Hausa *Chronicle of Abuja* expresses this view very nicely (Hassan and Na'ibi 1962:64):

> Now there is a practice which is common today in Abuja and indeed in all the Hausa lands; a very old practice called *Bori*, for which women are chiefly responsible. This is the propitiation and

58. See, for example, Tremearne (1912:254), Krusius (1915:292–97), Greenberg (1946:64–68), M. G. Smith (1954:20), King (1966:104), J. M. Nicolas (1967:19–21, 1972:45), Onwuejeogwu (1969:291), and Barkow (1971:72).

worship of devils which take possession of the human body. The performance of the various rites is always accompanied by much drinking of beer and of palm-wine until the devotees become quite intoxicated and dance and throw themselves about with wild howls and screams. In Abuja it is only the women who practise this; if you see a man here engaged in it, then you may be sure he is a stranger, for the men of Abuja greatly dislike this thing, but the women, even of the Chief's households spend much money upon it.

As a consequence of this relationship to pagan religion and the resultant disapproval of the Islamic community, *bori* is associated with women, prostitutes, homosexuals, the mentally disturbed, and other persons marginal to mainstream Muslim Hausa society and appears to serve as an emotional and therapeutic outlet for these socially, politically, and sexually repressed minorities.[59] Women, though not without considerable influence in their domestic circles (see, e.g., Cohen 1969: 51–64; Hill 1969; Barkow 1972), are cut off from positions of power and authority in the wider society. Legally they are inferior to males, and socially they exist in fragmented groups, cut off by their seclusion in *purdah* from the broader associations open to men. Prostitutes, alienated as they are from the respected value structure of Islamic morality, are yet another step removed from positions of social power. Homosexual men, who often live in the compounds of prostitutes, are likewise displaced from the dominant value structure of society. In this position of social marginality *bori* becomes an institution which gives greater cohesiveness to the lives of these people, and provides a therapeutic outlet for the mental and emotional strains engendered by their social situation. Indeed, formal initiation as a *bori* adept—a lengthy

59. The idea of these possession cults forming a therapeutic outlet of "marginal" groups is discussed at length in I. M. Lewis's *Ecstatic Religion* (1971). For the Hausa in particular, this theme runs throughout the work of J. M. Nicolas (1972) *Ambivalence et culte de possession*. Most commentators on the Hausa find merit in this idea. Faulkingham (1975:11) does not agree, based on his own research in Niger. He himself admits, however, that his research and the culture of the community in which he lived appears substantially different from much of hausaphone Nigeria. In particular he describes a spirit possession cult, the *'yam mushe*, existing alongside the *'yam bori*, which apparently has no counterpart elsewhere in Hausaland.

process known as *girka*—involves the removal of a mental or physical illness diagnosed as being caused by one of the spirits. There are definite bonds of shared affliction among the *'yam bori*.

In addition to this, the act of possession by a spirit in the course of the dancing involves the loss of the devotee's "sense" (*hankali*) and all that implies as the spirit takes control. The devotee is referred to as a "mare" (*godiya*) or, if a male, a "horse" (*doki*), which the spirits ride, controlling her actions as a rider controls his mount. The same verbal, *hau*, is used both for the spirits taking control of the dancers and for a horseman climbing onto his steed. In a similar fashion one also "mounts" a woman in the act of sexual intercourse. At the linguistic level, and especially if one notes the high incidence of homosexual men and prostitutes involved with the cult, there is a heavy aura of sexuality associated with these ecstasies of spiritual union.

This incontinent abandonment of self-control runs counter to one of the main foundations of Hausa virtue, namely that an individual (and especially a woman) should possess dignity, decorum, patience, and a proper sense of her position in the hierarchy of the social order. Spirit possession is a negation of this precept. The person afflicted by the *bori* spirits becomes frenzied and excited in the course of the possession. She loses propriety and decorum, moves in a violent and ungraceful fashion, rolls her eyes, and drools from the mouth. She engages in what would otherwise be completely frightening and unacceptable behavior, the actions of a madwoman (*mahaukaciya*). She is emotionally overheated and, in a very real sense, "loses her cool" in the passion of the moment. A proverb makes this feeling quite plain: *Ba a bori da sanyin jiki*, "There is no *bori* with a cool body," or more loosely, "There are no hysterics in an even temperament." Not only is proper decorum breached by these possession rites, but through their intercourse with the spirits they open up a highly disruptive, non-Islamic avenue of mystical power which threatens the proper order and balance (*lafiya*) of the Islamic community; and just as the moral balance of the community is disturbed, so the equipoise of health in the body is deranged by the influx of these *bori* spirits.

In chapter 3 the essential values of the Islamic community were delimited. These form the ideal values to which the Hausa aspire and are seen as setting the tone for the proper ordering of society. Implicit within this structure of values is divine sanction from Allah through the vehicles of the Prophet Muhammed and the holy Koran. These values represent the ideal state of "health" (*lafiya*) of the body politic. But this state of moral and religious order was not established without struggle. It was necessary to overcome the forces of darkness represented by paganism and unbelief through the holy war of Usman 'Dan Fodio. This battle has not been fully won and so a constant struggle—now mainly an inner, moral struggle rather than an outer, political one—must be waged. From without, the forces of paganism, witchcraft, spirit worship, and sorcery threaten and from within, the disruption of the moral *lafiya* of the community is threatened by the activities of women, especially prostitutes, and the deviant men who participate in the thinly veiled paganism of the *bori* cult. This chapter has described the struggle to attain the Islamic ideal, as well as the moral and metaphysical forces which threaten that ideal. In the following chapter it will be seen how these ideas of a broader moral *lafiya* find reflection at the individual level in the health and functioning of the human body, and how bodily balance is disrupted by the forces of illness.

V

Illness
and Its Causes

Lafiya ta fi ku'di.

(Health is better than money.)

HAUSA PROVERB

■ *Lafiya*, Health, and Illness

As we have seen, the Hausa word *lafiya* has a broad range of connotations referring to the proper ordering, correct functioning, and general well-being of human affairs. Although *lafiya* is often translated into English as "health," strictly speaking this is better expressed by the Hausa phrase *lafiyar jiki*, "well-being of the body," a more precise rendering of the concept of "physical health." Within the purview of Hausa medicine, *lafiya* refers to the correct, balanced, properly ordered state of the body. When that balance is upset *lafiya* is no longer present and a state of illness results. One is either healthy and has *lafiya*, or not healthy, and lacking *lafiya*. The Hausa expression used to convey this imbalance is *ba na da lafiya*, "I have no lafiya." *Lafiya* is a positive state of affairs and it is on the absence of this desired positive state that attention is focused. The absence of *lafiya* is a pathological state to be corrected by the application of an appropriate remedy.

Closely related to *lafiya* is *'karfi*, or "strength." A healthy man is a vigorous, strong man, and hence the term *'karfin jiki*, "strength of the body" is nearly synonymous with *lafiyar jiki*, "bodily health." If a Hausa says *ba na da 'karfi*, "I have no strength," or *jikina ba ya da 'karfi*, "my body has no strength," he is obviously unwell (*ba lafiya*). *'Karfi* and *lafiya* are interrelated concepts; one cannot exist without the other. The direct connection between the two is obvious from the large number of herbal tonics taken by villagers as prophylactics against weakness, to insure continuing *'karfin jiki.*[1] Indeed, if a man lacks strength not only does his own *lafiya* suffer, but also that of his household. In an agricultural society such as that of the rural Hausa, the ability to perform work in the fields is a necessity. Since farming is a principal occupation and source of food for nearly every village family, irrespective of whatever other crafts or economic endeavors they may be engaged in, the inability to farm changes a man's status and drops him outside his normal world of activities. His life is upset vis-à-vis his neighbors and he is no longer able to fulfill his expected role as a complete Hausa villager. Not only is he lacking in *lafiya,* but his entire compound is disordered as well. In the absence of *lafiya* and strength, a state of illness exists.

Two Hausa words are generally used to describe conditions of morbidity: *ciwo* and *cuta. Ciwo* is the more commonly used of the two words and refers to any pathological condition in the body that causes pain. It is the word most commonly used to describe "pain," "soreness," "aching," and the like. Usually, it is used to refer to pain or sickness in particular parts of the body, such as *ciwon kai,* "headache," *ciwon ciki,* "abdominal pain" or "stomach-ache," *ciwon kirji,* "chest pain," and so on. *Ciwo* implies a painful disordering of that particular part of the body and impairment of its normal functioning. It may also mean "an offense," "emotional pain," "a drawback," "a discouragement." *Cuta,* somewhat less commonly used, likewise refers to disrupted function of or injury to some part of the body. It has the additional meaning of "an offensive act," or "an underhanded deed." It exists as a verb form meaning "to do injury [either moral or physical] to," "to deceive," or "to cheat." The expression *ya cuce ni,* for example, may be translated as "he injured me" or "he did me wrong." Neither *ciwo* nor *cuta* may be properly translated into English as "disease," within the strict sense of that word as used in scientific medicine. These

1. These tonics have other purposes as well, also related to bodily strength. They are frequently used for *'karfin mutum,* "strength of the man," or *'karfin maza,* "strength of men (husbands)," both terms somewhat less explicit than the more direct *'karfin bura,* "penis strength." Such tonics are taken to insure general bodily strength, but with a special view toward insuring sexual potency. In a society where plural marriage is common and where all wives should be treated equally, impotence is not an insignificant fear.

Hausa terms refer to the signs (objective, physical manifestations) or symptoms (subjective feelings) that occur in the course of an illness. What the Hausa points out by these words is the "chief complaint," not the "disease" which may lie behind it.

In its original but now obsolete meaning, according to the *Oxford English Dictionary*, "disease" meant "absence of ease; uneasiness, discomfort, inconvenience, annoyance; disquiet, disturbance, trouble." In Hausa this is the state produced by the absence of *lafiya*, a state of "dis-*lafiya*," if one may coin such a term. Within the development of medical science, however, the meaning of the term disease narrowed considerably, eventually becoming "a condition of the body, or of some part or organ of the body, in which its functions are disturbed or deranged; a morbid physical condition; a departure from the state of health, especially when caused by a structural change" or, even more specifically, "any one of the various kinds of such conditions; a *species* [my emphasis] of disorder or ailment, exhibiting special symptoms or affecting a large organ." In short, "disease," as the term is used in modern scientific medicine, refers to an intellectual construction which lies behind or beyond the actual illness of any given patient. The same disease may produce widely different manifestations in different people (for example, renal cell carcinoma); conversely, similar signs and symptoms may be produced by vastly different diseases (for example, the innumerable varieties of anemia and their causes). As Hudson has aptly pointed out (1974, 1975), diseases are abstractions, but illnesses are processes in individuals.[2] Reading has summarized these distinctions as follows (1977:703–4):

> The terms *illness* and *disease* lack precision. Even though they are at times used almost interchangeably, there is a core distinction between them and it is this particular usage that will be emphasized here. Illness tends to be used to refer to what is wrong with the patient, disease to what is wrong with his body. Illness is what the patient suffers from, what troubles him, what he complains of, and what prompts him to seek medical attention. Illness refers to the patient's *experience* of ill-health. It comprises his impaired sense of well being, his perception that something is wrong with

2. See also the discussion of this distinction by Gilbert Lewis (1976, especially pp. 85–102).

his body, and his various symptoms of pain, distress, and disablement. *Disease,* on the other hand, refers to various structural disorders of the individual's tissues and organs that give rise to the
signs of ill-health. These are, for the most part, not accessible to
the patient and are not experienced by him. Disease may thus exist
for considerable periods of time without the patient knowing. Illness, in contrast, exists only by virtue of the patient's awareness
of it. Unlike disease, it is never present in the autopsy room.

Thus, generally speaking, one may say that Hausa medical thought recognizes illnesses (signs and symptoms), but has few (if any) concepts of
disease. Hausa medicine sees only medical "problems" or "ailments,"
each of which requires its own "medicine" or "remedy," (*magani*).

For example, let us take the problem of chest pain. In Hausa this
would be described as *ciwon kirji* ("chest pain"), or *gambasa* ("upper
epigastric pain"), perhaps with various qualifiers to describe the nature
and duration of the problem. Hausa medicine does not go beyond this
level. This is the "illness" that afflicts the patient; his "disease" is
merely the symptoms he presents. Scientific medicine, however, probes
more deeply. It searches for anatomical and physiological derangements
that can produce the patient's symptoms, and for pathological changes
in the cells and tissues of the body that can produce his physical signs.
A case of "prolonged chest pain" would have to be investigated to find
its cause from among a wide variety of underlying diseases: acute myocardial infarction, a dissecting aortic aneurysm, pulmonary embolism,
esophogeal reflux, pericarditis, pneumothorax, mediastinal emphysema,
acute pancreatitis, acute cholecystitis, acute gastritis, a perforated ulcer,
etc. None of these things exist as entities in Hausa traditional medicine.

Hausa medicine has not elaborated carefully delimited concepts of
disease because its foundations rest upon an uncertain knowledge of
the structure and function of the human body and because of a number of ultimately unverifiable presuppositions about metaphysical
causes of illness which permeate its texture. Western medicine was
once in a similar position, but progressed because it was able to abandon the speculative a priori assumptions about illness around which
Galenic medicine developed. Gradually, it jettisoned the intellectual
axioms of humoralism and turned instead to careful observation and
description of the clinical course of illness, correlating this with the

structural and functional derangements of the human body as demonstrated in postmortem examinations. As the foundations of the medical arts grew firmer in the sciences of anatomy, physiology, and pathology, they were joined by new developments in technology which rapidly improved the clinical examination of the patient. The result of this
process was the development of an impressive and highly detailed nosology of specific diseases which today has reached enormous proportions.[3] As the conceptual entities of disease emerged, medicine was able
to take more and more accurate aim in its therapeutic approach to the
sick. With specific disease, specific treatment became possible, a process vividly demonstrated by the rise of bacteriology in the nineteenth
century and the development of antibiotics in the twentieth century.
Scientific medicine is based on the premise that specific diseases lead to
generalized illness; Hausa medicine on the other hand, sees general
causes as producing specific complaints.

In his 1924 book *Medicine, Magic and Religion* (which in many ways
marks the beginning of medical anthropology), W. H. R. Rivers noted
what he believed to be the three major categories of the causation of
illness acknowledged by mankind (1924:7–8):[4] (1) human agency,
(2) the action of a spiritual or supernatural being or beings, and
(3) what we ordinarily call "natural diseases." He believed that scientific medicine was founded upon the last category, while the medicine
of primitive peoples fit mainly into the first two categories, with only
scant attention paid to the third. An examination of the notions about
the causation of illness held by the Hausa shows aspects of all three
classifications, but distributes their emphasis in a way Rivers might
not have anticipated.

In the Hausa view of things there are two basic etiologies of illness.
Either it is due to inanimate, unconscious forces in the physical environment, or it is the result of the intrusion of some conscious, malevo-

3. This process has been brilliantly described in Knud Faber's classic book (1930)
Nosography: The Evolution of Clinical Medicine in Modern Times. The enormous
proportions that this approach has reached can be seen in the fact that a standard
introductory textbook such as Robbins and Cotran (1979), *Pathologic Basis of Disease,* now runs to more than 1,600 pages.
4. It should be noted that Rivers here used the term "disease" in its looser sense
as a synonym of illness or sickness. For reasons noted above I have preferred to
retain "disease" for specific conceptual entities and have used "illness" or "sickness" for the more general condition of being out of health.

lent power. The former category consists of ailments that "just hap-pen," that are sent as the result of the ineffable will of God and may be loosely categorized as *ciwon Allah*, "illnesses of God," roughly com-parable to Rivers's "naturally caused ailments." The second category comprises those afflictions which arise from the influence of witchcraft (*maita*), sorcery (*sammu*), or evil spirits (*adjannu, iskoki,* etc.). Illnesses stemming from these sources are referred to as *ciwon miyagu*, "ill-nesses of evil." In this large category the implicit subdivisions of evil human influences and evil spiritual influences can be seen, correspond-ing to Rivers's first and second categories of causation. In order to un-derstand these paradigms for the explanation of illness, however, it is first necessary to understand something of the Hausa conception of the structure of the human body and the nature of its physiology.

■ Hausa Concepts of Anatomy and Physiology

The Hausa picture of the body and its construction is a fairly simple one, as befits a people with no autopsy practices and little practical rea-son for the study of anatomy.[5] Words exist for the major parts and ap-pendages of the body—a vocabulary sufficient for the needs of every-day use quite comparable to that existing in the language of a typical British or American layman. Even medical specialists such as the bone-setter (*ma'dori*) and the herbal healer (*boka*) utilize these terms; there is no specialist vocabulary common to the medical profession as one finds in scientific medicine and surgery.

The external covering of the body, the skin, is called *fata*—the same word that is used for hides and animal skins. Beneath this lies the mus-cle, *tsoka*—a word different from *nama*, the common term for meat and also the word used for animals that are hunted for food. The bones of the body are *'kashi* (pl. *'kasusuwa*), a term applied to animal as well as human bones. Running through the body and lying in the veins and arteries (which are not distinguished and are alike called *jijiyoyi*, a term also applied to tendons and ligaments) is the blood, *jini*, which is seen as filling up the body, giving it strength and power, and carrying

5. As Last (1976:126) has remarked for the Maguzawa, "No postmortems are done since no treatment is possible." On the general subject of primitive autopsies see the pessimistic views of Ackerknecht (1943, also 1971:90–94), and the more sym-pathetic approach of Davies (1965).

life. The internal organs—brain, heart, lungs, liver, etc.—are well known from the slaughter of animals and observations made in the course of butchering. These internal organs are related to one another through a rough-and-ready notion of their physiological functions, tied together largely through the intervening medium of the bodily fluids.

As might be expected, Hausa possesses a much more elaborate vocabulary for the topography of the external body than for its internal structure. *Kai* refers to the head taken as a whole and consists of the back of the head (*kwanya*, also referring to the brain inside), the forehead-temple (*goshi*), and the face (*huska*). Hair is called *gashi*. The face includes the cheek (*kunci*), nose (*hanci*), eye (*ido*), ear (*kunne*), mouth (*baki*), jaw (*mu'kamu'ki*), and chin (*ha'ba*). The mouth consists of the tongue (*harshe*, a word also used for "language" or "speech"), lips (*le'be*), teeth (*ha'kori*), and the uvula (*beli* or *hakin wuya*). The eye, one of the most distinctive features of the human countenance, has several components: the eyebrow (*gira*), the eyelid (*fatar ido*, literally "skin of the eye"), the eyelash (*gashin ido*, literally "hair of the eye") and the eyeball, or more specifically, the pupil of the eye, *'kwayar ido* (literally "the seed of the eye"). Bodily orifices, such as the nostrils or the auditory meatus of the ear, are frequently referred to as *'kofa*, the "doorway," as in *'kofar kunne*, "doorway of the ear." Fleshy protuberances are simply designated *fata*, "skin," as in the term for the earlobe: *fatar kunne*, "skin of the ear." The head is supported by the neck (*wuya*), which in its turn rests on the shoulders (*kafada*), a term that includes the upper regions of the chest, the clavicle (*karan karma*), and the scapula. The torso is divided into several regions: the *kirji*, or chest, with the xyphoid process of the sternum given the special name of *allo*, or "slate"; the ribs (*ha'kar'kari*); the armpit (*hamata*); the *kwi'bi*, or side of the body from roughly the shoulders to the hips, often including the ribs; the back (*baya*), which is distinguished from the lumbar region (*kugu* or *kwankwaso*); the hip (*kwatangwalo*); and finally the abdomen, or *ciki* (literally "inside"). The term *mara* is used to describe the pit of the stomach. The buttocks are called *duwaiwai*, and the anus, *tsuliya*. The appendages are generally given simple names: *hannu* refers to the entire arm, but particularly the hand; *'kafa* refers to the leg and especially to the foot. The term *gwiwa* is used to refer to bending joints, but particularly the knee, and *gwiwar hannu* (literally "knee of the arm") refers to the elbow. Other terms of importance for the lower extremities are *cinya* (thigh), *dambubu* or *'kwauri* (calf/shin of the leg), *dugadugi* (the heel), and *idon 'kafa,* the ankle, (literally "eye of the foot"), which refers specifically to the lateral malleolus of the fibula and the medial malleolus of the tibia, which protrude as bony bumps on each side of the ankle. The arm may be subdivided further into the forearm (*dantse*) and the wrist (*tsintsiyar hannu,* literally "broom of the arm"). *Tafi* refers to the palm of the hand (*tafin hannu*) or the sole of the foot (*tafin 'kafa*), and the digits are called *yatsa,* fingers being *yatsar hannu* and toes being *yatsar 'kafa.*[6] Fingernails and toenails are alike called *farce.* The sexual organs have a variety of names. The female breasts are *mama,* a term sometimes applied to the breasts and nipples of the man as well. The vagina is known by a wide variety of terms, the most polite being *farji* or *gato,* the crudest being *duri,* a term roughly equivalent to the English "cunt." Pubic hair is *zaza.* The term *gindi,* literally meaning "base" or "bottom" (as of a pot), is widely used as a euphemism for the genitalia of either sex. The clitoris is known as *belin gindi,* "uvula of the bottom." The penis is called either *bura* or the slightly more polite *azakari,* while the testicles are known as *golo* or *gwaiwa*—although this latter term is often used to refer to the condition of hydrocele.

From this examination of the Hausa vocabulary of the body it is obvious that their anatomical conceptions are limited. There is no extensive, detailed vocabulary of muscles, for example. They are all *tsoka.* Blood vessels, ligaments, and tendons are all string-like *jijiyoyi* inside the body. There is no extensive nomenclature of bones; all are *'kashi.* If it is wished to refer to a particular bone, it is designated as "the bone of . . . ," as in *'kashin baya,* "bone of the back," *'kashin 'kafa,* "bone of the leg," and so on. When one healer was informed that Europeans said there were 206 bones in the body and had a different name for each one of them, he was amazed, failing to see the utility of so many different names for the same thing. There simply is no necessity, given the strictures of Hausa culture, to possess a sophisticated anatomical vocabulary.

Similarly, Hausa notions about the internal body are rudimentary. The major internal organs all have names but, as the operation of these

6. The big toe is just that—*babban yatsa*—and the same term is applied to the thumb.

organs is hidden from view in a way that the external structures of the body are not, ideas pertaining to their functioning are quite mixed and are subject to a great deal of individual elaboration. Since nobody *really* knows what the liver does, for example, in the same way that they know what the tongue, a hand, a foot, an eye, or an ear does, any plausible description of its function is as good as another. If one asks the typical villager a question such as *Menene amfanin hanta?*, "What is the usefulness of the liver?" he is likely to get as a response *lafiyar mutum*, "well-being of the man." Anyone knows that everybody has a liver; if you didn't have one you would either be sick or dead. It is simply a part of the correct structuring of the body—to detract from it is to be less than whole, and this injures *lafiya*. Nonetheless, there are a number of general parameters of thought that circumscribe Hausa notions about the inner workings of the body and these may be said to constitute a simple system of ethnophysiology.

While all the internal organs of the body contribute to *lafiya*, perhaps the most important is the brain, which is known in Hausa as *kwanya* or *'kwa'kwalwa*. One man expressed its function quite simply by saying *Shi ne mutum*, "It's the man." In everyday experience the head is the most conspicuous part of the human body. The face displays those noticeable characteristics by which one identifies people and their moods. It is the most common site for tribal scarification and tattooing. The head houses the organs of sight, hearing, smell, speech, and balance. It is only natural, therefore, that the contents of the head should be deemed of paramount importance, that the brain should be the "chief" of the body. The brain is the seat of *hankali*, sense or judgment, as well as the subsidiary mental processes of memory (*tunani*) and thought (*tsammani*) which allow it to carry out its work. To be in full possession of *lafiya* a man must have *hankali*, the ability to think clearly and function in a normal manner. If the brain becomes "spoiled" (*lalace*, the same term that is used for the deterioration and decay of foodstuffs, etc.) or "jumbled" (*juye*) the individual is no longer able to function properly, and *lafiya* is absent. *Kwanya*, the brain, and *hankali*, judgment, are thus nearly interchangeable terms. For example, there was a senile old woman in the village who was very difficult to deal with and who was disoriented most of the time. When she left her compound to go to the market groups of children would run after her yelling

Kwanya! Kwanya! ("Brain! Brain!"), calling attention to her confused state of mind and lack of mental competence. Her son explained her condition by saying that "the spirits have brushed her," meaning they had rubbed all the sense out of her brain, causing her to go mad. When the brain is in a state of *lafiya*, therefore, a person has *hankali*. Absence of *hankali* results in madness (*hauka*), the principal and most feared disorder of the brain.[7]

If the brain, firmly ensconced high within the skull, holds sway over the thought, sense, and conscious mind of man, the heart (*zuciya*), located deep within the center of the body, is the focus of the swirling currents of emotion that dictate to the often turbulent unconscious mind. The Hausa proverb adequately expresses the importance of the heart: *Zuciyar mutum birninsa*, "The heart of a man is his *birni*," i.e., his "walled town," "fortified city," or "place of refuge." This centrality of the heart is manifested in numerous Hausa expressions: *ajiyar zuciya*, "sighing" (literally "laying down the heart"); *'karfin zuciya*, "brave, steadfast" (literally "strong of heart"); *zuciya biyu*, "uncertain, unsteady, doubtful, deceitful" (literally "two hearts"); *zafin zuciya*, "anger, deep emotional pain" (literally "heat of the heart"); *'bacin zuciya*, "vexation, sadness" (literally "spoiling of the heart"); *farar zuciya*, "happiness" (literally "white-hearted"); *ba'kar zuciya*, "anger, vile disposition" (literally "black-hearted"), and so on. While the brain is the seat of reason (*hankali*), the heart is often identified with life or the life-force itself (*rai*). If a man's brain is diseased and he goes mad, he is in deplorable shape, but still alive; if, however, the heart stops beating, there is no life at all. No wonder the Hausa say *Zuciya ta fi dukiya*, "The heart is worth more than wealth."

While the heart and brain stand somewhat apart, the other organs are systematically (if not always quite coherently) linked. This is particularly true of the digestive system. In the Hausa scheme of things there are two separate bodily pathways through which foodstuffs pass, one for solids and one for liquids (see Last 1976:142). Food passes from the mouth (*baki*), where it is chewed up by the teeth, down the throat (*ma'kogwaro*) and into the stomach (*tumbi or ciki*), from whence it passes into the intestines (*hanji*) and finally out of the anus (*tsuliya*)

---

7. Mental disorders are discussed more fully later in this chapter.

as feces (*kashi*). In the course of this process food (*abinci*) is gradually turned into blood (*jini*) and transported throughout the body to give it strength.

Fluids have their own, somewhat more complicated pathway. They begin their journey in approximately the same way as solids—into the mouth, down the throat, and into the inner body. Beyond this, however, the two pathways divide and, depending on the informant, the description of what occurs varies. Generally, however, fluids are said to pass through the lungs (*kuhu*), heart (*zuciya*), liver (*hanta*), and other organs into the bladder (*mafitsara*), from whence they are passed out as urine (*fitsari*).

In addition to ventilating the body, the lungs (*kuhu*) serve as the mechanism regulating thirst. In the normal course of things the lungs are filled with water and are moist. The passage of air into the lungs gradually dries them out, creating thirst (*'kishi*). When a man drinks water his lungs are moistened and thirst goes away. The function of controlling thirst is often also attributed to the liver (*hanta*). One informant explained the physiology of thirst and the liver's role in its regulation in the following manner. The liver is a kind of gauge inside the body, sitting in a pool of water. When this water is used up by the body or is passed out as urine the level of water around the liver gradually decreases, exposing it. As the liver emerges from the pool of water in which it lies it starts to dry out and the body feels thirst. The man must then drink more water to replenish the reservoir in which his liver is bathed. When the water level is again high enough to cover the liver the sensation of thirst subsides and the cycle is ready to begin anew.

Aside from water and urine, two other fluids exist in the body: blood (*jini*) and phlegm (*majina*). Blood is the single most significant factor influencing bodily strength. Since a cut made anywhere on the body produces blood, it is no surprise that blood is seen as filling out the body, imparting strength and life to all the organs, all the limbs. Most people will say that the blood "runs through the body" (*ya gudu cikin jiki*); others will say that when a man is moving his blood moves, but when he is lying down or sleeping, his blood also rests. Blood fills out the body's form and affects all its parts, but there is no unified conception of its movement such as exists in scientific biology. Lack of blood (*rashin jini*), however, is of extreme importance for it causes weakness and general lassitude (*kasala*), as does thin, watery blood (*jinin ruwa-*

ruwa). A man must eat enough food to avoid hunger (*yunwa*) and insure the right amount of strong, healthy blood in his body. Persistent
hunger can lead to the gradual debilitation of the blood and pervasive
tiredness. One man likened the blood in a man to the kerosene in a
lamp; if the kerosene gets low and runs out, the light goes out, just as
a man would "flicker" and then die if his blood were to dissipate and
all his strength ebb into nothingness. Another man likened the blood
in the body to the water in a borrow pit (*tafki*). If the dry season comes
and the water is not replenished, it will dry up and be of no use at all.
Similarly, if a man "dries up" (*ya bushe*) he is of no use for anything,
either: no strength, no life, no ability to do any kind of work. The
relationship between bodily strength and blood is clearly seen in the
belief that the spirit *Inna, Mai Shan Jini* (Inna, Drinker of Blood) is the
cause of paralyzed limbs. Either before or after birth the blood of the
victim is "drunk" by bloodthirsty spirits, leaving the limb withered and
"dry," just as the spirits "drink" the blood of sacrifices made to them.
Similarly, if the blood dies or is killed and turns from its normal healthy
color of bright red (*jawur*) to a sickly black (*ba'ki*), illness will result
and must be treated by the surgical removal of the useless dead blood.
The liver (*hanta*), spleen (*saifa*), and kidneys (*'koda*, pl. *'kodoji*) are
often thought to be instrumental in producing and regulating the body's
blood, having *amfanin jini* ("usefulness for the blood") as their physiological function—due no doubt to their dark red coloring.

Phlegm (*majina*), the other major bodily fluid, exists in small amounts
in three locations within the body: the head, the chest, and the lower
back. It aids in lubricating the nose, the lungs and chest, and the sexual
organs, respectively. If it increases too much it may result in head colds
(*mura*), congestion of the lungs and chest pains (*ciwon kirji*), lower
back pain (*ciwon kwankwaso*), or impotence (*mutuwar bura*, literally
"death of the penis").

Notions about the physiology of sex and reproduction are not highly
elaborated. The penis is called *bura* or *azakari*. *Maniyyi* (semen) resides
in the testicles (*golo*). During sexual intercourse the semen of the man
enters the vagina of the woman[8] and penetrates to the womb, where it

8. The common Hausa expression for a man having sexual relations with a woman
is *cin mata*, literally meaning "eating a woman," or *cin duri*, "eating a vagina."
Ci, "eat," has active, aggressive connotations which correlate with the superior
position and active role of the man. The comparable term for a woman having

mingles with the female fluids, sometimes referred to as *maniyyi* as well. Menstruation (*haila*) begins at marriage and continues until the woman becomes old and infertile, and "dries up" (*ta bushe*).[9] When the woman becomes pregnant (*tana da ciki*, literally "she has a belly-[ful]"), the flow of blood ceases and goes toward making up the structure of the infant. The embryo goes through several stages of development. In the earliest stage it consists of phlegm (*majina*), semen (*maniyyi*), and water (*ruwa*), transforming in the course of forty days to blood (*jini*), and after forty more days shaping into flesh (*nama* or *tsoka*). It becomes recognizably human at four or five months, after which time the developmental process consists of a gradual increase in size until the time of birth. Individual notions of how long the fetus remains in each of these stages vary, but the general conception is of a gradual transformation from a watery state of phlegm and semen, through a state of blood, into the fleshy stage, which then elaborates into a full human being.

The motive force behind this process is *ikon Allah*, "the power of God." Sura 22 of the Koran states:

> surely We created you of dust
>> then of a sperm-drop
>> then of a blood-clot,
> then of a lump of flesh, formed and unformed

---

sexual relations with a man is *shan mutum*, literally meaning "drinking a man." *Sha*, "drink," is used in Hausa for actions that have a submissive, subordinate connotation with regard to an act of incorporation or appropriation. For example, note the following expressions: *cin rana*, "eating the dry season," for undertaking seasonal labor; *cin riba*, "eating a profit," for making a profit; *cin kasuwa*, "eating the market," for making purchases in the market; conversely, the passive side of actions is seen in such expressions as *shan rana*, "drinking the sun," for being out exposed to the sun; *shan iska*, "drinking the air," for taking a stroll in the air or cooling off; *shan kasuwa* for "browsing in the market," etc. The meanings of *ci* and *sha* are explored in an article by Claude Gouffé (1966), " 'Manger' et 'Boire' en Haoussa."

9. One friend of mine, an inveterate rake, explained to me that old women were no fun to have sexual relations with because "they have no water in their vagina," (*durinsu ba ya da ruwa*), and went on to demonstrate all the noises made when the proper amount of "water" was present during the sexual act. See also Darrah and Froude (n.d.:17). Atrophic vaginitis is a common complaint of postmenopausal women.

that We may make clear to you.
And We establish in the wombs
what We will, till a stated term,
then We deliver you as infants.

In Islamic theology, as Watt has noted (1970:149): "God's creative
power is regarded as being present in the origination of every human
being. Moreover it is not restricted to origination, but also manifests
itself in the various transformations which occur in the course of development; thus God 'creates' each stage of the embryo from the previous one." This statement is fully in accord with Hausa beliefs; but
while God is the power behind the transformations, various factors can
affect the pregnancy: too much cold, bitter foods, attacks by spirits,
excessive intake of sweets, and so on. The pregnant woman must take
care not to disrupt the course of development by careless behavior while
God is creating (*halita*) the child in her womb; hence the Hausa proverb: *Duniya mace da ciki ce,* "The world is a pregnant women," i.e.,
nobody knows exactly how things will turn out.

Such, then, is the general nature of Hausa physiological thought. The
body consists of flesh (*tsoka*) and bone (*'kashi*) covered by skin (*fata*).
The seat of reason (*hankali*) is the brain (*kwanya*). The force of life
(*rai*) emanates from the heart (*zuciya*). Internally, food and water travel
through two separate passages and emerge as feces (*kashi*) and urine
(*fitsari*), respectively. Blood (*jini*) imparts strength and fills out the
body, while phlegm (*majina*) lubricates and cushions various sections
of it. When all these things are harmoniously integrated, *lafiyar jiki* is
the result; indeed, this harmonious balance is the normal state of the
body. Illness results only when some outside force impinges upon *lafiya*
and disrupts it. For example, in Hausa one does not say "I have caught
cold"; rather the expression is "Cold has caught me" (*Sanyi ya kama
ni*). The common question asked at a hospital when a patient comes in
is "What has got you?" (*Menene ya same ka?*), not "what have you
got?" It is to these forces of disruption that we now turn.

■ Environmental Illness: *Ciwon Allah,*
the Illnesses of God

Everyone has had the experience of not feeling well at some time or
another. Most of these ailments are minor irritations such as an upset

stomach, a head cold, or a slight touch of diarrhea; they are not physically devastating bouts of sickness. There are minor illnesses and major ones. Last, in the context of Maguzawa Hausa culture, has distinguished these as sicknesses occurring in situations of calm in contrast to those which arise as major crises.[10] While major illnesses are frightening and extraordinary, the minor irritations are simply a part of living in the world.

Like all people the Hausa are sensitive to the forces in their physical environment that affect them. They feel hot and cold, note wetness and dryness, enjoy the pleasures of good-tasting substances and dislike those that are bitter or putrid. Such everyday sensations and the observation of their effects on the body form the basic frame of reference the villager uses in understanding the ordinary illnesses that trouble him. These ailments and the influences which cause them are not unusual. They are a part of daily life and affect everyone at some time or another. These minor illnesses, usually short-lived, although undesirable are not extraordinary. They are *ciwon Allah*, "illnesses of God," which He in His inscrutable wisdom has seen fit to make a part of the normal order of the world.

Food is one of the most important aspects of daily life. A full belly insures strength, while prolonged hunger brings a weakness which may turn into major illness through gradual wasting of the blood. Good food (*abinci mai kyau*) is a source of pleasure and strength. It builds strong blood and banishes hunger. Bad food (*abinci mara kyau*) has the opposite effect. It results in abdominal cramps (*ciwon ciki*), nausea (*kumallo*), diarrhea (*zawo, gudawa*), and vomiting (*amai*). The causal link between what goes into the body and what happens there is obvious. This view also holds for the respiratory system, where the relationship between smoking (*shan taba*, literally "drinking tobacco") and respiratory ailments such as bronchitis and severe coughing (*huka*) is noted.[11] The relationship between drinking beer or taking amphetamines (*kafsu*, from English "capsule") and altered behavior is observed; both result

10. Murray Last (n.d.), "Tradition in Hausa Medicine," 11 pp., mimeographed.
11. The permissibility of smoking is an interesting point of debate in Islamic theology and law. Tobacco, being a New World plant, was unknown at the time of the Prophet and as a result there are no Koranic injunctions against its use. Strict Muslims follow the rule of "when in doubt, abstain," but many Hausa are ardent cigarette smokers even though they do not touch alcohol.

in a form of "temporary insanity" (*hauka*, the Hausa term for all mental disorders). Intestinal parasites, a wide variety of which are found in the Nigerian environment, are seen to stem from the ingestion of "eggs" (*kwai*) and are treated (as are many intestinal ailments) by the use of purgatives to force them out. Guinea-worm (*kurkunu*) derives from drinking stagnant bush water found away from human habitation.[12]

The maintenance of health within the internal body also depends upon the proper balance of sweet, sour, bitter, and salty substances. Eating too many sweet substances—such as sweet potatoes, sugar, bananas, or mangoes—can cause the production of excess phlegm (*majina*), leading to sickness (Last 1970). Bloody urine (*fitsarin jini*) may be caused by eating too much tamarind fruit, which is noted for its sourness.[13] Concern with such matters is especially important for pregnant women. Bitter substances, such as the *gauta* tomato (*Solanum melongena*), which are normally used as remedies for stomach upsets, are forbidden to pregnant women for fear they will spoil the pregnancy. Similarly, pregnant women are forbidden to take much sugar or salt, for fear that it will cause closure of the vaginal opening and difficult childbirth. This is said to occur when the sugary or salty substances cause a web (*yana*, such as might be found forming on the surface of a bowl of gruel) to grow over the vaginal introitus and result in prolonged labor, a condition known variously as *gishiri* (salt), *zaki* (sweet), or *dankali* (sweet potato).[14] Too much salt may also cause the regrowth of the uvula (normally excised a few days after birth), leading to blockage of the throat, difficulty in swallowing, and ultimately death if untreated by surgical removal.[15]

12. The influence of public health education campaigns can probably be seen here.
13. The word for tamarind fruit (*tsamiya*) is actually derived from the Hausa word for sour (*tsami*). Bloody urine is also known as *tsagiya*; the most common cause for this condition is urinary schistosomiasis. Bloody urine in men is often attributed to a venereal disease (*jan sanyi*, "red cold") caught from women.
14. This condition is treated by cutting the anterior vaginal wall, which often leads to serious gynecological complications. See especially Last (1976:131–36) and Darrah and Froude (n.d.:15–16). *Gishiri* is also the term used for the white salts found on the bottom of water pots. *Zaki* or *faya* is used for the amniotic fluid and breaking of water at the onset of labor.
15. See Darrah and Froude (n.d.:24). This cutting of the uvula may produce tragic results. The complications of this procedure are frequently seen in the emergency rooms of hospitals in northern Nigeria. See also Fleischer (1975).

Diseases of the sexual organs are universally regarded as venereal in origin and are called in Hausa *ciwon mata*, "sicknesses of women," or *ciwon karuwai*, "sicknesses of prostitutes." Of these there are many. The most common is gonorrhea, (*ciwon sanyi*),[16] which is rampant in northern Nigeria and is characterized in men by painful urination and the excretion of a milky, pus-filled discharge. *Jan sanyi* refers to bloody urine, believed to be caused by sexual relations with a diseased woman. *Tunjere*, syphilitic ulceration of the sexual organs, is now rarely seen in the north due to effective public health measures. *Gwaza* refers to scrotal ulceration. *'Da'dali* is a venereal complaint of the abdomen, a "knotting" of the belly, believed to be caused by sexual relations with Fulani women. The most serious venereal complaints, however, are *yankan gashi* and *basur*. *Yankan gashi*, "cutting of the hair," results from intercourse with a woman who has infected pubic hairs or a diseased vagina. If this is the case, her pubic hairs will rub against the head of the penis or her vaginal walls will become knife-like, resulting in laceration of the penis and concomitant sores, or even its very amputation! *Basur*, a term more commonly applied to rectal disorders such as hemorrhoids, is a disease in which the penis is perforated on all sides by sores which penetrate through to the urethra. The result of this unfortunate condition is that when the man urinates his urine sprays out in all directions, like water from a pipe drilled through with holes. All these venereal diseases seem to be the natural result of the activities of the sexual organs. If the penis is diseased, it must have become so from where it has been: *wurin mata*, the place of women. Since the position of women in all Muslim societies is inferior, venereal diseases are only one further example of female perfidy. Prostitutes (*karuwai*) who

16. Literally translated this means "diseases of wet cold." As will be seen below, *sanyi*, damp coldness, is a major cause of illness in the Hausa system of aetiology. *Sanyin mata* (literally "coldness of women") is, however, always distinguished as a separate thing from normal environmental *sanyi*, the cause of so much internal sickness. One can postulate that because *sanyi* is such a pervasive explanation for internal ailments it was taken as an intervening agency applied to venereal complaints; that is, because *sanyi* is the cause of internal ailments, venereal diseases are due to the same sort of *sanyi* residing inside women. This is substantiated by the notion that *amosanin ciki* a "rheumatic" ailment of the abdomen, is thought to be transmitted sexually from a woman to a man as well, as is *gwaiwa*, scrotal hydrocele.

abandon the proper role of female behavior spread illness throughout society.

The most pervasive causes of illness in the Hausa scheme of things, however, are the effects on the human body of variations in the physical environment: heat and cold. *Sanyi* is the Hausa word meaning wet, damp cold—the penetrating kind of cold that goes "right to the bone," such as *sanyin fadama*, the unpleasant wetness associated with working in a marshy or irrigated field (*fadama*) close to a river. *Zafi* means "heat," and is also a common word for "pain," such as that from a burn, a cut, or the pain of forced, bloody stools—an alternative word for *ciwo* when the latter has primary reference to sensations of pain rather than a state of disease. The interactions of *sanyi* and *zafi* in the body are major factors bringing sickness.[17]

The blood, in particular, is subject to the pernicious influences of *sanyi* and *zafi*. Too much cold or too much heat leads to the buildup of *mataccen jini*, "dead blood," a prominent cause of ailments, in the Hausa view. As an example, pain in the lower back is frequently attributed to *mataccen jini*, caused by the heat of the sun killing the blood while farmers are stooped over in the fields cultivating the ground. Such conditions are treated by surgical cupping (*kaho*) to remove the black, dead blood—one of the routine tasks performed by village barbers (*wanzamai*). Periodic performance of this procedure is deemed a prudent health measure, for an accumulation of dead blood can lead to more serious ailments, such as *kasala*, a state of persisting tiredness seen as the result of the gradual weakening of the blood.

Kasala left untreated can lead to other, more serious disorders of the

17. Two other words are related to *sanyi* and *zafi* and merit at least cursory mention. *'Dari* is a Hausa word also meaning "cold," but it refers primarily to the coldness brought by the winds of harmattan. As such it refers to "feeling cold," and would be used in questions such as "Are you feeling cold?" (*Kana jin 'dari?*). Were *sanyi* to be used in such a question it would be asking if one "had a cold," as a head cold (*mura*). *Zafi* refers mainly to unpleasant heat—pain from a burn, *tuwo* that is too hot to eat (and burns the fingers in the attempt), or the oppressive heat of the sun at midday which hinders work in the fields. *'Dimi* means "warmth," and refers to the warmth of sitting around a fire in the cold season, drinking in (*shan 'dimi*) the heat of the glowing embers. *Zufa*, likewise meaning "heat," refers to perspiration as well, and is generally employed for the unpleasant wet heat of the time just before the onset of the rains.

blood: *farin mashashara* ("white fever") or *shawara. Farin mashashara* is a condition in which the body turns white from the gradual death of the blood, a process that can be noted especially in the palms of the hands. The lack of enough healthy blood results in extreme, prostrating tiredness, the inability to do any work, and a gradual wasting away. It is seen as either a synonym for, or an advanced state of, *shawara,* an ailment characterized by all the clinical symptoms of acute hepatitis: severe fatigue, dark reddish urine, and jaundiced discoloration of the eyes to "yellow" (*rawaya*), "green" (*'kore*), or "scarlet" (*jawur*). In fact, the jaundiced condition of the eyes is such an obvious symptom that the ailment is often called *shawara ta ido,* "*shawara* of the eye." *Shawara* is one of the most feared ailments facing the Hausa villager, for its devastating effects completely sap his strength and hinder him from working. In fact, any state of extreme tiredness whose apparent cause (such as prolonged work in the fields) is not obvious may be referred to as *shawara,* and a herbal tonic is usually employed to bring back *'karfin jiki,* "strength of the body." The additional fact that there is no effective treatment for hepatitis in the arsenal of scientific medicine leads the Hausa to conclude that herbal remedies are the only effective treatment. The large number of such medicines in the Hausa pharmacopoeia underscores the importance of healthy blood and concomitant strength in the Hausa conception of bodily well-being.

If the penetration of wet cold into the body kills the blood, it has the opposite effect on phlegm (*majina*), causing its increase. Normally, *majina* exists in small amounts in the head, chest, belly, and lower back, serving essentially as a lubricant. The penetration of *sanyi* into the body results in the increase of *majina,* with disruption of the body's functioning where cold has entered. Increased *majina* causes head colds (*mura*), chest colds (*mura ta kirji*), lower back pain (*ciwon kugu, ciwon kwankwaso*), stomach upset (*ciwon ciki*), growling of the stomach (*kukar ciki*), flatulence (*tusa*), dysentery (*atuni*), and may lead to impotence in men by spreading out to affect the penis, scrotum, and testicles. *Atuni,* severe dysentery (also called *'Dan Kanoma,* particularly when accompanied by bloody mucous discharges) is seen as resulting primarily from the buildup of excess *majina* in the bowels and belly. To prevent this disorder, which is greatly feared, the typical villager will dose himself periodically with a purgative (*maganin zawo*) to force the gradually increasing phlegm out of his body and ward off sickness.

Even as *sanyi* kills the blood and causes phlegm to expand outside its proper parameters, so it affects all the internal organs of the body. It causes swelling (*kumburi*) which may manifest itself in many areas: in the jaws (*hangun*, "mumps"), as rashes and pimples (*kuraje*), as large festering boils on the lower back and buttocks (*maruru*), as blisters or shingles (*bulala*) over the chest, etc. It is the most important cause of fever (*jante, zazza'bi, mashashara*). So pronounced are its effects on infants and small children that illnesses of all sorts are lumped together under the names *tafiyar ruwa*, "going away in the wet season," and *damina*, a word which is itself the Hausa name for the rainy season of the year, a period when *sanyi* is omnipresent. When *sanyi* penetrates through the flesh and embeds itself in the skeleton it causes aching of the joints, pain in the knees and hands, arthritis, and rheumatism—all known in Hausa as *sanyin 'kashi*, "cold in the bones," or *amosanin 'kashi*, "*amosani* of the bones."

Amosani is the Hausa term referring to the most long-lasting and disruptive effects of *sanyi*. The Hausa dictionaries by Abraham and Robinson define *amosani* as "rheumatism," but this does not really do justice to the concept involved. *Amosani* may occur in the joints and bones as *amosanin 'kashi*, in the head as *amosanin kai*, in the abdomen as *amosanin ciki*. As *amosanin kai* it may linger and grow in the head, causing scalp irritations, headache, loss of teeth, deafness, and ear disorders (*ciwon kunne*).[18] It can lead to eye disease (*ciwon ido*), cataracts, and eventual blindness. *Amosani* of the abdominal region is a major cause of gastrointestinal ailments. *Amosanin ciki* is given various names and is described in various ways, one of the most common being *'kabar ciki*, "anger in the belly." *Ciwon ciki* due to *amosani* is described by such phrases as *cikina yana yawo*, "my belly is walking around," or *cikina yana motsi*, "my belly is churning about." The idea of twisting, turning, loosening, and constriction is very important in describing *amosina*. One healer, while examining a little girl, palpitated her abdomen and upon finding it tight and hard with a lump on one side promptly said the condition was due to *amosani*. *Amosani* could perhaps be best described through analogy as an "infection" of the body by damp cold, with resulting morbidity accompanied by aching, throb-

18. The translation of *amosani* as "dandruff, scalp disease" in the recent (1977) *Modern Hausa-English Dictionary* is clearly inadequate.

bing, twisting, and turning sensations in the afflicted region. In men *amosanin ciki* is feared because in addition to the stomach disorders and discomforts it normally brings, it can descend to the scrotum and affect the testicles, causing *gwaiwa*—hydrocele or scrotal elephantiasis.[19] *Amosani* in women can lead to an affliction known as *kwantacce* (literally "lying down") in which a pregnancy "lies down" inside the mother, going into a dormant stage in which development stops. Such conditions may persist indefinitely and are a common explanation for infertility in Hausa women. Proper treatment with herbal remedies may cause the fetus to shake off his lethargy and resume development, resulting in a normal birth weeks or months (or perhaps years) beyond the normal terms of nine months.[20]

The effects of heat (*zafi*) are felt mainly on the external body and are generally not as important in pathological explanations as are the effects of cold (*sanyi*). As an alternative word for pain (*ciwo*), but also meaning heat, *zafi* is most often confined in semantic usage to manifestations on the exterior of the body: for banging a finger inadvertently with a hammer, a cut, a burn, for rectal disorders (*basur, atuni, 'Dan Kanoma*), etc. Diseases which manifest themselves as painful rashes and eruptions on the skin, such as smallpox (*agana*), chicken pox (*karambau, 'kyanda*), or measles (*ba'kon dauro, 'kyanda*), are often described as being caused by *zafi*—establishing a relationship between sensations of pain on the skin and body surface with heat. Meningitis (*sankarau*),[21] which sweeps through West Africa during the hot season in cyclical epidemics,[22] is sometimes attributed to the pernicious effects of heat on the body, an obvious correlation between the seasonal nature of the disease and Hausa physiological concepts.

Zafi is also related to leprosy (*kuturta*), and *zafin kuturta* is sometimes given as a reason for eruptions on the skin. Indeed, lying within

19. It is said that this condition can be contracted venereally from a woman who herself suffers from *amosanin ciki*, or from a woman who has had sexual relations with a man suffering from *gwaiwa*.

20. Spirits are also seen as a frequent source of interference with pregnancy and as a cause of infertility. See Last (1970).

21. From the verbal *sankare*, meaning to stiffen, stretch out, referring to the stiffening and straightening of the neck, one of the principal symptoms of cerebrospinal meningitis. See Last (1976:131).

22. Cf. Whittle and Greenwood (1976). Meningitis is very often associated with spirits as well.

the Hausa framework of notions about the body is one of a gradual progression of "skin types" or "body types," ranging from healthy to leprous. Some people just have bad bodies (*jiki ba kyau*) as the result of God's handiwork. Something of this is expressed in the Hausa proverb that says *Da haka muka fara da kuturu ya ga mai-kyasfi*, " 'So we began,' said the leper when he saw the man with ringworm." Leprosy is something God puts into everyone's body while they are being created in the womb; only in some does it manifest itself as the actual ravaging form of the disease, and many disruptions of the skin may be attributed to leprosy in some form or another. Ulcerating sores that linger and refuse to heal, called *'kasala*, are one example of the phenomenon of "leprosy" coming out of the body in mild form.[23]

There are, of course, numerous other beliefs concerning leprosy. It can be transmitted through a mother's milk to her children.[24] If a man has intercourse with a menstruating woman and she conceives, the child will be a leper (*kuturu*) or an albino (*zabiya*). Goat meat aggravates leprosy, so lepers refuse to eat it or to drink goat milk. If one eats with a leper he should allow him to finish last so that any leprosy left in the bowl will be reabsorbed into his body and not communicated. The urine of toads (*fitsarin kwa'do*) may lead to leprosy if it gets on the body. If one sleeps in the same room with a leper (which is generally regarded as unpleasant), he should make sure the leper leaves first in the morning, since the affliction comes out at night and spreads over the doorway as a web (*yana*) which may entangle the first person going out. Lepers are reputed to be hot-tempered and sexually prolific—both correlates of excessive heat (e.g., Darrah and Froude n.d.:28).

In general, however, leprosy is regarded as a not quite comprehensible manifestation of *ikon Allah*, the power of God, and is accepted as such. The fact that everyone is a latent leper goes far to explain the tolerance with which they are treated. Among the Hausa there is no

23. This is perhaps one reason why the statistical incidence of leprosy in northern Nigeria is reported to be so high (up to 600,000 cases). Leprosy attendants frequently classify any severe skin ailment as a manifestation of the ravages of *Mycobacterium leprae*. On leprosy in northern Nigeria see Shiloh (1965).
24. The relationship between a mother's milk and many infant health problems is universally acknowledged by the Hausa, and infant mortality is often attributed to *ciwon nono*, milk sickness. A wide variety of herbal tonics (usually white) are used in the treatment of such difficulties.

fearful horror of the contagiousness of the disease such as commonly exists in the Western mind, and the practice of almsgiving (*sadaka*) enjoined by Islam as a means of caring for the unfortunate works toward creating a tolerant (if not always very supportive) atmosphere. Children often make fun of their stumpy limbs and collapsed faces, but lepers are still a part of life, have friends in the village, smoke, talk, laugh, share kolanuts, and go on farming as best they can.[25]

Such, then, is the general nature of *ciwon Allah*, "diseases of God." These afflictions are a part of everyday life, stemming from the interaction of man and his environment, the food he eats, changes in heat and coldness—results of the structuring of the world by God. "God is powerful over everything, chastising whom He will, and having mercy on whomsoever He will, and unto Him you shall be turned" (Koran XXIX, 19ff.); but there are other forces at work in the world as well.

■ *Ciwon Miyagu:* The Illnesses of Evil

Because *lafiya* in its most general sense is a correlate of the moral order of the world and describes a metaphysical state of "correct being" as well as a condition of good physical health, it can be disrupted by the intrusion of occult powers as well as by forces from the physical environment. These conscious, malevolent forces which interfere with *lafiya* to bring illness are the causes of *ciwon miyagu*, the "illnesses of evil." These powers are witchcraft (*maita*), the power of the curse (*kambum baka* or *baki*), sorcery (*sammu*), and the spirits (*aljannu, iskoki*). None of these are physical causes of illness in the same way that hot, cold, excess bitterness, or too much phlegm are (although they do indeed produce effects on the physical body); rather, they are metaphysical counterparts of the physical causes of sickness, emanating from outside the *jama'a* of Islam to afflict individuals and disrupt their bodies, just as they disrupt the proper moral order of the Islamic community. Within this general classification of "illnesses caused by evil forces," two general subcategories may be noted, corresponding to Rivers's categories of illnesses caused by human agency and those

25. One of the social centers of the village in which I lived was the fire next to the lorry-park where Jibril the Leper sold kolanuts, talked with his friends, and engaged in gossip with *Sarkin Tasha* (the chief of the lorry-park) and his cronies, me among them.

caused by spiritual beings. The human agencies that cause sickness may be further subdivided into those powers inherent in the individual (witchcraft, *maita*) and those which are acquired (sorcery, *sammu*).[26]

Witchcraft is an evil power inherent in an individual, imbibed through the mother's milk or inherited as a kind of "ice" or "flint" (*kankara*) in the belly. As was noted in the preceding chapter, the most common manifestation of this evil power is the ability of the witch to seize the soul (*kurwa*) of an individual and by thus attacking it to disrupt the link between the life force (*rai*) and the soul, causing the victim to sicken and eventually to die. The principal sign of such a witch attack is epistaxis (*ha'bo*), especially when accompanied by severe illness. The soul being a kind of spirit, and thus a kind of "air," it is not surprising that an attack on the soul by a witch should be associated with nasal and upper respiratory symptoms. In the *bori* dances the possessing spirit is expelled at the end of the séance by a series of sneezes. Similarly, under ordinary circumstances (and in a somewhat jocular fashion), sneezing is regarded as a sign of a witch attempting to draw his victim's unwilling soul out of the body. An appropriate Islamic blessing such as *Alhamdulillahi!* ("God be praised!" or "Gesundheit!") should be uttered as a countermeasure to protect the soul. In cases of mental illness diagnosed as being due to an attack by an evil spirit, a common method of treatment is the use of *sha'ke*, a hot, peppery medicinal snuff which is blown up through the nostrils into the nasopharynx in order to induce violent sneezing and thus cause the expulsion of the offending spirit. Witches themselves are said to eat enormous quantities of pepper to fuel their inherent "hotness," a habit which no doubt enhances their spiritual power to extract the souls of their victims.[27] Since the witch captures and then slaughters the soul of his victims (just as a pagan slaughters a sacrificial goat or fowl and then offers the blood to the spirits), it is appropriate that the prey of the witch should show a gushing of blood at the moment of his spiritual slaughter.

26. These two terms are used in the sense described by Middleton and Winter (1963:3).
27. Some informants said that this heat was so strong that witches could be identified by observing the columns of smoke that emanated from their heads. This smoke was observable only if one had access to an appropriate medicine that made it visible.

The witch is said to possess wild, furtive eyes, always on the look-
out for souls to attack (especially children, whose souls are weaker and
thus more vulnerable). The power of the witch is manifested not only
in his stealthy glance, but also in his speech. He has the power to utter
an effective curse, *kambum baka* or *baki* (literally "mouth"). The expressed desire of a witch that misfortune should befall someone causes
that thing to happen; consequently, an action that coincides ex post
facto with a previously uttered imprecation may be viewed as a sign
of witchcraft. Among the Maguzawa both blessings and curses are
taken seriously (Krusius 1915:298), and among Muslims curses are
technically actionable offenses under Islamic law, nor should the importance of the Word or Speech of God in Muslim theology be overlooked in this respect (O'Shaughnessy 1948:30).

In village Muslim thought, witchcraft (*maita*) is nearly synonymous
with pagan sacrifice and spirit worship (*tsafi*). Since the Maguzawa
offer the lives of goats and fowls to their spirits, in violation of Koranic
injunctions against such idolatry, it is but a short jump to viewing them
all as witches, preying upon the souls of others. Even though an individual pagan may be treated with tolerance by villagers, attend markets
freely, and suffer minimal obvious discrimination, there is always a
lingering suspicion and a recognition that he is not part of the proper
order. He is a moral outlier as well as a residential one.

In theory, when a witch attack occurs the offending witch should be
identified and forced to release the soul of his victim. The procedure
most usually described for this is to make the witch step over the body
of his victim, thus returning to the owner the soul that was stolen
from him. The witch may be identified by having the sick person recall
all the people he has been in contact with recently, reciting their names
while under the influence of a medicinal spell, or by some other means
(Trimingham 1959:116–17). In reality, however, witchcraft accusations
are rare in Hausa villages.[28] While everyone acknowledges the fact that
witches exist, few are ever identified by name, except perhaps in jokes.
Most of the combat with witches takes place on a metaphysical plane;
people wear medicinal charms (either Koranic or herbal) to ward off
evil influences such as witches. In cases of illness where witch attacks

28. This is my own observation, as well as that of D. P. L. Dry (1950:183, 1953:
223), Last (1970), Barkow (1974:8–9), and Faulkingham (1975:18–21).

are diagnosed by herbalists, the general practice seems to be to give the patients medicines to ensure their recovery and to negate the power of the witch at a distance, rather than to undertake a long process of divination or investigation to identify the witch specifically. Indeed, it would seem that the significance of witchcraft is diminishing and becoming less individual in its import, now being amenable (as are many of the illnesses caused by evil) to "broad spectrum" therapy.[29]

While witchcraft is a power inherent in the individual, sorcery (*sammu*) is an acquired technique. In theory, at least, anyone may attain a knowledge of sorcery or obtain the requisite ingredients to cast a spell or prepare a sorcery poison. It is really a kind of "medicine" (*magani*) which may be obtained for evil purposes and, depending upon one's access to the specific occult knowledge involved, can be used to cause any number of horrible afflictions: infertility, madness, leprosy, withering of limbs, blindness, unwanted abortion, and so on. It is an illness-causing rather than an illness-preventing kind of "medicine," a "black medicine" rather than a "white medicine."[30]

Although the term *sammu* is derived from the Arabic word *simm*, or "poison," it is not a poison in a physical sense, but rather in a metaphysical one. This sorcery poison does not have to be ingested by its victim, or even applied to his body. It merely must come into contact with his sphere of living through a piece of clothing, a portion of hair or fingernails, a footprint on a path, or a place where he has urinated; it only has to affect the victim's soul in order to be effective. At this level the distinction between the modes of action of witchcraft and sorcery becomes almost indistinguishable. For example, one generally acknowledged technique used by sorcerers among the Hausa is called *harbin kasko*, or "shooting in a bowl." In this technique the sorcerer prepares a small bowl of water and then, by using the proper medicines or reciting the proper incantations, summons up the image of the victim's soul within the water. He then shoots the water with a needle or arrow, striking the soul and causing illness to its owner. The sorcerer may use medicines to wash out his mouth, giving him the same powers

29. This is no doubt due at least in part to the fact that accusations of witchcraft have no status in Islamic law. See also Faulkingham (1975:18–21).
30. Although I cannot recall anyone ever having made this distinction between "black" and "white" medicine as regards sorcery, it certainly fits in with Hausa color symbolism and also with English notions of "black" and "white" magic.

of cursing ascribed to witches, or by the proper techniques he may gain control over spirits and cause them to do his bidding, wreaking havoc on his enemies. The idea of the *dodo* (described previously), an evil spirit working in harness with a master to secure him wealth in return for the lives of others, is very close to this concept.

Although these two categories of human action—witchcraft and sorcery—are acknowledged as possible causes of human illness, the most common malevolent influences causing sickness are the spirits. As was pointed out earlier, there are an infinite number of spirits in the Hausa pantheon, and these are known by various names: *iskoki* ("winds"), *aljannu* (*djinn*), or *inuwoyi* ("shades"). Although there is an elaborate social and occupational hierarchy of spirits, broadly speaking they may be grouped into two categories: white spirits (*farin iskoki*) and black spirits (*ba'kin iskoki*). These correspond roughly to Muslim spirits (*iskoki masu salla*) and pagan spirits (*iskoki mara salla*), respectively. In Hausa color symbolism white generally means "good or pleasing" and black means "evil or undesirable." This same classification is also basically true as regards the spirits; however, the extent to which a person is involved with the spirits has a great bearing on the way in which they are conceptualized. In general, Muslim villagers want as little to do with spirits as possible. They are widely acknowledged as existing, and the Koran specifically recognizes the existence of the *djinn*, but the connotations of spirits with paganism make them basically undesirable entities. All spirits are capricious—not to be trusted—and this applies to white as well as black spirits. It is said that one can meet a white spirit in the bush and receive its blessing, thereby obtaining wealth, power, and popularity, but most people would rather not have such an experience. The spirit could just as easily cause madness. *Bori* devotees, herbal healers (*bokaye*), and others claiming to have intimate relations with the spirits may state that *all* the *bori* spirits are white spirits and that they establish their peculiar relationships with people in order to help them by revealing medicines as aids in the conquest of sickness. Since many *bori* spirits are in fact associated with very debilitating sicknesses, this is obviously an attempt at legitimating their activities in terms of Islamic morality. Sometimes the *bori* spirits are classified as white or black depending on the color of the clothing they wear. Because in pagan religion and also in some *bori* rites each spirit has a specified sacrifice of a different colored fowl or animal,[31] precise attempts at classifying specific *bori* spirits as white or black are difficult. In general, however, black spirits—regardless of whether or not they are given specific names—are seen as causing illnesses, especially devastating ones, whereas white spirits are more benign. The illnesses caused by black spirits, such as raving mania, are very difficult to treat, while an illness caused by a white spirit is much more susceptible to a cure. Which spirit is actually causing the problem may not even be known until such time as the effects of the treatment are seen.

The spirits cause illness by coming in contact with the body of their victims. They "touch" (*ta'ba*), "rub" (*shafe*), or "beat" (*buge*) them, each word carrying a slightly more serious implication for the course of the illness. Senile old women, for example, are regarded as being "a little touched," but epileptics in the midst of their fits are seen as having been "beaten" or "struck" by the spirits. Certain hunter spirits who live in the bush, such as *Gajere* ("the short one") are associated with an illness called *harbin daji* or "shooting in the bush." In such a case a villager working in his fields or trekking through the bush is "shot" and wounded by one of the spirit's invisible arrows. A sickness results, characterized by pain in an extremity, general swelling of the limb or the body, sores or rashes, severe fever, and loss of strength. In cases of madness the spirit is seen as having taken up residence in his victim's body; hence efforts are made to induce the expulsion of the spirit by the insertion of unpleasant substances into the nose and the inhalation of foul medicinal smoke.

Spirits may linger in the subconscious mind during dreams. It will be recalled from chapter 4 that dreams are commonly explained by the Hausa as being due to the nocturnal peregrinations of the soul around the world as its owner sleeps. Nightmares may be caused by the attempts of witches to capture the soul. Similarly, spirits can affect the soul and cause other kinds of dreams, which may be important omens

31. Greenberg (1946:30–39) gives a long list of the spirits and their sacrifices. For example, Gajimare requires the sacrifice of a sheep with a black navel; Inna requires a white chicken or white female sheep; Duna rquires a black cock or a black goat; 'Ka'kari requires a red and white goat; 'Dan Musa requires a speckled cock, etc. See also Besmer (1983:62–120).

of the future. In women, dreams about water (*mafarkin ruwa*) are particularly ominous, indicating that a water spirit has come to affect the fluids of her womb and cause infertility (*kwantacce*, literally "lying down," a dormancy of a pregnancy which may last months or even years). Dreams in which a woman has incestuous or profligate sexual relations may be the sign of a spirit coming to plague her and likewise cause sterility. Such dreams are called *namijin dare*, "husband of the night." Similar dreams of succubae by men may result in impotence, known vividly in Hausa as "the death of the penis," (*mutuwar bura*); and (not surprising), water spirits such as the *bori* spirit *Sarkin Rafi* can cause bed-wetting (*fitsarin kwance*), especially in adults.[32]

In general, spirits function as ultimate explanations for illness, distant causes for illnesses that are otherwise puzzling. They effect their damage through a derangement of an intermediary bodily structure or function. They may cause withered limbs by drinking the blood normally present in that limb, causing it to atrophy. They cause madness by removing a man's "sense." They cause female infertility by disturbing the fluids in her womb, by "tying up" her blood vessels or "wrapping up" the fetus so that it cannot develop. Healers in particular, when pressed, can offer any number of ways that spirits can affect the body to cause illness. In general, however, the way in which the spirits act is of less importance than the overriding fact that they are in some way responsible for the illness, an illness that in many cases is frightening or puzzling in nature.

Depending on the circumstances and the people involved, nearly any ailment might be diagnosed as being caused by a spirit. In most cases, however, illnesses attributed to spirit attacks are serious ones. They tend to be highly debilitating neurological, neuromuscular, or personality disorders such as headaches (*ciwon kai*)—especially severe, crippling ones of the migraine variety—epilepsy (*farfadiya*), hunchback ('*kusumbi*), withered or paralyzed limbs (*sayi, ciwon Inna*), elephantiasis (*tindimi*), and birth defects, which may also be ascribed to the whimsy of God as He creates the child. Epidemic illnesses such as meningitis (*san'karau*), measles (*ba'kon dauro, 'kyanda*), and in former times smallpox (*agana*) are said to result from the marauding actions of

---

32. In children bed-wetting is seen simply as a manifestation of their undisciplined childishness.

spirits. Blindness (*makanta*), leprosy (*kuturta*), deafness (*kurmanci*), and deaf-mutism (*bebenci*) may all be caused by spirits as well.

In short, any long-lasting, enfeebling, pathological condition of the body may be attributed to the penetration of the body by malevolent forces, especially if it falls outside the range of those ailments readily explained by more apparent causes, such as cold or heredity.[33] For example one villager, Hassan, had a lovely wife named Hajara, who suffered from generally poor health and tiredness during her pregnancy. He arranged for her to go to the hospital at Malumfashi for treatment. She remained with relatives for over a month as an outpatient, but felt no better. Seeing no improvement, he decided she was suffering from spirits and let one of the local herbalists treat her instead. The rest of her pregnancy was uneventful and she delivered a baby boy, much to her husband's delight.

Certain *bori* spirits are associated with specific illnesses, so much so that I. M. Lewis (1971:82) has referred to the *bori* pantheon as a veritable "medical dictionary."[34] One of the most notable of these spirits is *Inna*, "mother" or "maternal aunt." She is also known by a number of other names such as *Bafilatana*, "Fulani woman," *Uwardaji*, "mother of the bush," *Uwargona*, "mother of the farm," *Doguwa*, "tall woman," and *Uwargari*, "mother of the town." *Inna* is the primary cause of paralysis and withered limbs, and *ciwon Inna* ("sickness of Inna") is a synonym for this affliction. So strong is this association that one healer and *bori* adept described three different aspects of Inna that could manifest themselves in human illness. Paralysis of the left side was caused by *Inna Ta Daji* ("*Inna* of the bush"), an interesting association of left-handedness with the uncontrolled forces of the wilderness. Right-side paralysis was caused by *Inna Ta Gida* ("*Inna*

33. An example of this latter condition was a family of deaf-mutes who lived in the village, all obviously suffering from the same affliction, which had appeared in several generations. This was simply regarded as *gadonsu*, "their inheritance," and that sufficed for an explanation.

34. It is in this aspect of Hausa medical thought that they perhaps come closest to developing a notion comparable to that of "disease" in scientific medicine. The spirits could be likened to invading pathogenic microorganisms. Tremearne (1914: 20) noticed this when he wrote of *bori* initiations, practices, and ceremonies as a kind of "inoculation" against the spirits, and concluded "if for *bori* we read bacillus, we shall find that the Hausa tabus are at least as intelligible to us as are our sanitary regulations to certain alien denizens of the London slums."

of the household"), an association of domesticity and the village with the right side of the body.[35] Paraplegia was caused by *Inna Ta Kwance* ("*Inna* the recliner"). A great drinker of blood (or milk, hence her characterization as a Fulani milkmaid), *Inna* sucks the blood out of limbs and bodies and causes atrophy, weakness, and paralysis.

The spirit *Mallam Alhaji*, "the pilgrim," likewise causes specific illnesses. He is an elderly Muslim spirit who wanders around fingering a rosary, muttering to himself and coughing. He may cause an interesting kind of madness called *hauka ta karatu* or "reading madness," which stems from excessive reading and study of the Koran and theological works to the point that, in Shakespeare's words

> the native hue of resolution
> Is sicklied o'er with the pale cast of thought,
> And enterprises of great pith and moment
> With this regard their currents turn awry,
> And lose the name of action.
> (*Hamlet* III, 1, 84–88)

An individual suffering from this ailment puts all his energies into study, neither eating, drinking, nor sleeping, living only for religious study, until he goes mad. More commonly, however, *Mallam Alhaji* is said to bring bronchial and respiratory ailments, manifested by severe coughing (*huka*). Another spirit, called *'Dan Tosho* or "the old man," also causes these latter illnesses and may be conflated with *Mallam Alhaji* to form one nebulous character with two names—a process not uncommon in the pantheon of the *bori* spirits.[36]

Many examples of the relationships between spirits and specific kinds of illnesses could be given. A representative sampling of *bori* spirits, their possession characteristics, and the sicknesses associated with them are given in table 2. It should be pointed out that in practice one ailment can fade into another and many of the disturbances asso-

35. The significance of "right" and "left" in Arabic and Muslim thought is discussed in Chelhod (1973). His essay may be profitably compared with the others that appear in that same volume.
36. This process can be seen in the numerous subheadings and epithets of each spirit in Greenberg (1946), and by studying the various appellations of the spirits in the extensive *bori* liturgy published by King (1966, 1967). Besmer (1983) is the best discussion of *bori* in Hausaland.

ciated with these spirits are vague from the outset, so there is a great amount of latitude in the diagnosis and treatment of any given case. In fact, after observing herbal practitioners who specialize primarily in the treatment of spirit-induced illnesses, one comes to the conclusion that the basic diagnosis of a particular trouble as spirit-related is the major element of importance, not the identity of the individual spirit. Only those patients so seriously stricken as to seek initiation into the *bori* cult through the formal process of *girka* are likely to pay much heed to the identity of the specific spirit; and, in any case, after initiation they will be able to converse with many other spirits while in the state of possession, as well as the one who caused their own personal misfortune. There is, no doubt, a sense of relief if a name can be placed on the spirit afflicting the patient. The name conveys to the patient a sense of his affliction being known to the therapist and hence somehow under his control. The illusion of knowledge can be a powerful placebo; but even in the West the name of the disease is not nearly as important to the patient as is the question of whether or not his physician can correct what is wrong with him.

There remains one other way in which a spirit can cause illness. This is the instance of a "soul attack." The Hausa concept of the soul (*kurwa*) and its relationship to the life force (*rai*) of the body was discussed earlier. In the case of a witch attack, the soul is captured and later slaughtered, breaking the link between the soul and the life force, ultimately leading to the demise of the patient. This link between the two entities is also broken at death, and both the soul and the force of life return to Allah, who sent them originally. On occasion, however, instead of returning promptly to God, the soul may linger around its own familiar haunts to plague a member of its family and cause sickness. The common signs of such an attack are prostration, disinterest in one's normal affairs, an inability to eat and drink, and so on; but the important criterion is that it occurs in the aftermath of a recent death. This problem is reported by villagers to be much more common among the Maguzawa than among themselves.[37] and to be especially troublesome at the death of brothers, twin brothers being particularly susceptible.

37. From the Muslim point of view it is easy to understand why the soul of a pagan would be less interested in ascending to confront a wrathful God; the prospects of entering paradise would seem slim indeed.

Table 2   A Sample of *Bori* Spirits.

Name of Spirit	Meaning	Possession Characteristics	Illness Caused
Inna Uwammu	Mother maternal aunt, our mother	Dances holding an arm curled up at her side	Withering of limbs, paralysis
Uwargona	Mother of the farm		Swellings, especially of the belly
Danko 'Dan Musa	Son of Musa, a snake	A snake spirit, he writhes on the ground on his belly	Stomach and other internal disorders
Gajere	The short one	A hunter spirit, he carries a bow and arrow or spear and stalks his prey	"Shooting in the bush," various sores and illnesses, swellings of the body
Gajimare Mai-shan-ruwa	The rainbow water-drinker	A snake spirit, appears arched over like a rainbow	Various afflictions: stomach trouble, mental illness, nosebleeds
Yaya	Elder sister, senior wife	Dances rubbing arms, scratching	Rashes, itching, scratching
Mai-Dariya	The laughter	Wild, uncontrolled, hysterical laughing	Mental illness characterized by hysterical laughter
Malam Alhaji	The pilgrim to Mecca	Walks about bent over with a shuffling gait, fingering a rosary, muttering and coughing	Mental illness, coughing
'Dan Tsoho	The old man	Acts in a senile fashion, coughs a lot	Coughing
'Kunau	The burner (?)	Moves about holding his abdomen	Stomach and abdominal pain
Kuturu	The leper	Crawls along on his hands and knees with legs and hands curled up, begs for alms	Leprosy

Table 2 A Sample of *Bori* Spirits (continued).

Name of Spirit	Meaning	Possession Characteristics	Illness Caused
Kurma Bebe	The deaf one, the deaf-mute	Uses rudimental sign language, attempts to talk in a high-pitched, squeaky voice	Deafness, mutism
Makaho	The blind one	Wanders about like a blind man, led by a boy with a long stick	Eye troubles, blindness
'Dan Galadima	The noble youth	Acts like a gambler, throwing cowry shells; should be a fancy dresser	Various afflic-tions, including wanderlust, pa-ralysis of the hand
Kure	The hyena	Rolls about, bangs his head on the ground, throws dirt into his face and eyes	Headache
Sarkin Rafi	Chief of the river	Wild striding steps in-terrupted by falls, searching for water, pouring dirt and water over his head	Various ail-ments: mental illness, chest pains, bed-wetting
Nakada	The striker, the over-thrower	Wild, uncontrolled ac-tions; may simulate in-tercourse with a phallic pole or masturbation; acts as though eating his own feces	Severe mania and mental dis-order; greatly feared
'Dan Uda	Son of the rams	A Fulani spirit	Mental illness, especially of the type where the victim wanders off into the bush

Note: There appear to be some local and regional differences in the names and attributes of many *bori* spirits. This list differs in some respects from other lists found in the published literature for this reason.

This notion appears to be an interesting cultural interpretation of the process of grief. That it is said to be much more common among the Maguzawa than the Muslim villagers is an attestation both to the extent to which Islam has undermined old beliefs regarding the soul, and to the relative strength of kinship ties within the two different groups. In this light it is worth discussing the nature of mental illness and considering to what extent it may arise naturally, independent of attacks by souls, spirits, or the occult poisons of sorcerers.

■ Emotion, Mentation, and Madness

The Hausa language possesses a number of words and phrases descriptive of mental processes and inner states of the mind. In general it is not a sophisticated vocabulary. Happiness and joy are expressed by the phrase *farin ciki* ("white inside"), while sorrow, grief, and unhappiness are expressed by *ba'kin ciki* ("black inside"), in line with the general Hausa scheme of symbolic color classification. There are words expressing positive emotions such as gladness (*murna*), pleasure (*da'di*), affection or desire (*so*), and loyalty (*biyayya*), as well as a range of words expressing negative emotions such as anger (*haushi*), jealousy (*kishi*), fear (*tsoro*), longing (*bege*), and loneliness (*kewa*). Other words describe mental activities such as thought (*tsammani*), memory (*tunani*), forgetfulness (*mantuwa*), and reflection (*waswasi*). All these mental processes are performed by the brain. When the brain is functioning properly it produces *hankali*, or "sense." This word has meaning both as a process—the ability to function normally, to piece ideas and thoughts together coherently—and also as regards the content of those thoughts. The word applies not only to rationality or lucidity in the clinical sense, but also to common sense, the ability to exercise good judgment and to interact properly with one's social environment. If a man possesses *hankali* it means that his brain is intact and also that he can use that brain to carry out his proper social role.

The Hausa word *mahaukaci* (f. *mahaukaciya*, pl. *mahaukata*) means "madman" or "crazy person." It refers to one characterized by *hauka* ("madness") and is related to the verbal *haukace*, meaning "to go crazy, insane." The word *hauka* is generally translated in dictionaries as "madness" or "insanity," and it implies a loss or disorientation of self-control leading to disordered behavior. Etymologically, the word *hauka* may originate from *hau,* meaning "mount" or "climb," and *kai,* the word for "head." This "mounting of the head" is best exemplified by the possession state of *bori* (which is regarded as a form of "madness") where the spirits "mount" the dancers, who are referred to as "horses" (*dawaki*) which the spirits ride. The spirits are thought to take command of the dancers, who lose their self-control and "become" the spirits who ride them, assuming the characteristics of their temporary masters. The spirits are believed to exert their control by virtue of having mounted the dancers' heads, where they reside until they are expelled by sneezing at the end of the dance.

Manifested as a loss of self-control, "madness" (*hauka*) thus includes the permanent derangement of the lunatic, the temporary loss of self-control to the spirits in *bori,* and other forms of disordered behavior, especially if accompanied by an altered mental status. Thus, epileptics are "mad" when smitten by the spirits both during their seizures and in the post-ictal state. Spastics or people with palsies are often referred to as "mad" because of their disordered movements, especially if they suffer from altered mentation as well as neuromuscular dysfunction. The mentally retarded likewise are "mad," especially if they cannot follow simple social cues or if they have lost control of bowel and bladder function. People who lose their self-control while drunk or after taking illicit drugs have also become "mad," albeit temporarily. Similarly, someone who is beside himself with inconsolable grief or has been captured by a livid rage has likewise gone "mad" for a time. Something of this temporary loss of control can be seen in the use of "going mad" in expressions such as *tukunya tana hauka,* "the pot is going mad," when referring to a cooking vessel which is boiling over.

Above all, *hauka* refers to the absence of *hankali,* a deranged state of mind; but there are variations and gradations of this condition. That there are variations in individual behavior and adaptation to the social environment is obvious to everybody; as the proverb says, *Hauka, kowa da irin nashi,* "Craziness, everybody has his own kind." Hausa views of madness thus fall along a spectrum of people who have all lost self-control and become to some degree disoriented.

At the mildest end of this spectrum lie such people as the irresponsible village youth, who rides a bicycle wildly and recklessly through the village streets, careening in and out of groups of children, dodging chickens and sheep. Exuberant children spinning around playing silly

games and getting dizzy may be characterized by laughing adults as
"crazy" in this sense. In a more serious way drunkards, drug abusers,
and especially lorry drivers who get high on amphetamines or cannabis
are "crazy." Senile people likewise are *mahaukata,* as are epileptics,
spastics, the mentally retarded, people with severe speech impediments,
and people with neurological problems that cause palsies, tremors, or
choreiform movements. The most feared end of the spectrum is composed of those whose behavior and personal characteristics cut them off
completely from the rest of society: madmen or madwomen who amble
about naked, mumbling, sleeping in the markets or by the sides of the
roads, scrounging for food in the leavings of trash heaps, and drinking
from stagnant borrow pits; or maniacs, violent psychotics, and other
wild, uncontrolled persons whose presence may threaten the peace and
order of village life. The spectrum thus ranges from mere silliness and
moral recklessness or irresponsibility, to disturbances of motor and
mental function of varying degrees, to the frightening specter of total
derangement, abandonment of recognizable humanness, and descent to
a level of merely animal existence.

In close relation to *hauka* lies another word that also implies a loss
of *hankali: wauta* or "foolishness." While *hauka* refers to loss of *hankali* in the sense of "loss of reason" or "mental derangement," *wauta*
refers to loss of *hankali* in the sense of "loss of common sense." *Wauta*
refers to foolish or poorly considered acts that temporarily go beyond
the proper bounds of behavior or propriety, rather than a deranged
state of mind. For example, on one occasion a laborer was brought before the village headman as the result of a quarrel. In the course of
things he became angry and punched the village chief in the face. This
was described by my friends as a classic example of *wauta,* "foolish
behavior," or *sakarci,* "senseless action"—and indeed it was, for the
assailant paid for his misconduct in the district lockup.

The verbal *wautu* means "to be guilty of foolish conduct"; and
wautad da means "to make a fool of" or "to treat as a fool." One can
make a fool of somebody; one cannot make a madman of somebody
(without the use of sorcery). The process of "going mad" (*haukace*) is
something one does by oneself. A *wawa* is a fool, a person who lacks
judgment and intelligence, but he is not a madman, *mahaukaci.* The
term *wawa* is never used to refer to bush lunatics or market madmen,
those naked, pathetic creatures who wander from village to village

scrounging whatever subsistence they can. Such *mahaukata* have lost
control, modesty, even reason itself, and they manifest far more than
poor judgment—they display no observable rationality at all, living
little better than beasts. While the *mahaukaci* is often feared, the *wawa*
is frequently an object of amusement. The *Wawan Sarki* or "king's
fool" is the *gauji*, the court jester of an emir, a silly prankster.

Wauta implies going beyond the proper bounds of common sense or
decorum, and because the fool is one who does this, the word *wawa*
is also used as a modifier which carries the sense of "foolish or improper
excess." This usage is found in such expressions as *wawan barci*, "fool
of sleep" (a very deep sleep); *wawan ci*, "fool of eating" (a greedy appetite); *wawan nisa*, "fool of distance" (an exceptionally long way,
especially on a journey); *wawan sawu*, "fool of a track" (a false track
or false scent in hunting); *wawan zama*, "fool of sitting" (sitting in-
decently exposed, or selling something at a ridiculously cheap price in
the market); *wawan kiwo*, "fool of grazing" (referring to an animal that
wanders off while grazing in the countryside) or *wawan yawa*, "fool of
largeness" (that is, a ridiculously large amount or extent). These expressions also imply that the person involved is somehow "made a fool
of"—by sleeping so heavily, by eating so much, by starting out on a
ridiculously long journey, or by exposing himself to public ridicule by
the manner of his sitting—in short, by behaving recklessly or abandon-
ing common sense.

To define the differences sharply, one might say that *hauka* involves
the abandonment of reason, the loss of self-control, and disorientation,
while *wauta* implies the use of silly reasoning, faulty judgment, flawed
common sense, and the disregard of Hausa social standards. A *mahaukaci* may very well perform acts of *wauta*, but everybody who does
something foolish is not necessarily a madman.

There is, of course, clearly some middle ground in the use of these
terms, especially in the "soft" meanings of everyday parlance and
poetic hyperbole. Someone who persistently displays bad judgment
and unacceptable social behavior may be called "crazy," even though
he is not obviously psychotic; but the core meaning of mental disorientation—even temporarily—and loss of self-control belongs to
hauka alone. The absence of *hankali* ("sense") is madness; if *hankali*
is present but flawed, the result is *wauta*.

Wauta is basically a category unto itself. *Hauka*, on the other hand, is often broken down into subcategories of madness. These tend to be brief clinical descriptions of patient characteristics, generally of the more striking and serious forms, for these are the most devastating and most feared. Discussions of "kinds of madness" depend a great deal on the individual discussing them, but among the more common kinds of madness one could name would be the following:

1. *Haukar zagi*, "abusing madness," where the individual's behavior is marked by quarreling, swearing, insults, and general troublemaking

2. *Haukar ba duka*, "violent madness," where the affected individual physically assaults others

3. *Haukar shiru kawai*, "madness of complete silence," where the patient withdraws from everyone, becomes listless, hard to arouse, and uninterested; the severely depressed patient

4. *Haukar dariya*, "laughing madness," where the patient laughs hysterically and uncontrollably; the expansive, hyperemotional side of manic-depressive psychosis, for example

5. *Haukar surutu*, "babbling madness," where the patient rambles on and on incoherently, as in senility or delirium

6. Neurological "madness," which would include such afflictions as grand mal-type epilepsy (*farfadiya*), spasticity, tremors, etc.

7. *Haukar kwana kasuwa*, "sleeping-in-the-market madness," where the patient abandons home and family to wander aimlessly, scrounging for food, sleeping in the streets or in the empty market stalls. The village which formed the focus of the present study had one such madwoman, Dala, a Maguzawa girl who had left her family's homestead to wander naked in the market, laughing and talking to herself, sleeping where she could. Each time her family took her home she ran away again, until they finally gave up and left her to her ways.

8. *Haukar tafiyar daji*, "bush-wandering madness," where the individual leaves home and family to wander off into the bush away from the civilization of the village. Many times they wander the roads from village to village, sleeping where they can, eating what they can find. They are wild and uncared for and show up silently and suddenly, presenting a naked, frightening, unkempt appearance as they walk through the dusty village streets. They are avoided by villagers when they show up, if not driven away. This kind of madness is the most feared and, like sleeping-in-the-market madness (to which it is obviously related in terms of its manifestations), is generally regarded as incurable.

Hausa ideas about the causation of mental illness are fluid, as they are regarding the classification of mental disorders; however, at least eight modes of causation can be discerned:[38]

1. *Dukiya ta watse*, "destruction of property," mental illness resulting from a great personal blow, such as the death of one's family or the destruction of all a man's possessions in a fire or other catastrophe. Hausa recognize the existence and importance of emotions in people's lives. While equanimity and balance are highly regarded as the proper aspects that a person should show the world and contribute to the striking picture of composure and dignity that an outside observer sees, the various small swings of mood that everyone experiences are well known and are recognized in daily speech. When circumstances disrupt a person's mental and emotional composure the common way of describing it is to say *Ba na da lafiya yau; hankalina ya kwanta*, "I have no *lafiya* today; my sense has lain down." This expression is used to describe temporary stress, fatigue, or depression. Similarly, words such as *'dimua*, "losing one's way," *rigima*, "uproar, tumult," and *damewa*, "confusion, worry," are used to describe the common kinds of upsets and pressures that everyone faces from time to time. It should not be surprising that, since these factors are recognized in the minor crises of life, it is also recognized how powerful they can become in the face of major devastation. In such a case the overwhelming emotions of grief or terror can make someone mad by causing his sense to leave. *Hankalinshi ya tashi*, "His sense has left," it is said, using the same verb form as for someone getting up and setting out on a journey.

2. *Jini ya juye*, "turbulence of the blood," in which it is thought that the blood in the head becomes a seething, swirling mass, disordering the person's thoughts and actions. Dizziness (*juwa*) and temporal headaches (*jiri*) are also ascribed to milder versions of this condition.

3. *'Kwa'kwalwa ta fashe*, "breaking of the skull," refers to mental derangements appearing in the aftermath of physical trauma, such as receiving a blow on the head from a rock or stick, or injuries received in a motor crash. The cause-effect relationship is obvious in this case. The man's brain has been injured; therefore his sense cannot function properly.

---

38. The following list is similar to the one presented in J. M. Nicolas (1972:366–67), but differs in some respects.

4. *Farkon haifuwa*, "beginning with birth," i.e., congenital kinds of mental disorders. These include mental and neurological disorders which have always been seen in the individual since he was a child. They may be ascribed to Allah, to the actions of spirits acting on the unborn child in the womb, or to some affliction obtained through the mother's milk.

5. *Cuta ta ke sawa*, "those brought about by sickness." This category includes mental disorders arising in the aftermath of severe physical illness, such as high fever with delirium or cerebrospinal meningitis. The madness in this case is seen as a residual effect of the original sickness.

6. *Giya da kafsu*, "from beer and amphetamines." These disorders are seen as arising from continual use of alcohol and abuse of drugs, unfortunate but increasing problems in rural Hausaland.

7. *Sammu*, "sorcery," a common explanation for severe mental illness such as the sleeping-in-the-market or wandering-in-the-bush variety.

8. *Ba'kin aljannu*, "evil spirits," the most widely accepted causal factor for mental illness.

The fluidity and haziness of Hausa medical beliefs are most obvious in their ideas about mental illness. Here, at the interface of mental and physical health, the junction of social and individual well-being, aspects of both natural causation and the forces of evil intermingle. Indeed, this is the case even in scientific medicine, where the proliferation of psychiatric models for the classification and treatment of mental disorders has reached confusing proportions. Siegler and Osmond (1976), for example, describe eight different models of mental illness and discuss their differing implications for psychiatric treatment. An understanding of mental illness has not yet been reached that would place psychiatry on a level of explanation and treatment comparable to that of internal medicine or surgery. For the Hausa, this causal fluidity has obvious consequences when the patient begins to seek treatment for his or her affliction, for a number of sources for therapy are available. The nature of these remedies and the sources from which they may be obtained form the subject of the next chapter.

VI

Medicine and Medical Practitioners

Mai-ciwo ba ya rena magani.

(*The sick man does not despise medicine.*)

HAUSA PROVERB

■ *Magani:* The Concept of "Medicine" in Hausa Thought

In English when we think of the word medicine we think of it generally in one of two ways. It is envisioned either as a substance used in curative treatment, that is, a medicament, or as a branch of knowledge:

> that department of knowledge and practice which is concerned with the cure, alleviation, and prevention of disease in human beings, and with the restoration and preservation of health. Also, in a more restricted sense, applied to that branch of this department which is the province of the physician, in the modern application of the term: the art of restoring and preserving the health of human beings by the administration of remedial substances and the regulation of diet, habits and conditions of life; distinguished from Surgery and Obstetrics. (*Oxford English Dictionary*)

The Hausa concept of *magani* includes both of these senses, but it also includes much more. To translate *magani* into English simply as "medicine" is to convey only a portion of the range of meanings this word has in Hausa usage. In order to understand some of the more puzzling aspects of Hausa medical practice, this range of meanings must be explored.

Lafiya is a Hausa word generally translated as "health." As has been pointed out in previous chapters, however, *lafiya* embraces a range of meanings that extends beyond the English notion of "health" to include the proper ordering, correct structuring, and general well-being of the social order and the individual's relations within it, as well as the state of wellness in the human body. When an individual is ill he has no *lafiya*; but similarly, when affairs in a village are in turmoil and times are bad one hears expressions like *Gari ya lallace, ba mu da lafiya,* "The town has spoiled, we have no *lafiya,*" and it is the social or moral order which has been disrupted in this case, not bodily functions. That which corrects either of these situations and brings about the right state of affairs is *magani,* "medicine."

Magani is a "remedy," a "corrective," an "active restorer of a disrupted state" or a "prophylactic against trouble." *Magani* is thus perhaps best defined as "that which restores *lafiya,*" or "that which ensures *lafiya.*" As such, *magani* can refer to anything which corrects or prevents an undesirable condition.

The mud plaster used in roof repair during the dry season is called *maganin ruwa* or "medicine for [rain]water." Blankets are *maganin 'dari* or "medicine for cold"; insecticides are *maganin sauro,* "medicine for mosquitoes"; food may be called *maganin yunwa,* "medicine for hunger." A sharp, pointed stick may be referred to as *maganin barawo,* "medicine for a thief."

Not surprisingly, given this supple range of meaning, *magani* is a favorite workhorse for Hausa proverbs: *Dukiya maganin 'kan'kanci,* "Wealth is the medicine for ill-treatment." *Yunwa maganin mugunyar dafuwa,* "Hunger is the medicine for bad cooking." *Maganin tsoro barci,* "The medicine for fear is sleep." *Ajiya maganin wata rana,* "Laying aside is the medicine for the future." *Gida biyu maganin gobara,* "Having two houses is the medicine for house fires." *Barin kashi a ciki ba ya maganin yunwa,* "Refusing to defecate is not the medicine for hunger." *Maganin gari da nesa tafiya,* "The medicine for a distant town is walking." *Maganin kiyaya rabuwa,* "The medicine for hatred is separation." *Maganin maki gudu ban kashi,* "The medicine for a slackard is a beating." *Yawan rai maganin aloba,* "A plenitude of life is the medicine for pestilence." *Hakuri maganin duniya,* "Patience is the world's medicine." And, of course, the ultimate Hausa proverb: *Allah maganin kome,* "God is the medicine for everything."

"Medicine," in this view, thus encompasses practically the whole range of human activities, since it can include any act which results in the restoration, maintenance, or creation of order and balance. It may refer to a substance administered as a drug or to an action performed for a therapeutic purpose. It refers to actions or substances that are used therapeutically or prophylactically to restore or enhance an individual's physical, mental, or social health. Thus, *magani* can be the application of a cupping horn by a barber or the splinting of a broken limb by a bonesetter. It can be the herbal powder given by a healer to remedy an illness or a Koranic charm worn to ensure (it is hoped) success as a market trader, sexual attractiveness, or popularity. In common usage *magani* generally refers to *substances* which are thought to possess powers that can bring these things to pass.

Hausa medicines include substances of animal, vegetable, and mineral origin, as well as texts taken from the religious and esoteric literature of Islam.[1] They may be administered in almost any manner: by drinking them as a medicinal gruel (*salala*) or tonic (*tsimi*), by washing with them, by taking them as powders in food, by inhaling them as vapors from a steaming mixture or smoke from a fire (*turare*),[2] by enema (*guguci*), by burying them in one's house (*kafi*),[3] or by wearing them around one's neck in a leather pouch called a *laya* or around the waist in a belt called a *guru*. Often several such modes of administration are combined. As Robinson noted with frustration (1900:142–43):

> We took with us a very large supply of English medicines, many of which we found it quite impossible to use with any effect, owing to the reluctance of the patients to submit to any lengthy course of treatment. They seemed to think that it could only be due to the incapacity of the doctor if a disease of many years' standing could not be cured in a day. As in most instances the applicants for medicine were unable to read, it was necessary to give them verbal

1. Hausa medicinal plants are dealt with in detail in Adam et al. (1972). A long list of Hausa *materia medica* is given in G. Nicolas (1975:405–7). Pharmacologic evaluations of Hausa medicines are given in Parrott (1970), Etkin (1980, 1981), and Etkin and Ross (1982). Additional information on Hausa ethnobotany may be found in Dalziel (1916, 1937).

2. *Turare* is used to refer to any vapor or scent, including perfume, the vapors of gasoline, aerosol insecticides, etc. It also is used for medicinal substances placed on fires, in distinction from the normal word for smoke, *hayaki*.

3. *Kafi* refers to a hut made of cornstalks or to a stockade constructed around a town (*kafin gari*), as well as to a medicine buried in the ground inside the entry-hut of a compound to protect it, or a charm buried inside the walls of a town to ensure its invulnerability.

instructions as to how their medicine was to be taken, the result
being that the patient, often forgetting the instructions which he
had received, would occasionally have recourse to an empirical
method of treatment which was not always productive of the best
results. During our stay in Tunis,[4] one patient returned after the
lapse of several days to complain of the medicine which had been
given to him, and on being questioned as to how he had used it,
stated that he had first drunk some of it, and then finding its taste
disagreeable, had washed himself with the remainder, the results
of either operation proving equally unsatisfactory.

The advent of scientific medicine has added another method of administration to this list of therapeutic techniques: injection, known in
Hausa as *allura* or "needle." It is not uncommon for individuals having
access to an old syringe and a set of used needles to set themselves up
in the business of giving injections. These practitioners are very popular, the pain of the injection being an indication of the strength of the
medicine used (in the Hausa view). These medicines may be pirated
antibiotics, aspirin tablets mixed with well-water, or herbal remedies.
Generally they are given under unsterile conditions and can lead to a
wide variety of complications ranging from local inflammation to ab-
scesses, necrosis, gas gangrene, and even death (Fry 1965). In spite of
the potential consequences of illicit injections, the procedure is the most
common and best understood therapeutic practice of modern scientific
medicine. In an area where access to high quality medical care is virtually nonexistent, it is hardly surprising that the external features of
such care should be popularized.

■ Medicine Sellers: The *Magori* and the *Kantankar*

The largest portion of traditional Hausa therapeutics consists of the
administration of herbal medicines designed to cure specific disorders
or to ward off illnesses and the agents causing them. Herbalism is the
essence of *maganin gargajiya*—"traditional medicine"—which can be
contrasted to *maganin zamani*, "the medicine of modern times," or

4. Robinson is speaking here of his experiences among the Hausa-speaking community in Tunis which, in this regard, are quite applicable to the Hausa heartland
in northern Nigeria.

maganin asibiti, "hospital medicine." Hausa bontanical lore is extensive, and well over a thousand plants, trees, and shrubs have been listed in Dalziel's *Hausa Botanical Vocabulary* (Dalziel 1916). Any part of a plant may have medicinal uses: the roots (*saiwa,* pl. *saiwoyi*), chips (*sassake*) hacked from the bark and underlying wood, the sap (*ruwa*), fruit (*'ya'ya*), leaves (*ganye,* pl. *ganyaye*), flowers or blossoms (*fure,* pl. *furanni*), and the seeds (*kwayoyi,* a term also applied to the pills dispensed at hospitals and infirmaries). Other items from the natural environment such as animal droppings, insects, honey, twigs from the nests of birds, feathers, or animal skins may be used medicinally because of their reputed therapeutic powers.

Many herbal remedies and the plants from which they are made are common knowledge. Individuals and families often have their own special recipes for medicine which they pass on from generation to generation. There are, however, individuals who make herbal medicines their specialty. These are the *magori,* an itinerant medicine salesman usually preoccupied with love philtres, aphrodisiacs, and similar medicines; the *kantankar* or *mai-saidda magani* ("the medicine seller"), also known as the *'dan ganye* or "son of leaves," who sells medicines on a regular basis in the markets of the area in which he lives—the rural Hausa equivalent of the pharmacist or dispensing chemist; and the *boka* or "herbal healer," who acts as a consulting physician. At this point our concern is with the first two; the *boka* will be discussed later.

Aphrodisiacs comprise a large share of the Hausa pharmacopoeia. Collectively they are known as *gagai,* but there are many other names as well: *maganin mata,* "medicine for women"; *maganin aikin dare,* "medicine for the night's work"; *maganin burar gajiya,* "medicine for a tired penis"; *maganin cin da'din duri,* "medicine for the pleasant 'eating' of a vagina," etc. The components of these medicines consist of a wide variety of materials—roots, wood chips, herbs—most of which bear a striking resemblance to an erect penis or have aromatic properties of some sort. Hot, spicy materials (*kayan yaji*) are especially favored ingredients of these compounds because they are thought to increase male sexual potency and at the same time to ward off the ill effects of cold.

Other "social" or "magical" medicines hawked by the *magori* are things such as *maganin 'karfe* ("medicine for metal")—amulets and potions supposed to prevent the body from being cut by knives, hoes,

or weapons in war—*maganin farin jini* ("medicine for 'white blood,'
that is, popularity) or *maganin tarawar ku'di* ("medicine for attracting
money"), both thought to increase one's success in business—a wide
range of compounds for almost any desired purpose.

The *magori* is a generally disreputable character. Ill clad, often
dressed in ragged skins and carrying a bag of medicines slung over his
shoulder, he walks from village to village crying out his wares and singing descriptive (often ribald) songs to attract business. Of low social
status, he seldom spends much time in any one place, being here today
and gone tomorrow—a convenient habit considering his line of work,
where the failure of an aphrodisiac or the sudden down-turn in a
client's business fortunes might lead to unpleasant encounters with
dissatisfied customers.

The market medicine seller (*mai-saidda magani* or *kantankar*) is a
somewhat more respected person, usually being an inhabitant of the
area in which he lives and works, a part of the community rather than
an itinerant peddler. He may make his living partly from his sales of
herbal medicines in the market and the rest from a small farm, or he
may rely solely upon his ability to sell *magani* in the marketplace—in
which case he is almost certainly poor. Like other village traders he
brings his wares to the marketplace on market day, unrolls his tarp or
bundle in his stall or under the shade of a tree, and waits for business
to come to him. In most cases the medicines he sells are bits of bark
and wood or roots of plants familiar to his patrons. Rather than seek
out these items in the bush themselves and go to the trouble of digging
up roots or chopping the bark off trees (which can be very laborious
work), they come to the market medicine seller to ask for a particular
ingredient: *sassaken minjiriya*, for example, wood chips from the coral
tree, *Erythrina senegalensis*, widely regarded as a cure for *shawara*
(jaundiced fatigue). The herbalist then digs into his mounds of medicine, pulls out a few strips of the requisite bark, several sections of
roots, a handful of leaves—whatever is necessary—ties them up with
a bit of twine or a piece of hemp, and gives them to the customer, who
tenders ten or twenty kobo in return. In other cases a person may ask
for a remedy for a specific complaint, such as *ciwon ciki* (gastrointestinal distress). The herbalist will then gather the ingredients for the
remedy he recommends, together with verbal instructions as how best
to use it. If he is out of a certain substance he may agree to look for it

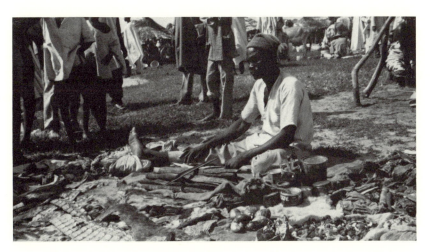

10. *A medicine seller in a village market.*

and set it aside the next time he goes out medicine collecting, bringing it for his customer on a subsequent market day. At the end of market he will pack up his wares and return home, going to another market on a following day, or perhaps out into the bush to collect more medicines.

In general the market medicine seller serves as a source for the raw ingredients the general populace uses in making up their own cures— as a sort of pharmaceutical supply house for home use. Home remedies are very popular. Since strength (*'karfi*) is one of the most obvious ways that a villager monitors his health, the maintenance and cultivation of strength is one of his more pressing concerns. A major aid in ensuring strength is *maganin 'karfin jiki,* "medicine for bodily strength," which nearly every man utilizes from time to time. These medicines are usually herbal concoctions known as *tsimi,* made from steeping roots or wood chips in clay pots full of water. The resulting liquid contains many different ingredients and is usually quite pungent. Each of these individual ingredients may have its own medicinal use, thought to combine with the others to produce a highly valued synergistic effect. In explaining his personal recipe for a *tsimi,* which was held in high repute locally, one old man sorted through an enormous pile of roots and wood chips gathered for his brew and pointed out each ingredient individually, naming medicines useful in the treatment of back pain, snakebite, fever, "internal strictures" (*amosani*), urinary disorders, impotence, the ill effects of cold in the body (*sanyin jiki*), for inducing popularity and sexual attractiveness, avoiding the cutting effects of knives and hoes, afflictions caused by spirits, swellings of the body, teething ailments in infants, and venereal disease, as well as for preventing fatigue and ensuring strength. Such tonics function rather like vitamin supplements in the popular Euro-American perception, serving to maintain bodily health, increase vigor, and prevent illness from catching someone.

The ingredients for these tonics are found in the bush, and the process of collecting medicines is arduous. The herbalist usually sets out shortly after daybreak, as soon as he has finished eating his morning *tuwo* or drunk his hot *kunu*, a tasty, tart gruel. He will take with him one or two implements—usually an axe (*gatari*) or a short, sharp hoe (*magirbi*) different from the hoe used for cultivating the fields (*fartanya*)—as well as a large canvas or heavy plastic bag. He then trudges out into the bush, frequently miles from the village, to those locations where he has found trees, herbs, shrubs, and plants of the kind he wants. Often the location of the tree is important. Trees close to a river may have more powerful properties in the treatment of certain maladies than those located away from a river. Remedies designed to increase the flow of a mother's breast milk, for example, or to cure urinary disorders, are better if found close to a flowing source of water. Plants growing high on a hill are preferable to those growing down low if one is seeking medicines effective against evil spirits. Depending on what he is seeking—bark and wood chips, roots, leaves, flowers, seeds, or fruit—the herbalist will then set about stripping the bark or digging up some of the roots, or taking whatever else is needed.

Before beginning, an invocation to the tree is frequently (but not necessarily) made—usually the opening of the *fatiha*, the first sura of the Koran: *Bismillahi-rrahmani-rrahim*, "In the name of God, the merciful, the compassionate," perhaps followed by a short exclamation such as *Allah shi taimake mu*, "May God help us." Sometimes the medicine collector will take time to praise the tree, saying how powerful its medicinal properties are, how they exceed the powers of the evil spirits (*aljannu*), the "invisible men" (*mutanen 'boye*), healers (*bokaye*), the powers of witches, sorcery (*mayu, sammu*), and all the illnesses (*ciwo*) plaguing people. On some occasions much more elaborate ceremonies may be undertaken. One herbalist, 'Dam Baba, once lit a huge bundle of grass after making a long invocation to a *shirinya* tree (*Ficus sp.*) and circled it three times with the flames burning, scorching the trunk, after which he began the process of chopping off sections of the bark. He stated this was so the fire would enter the tree and enhance the medicine, which would follow the illness and "burn it out" of the patient's body when it was administered.

The preliminaries completed, actual collection of the medicine then begins. The ground is dug away from the roots and they are chopped out with the axe and then cut into small sections for easy transport. In the case of a small tree, the whole thing may be uprooted, chopped to bits, and stored in the sack. Bark is stripped either by hacking it off with an axe or a hoe or by beating the tree all around with a large piece of wood to loosen the bark, and then flaking it off. Depending on the scarcity of the material, how far one has traveled to obtain it, and similar factors, an entire tree may be denuded in one of these expeditions.

All the medicines thus obtained are thrown together in a hodgepodge in the bag and separated upon returning home. A herbalist has extensive knowledge of the plants in his pharmacopoeia and can distinguish them by sight, texture, and smell. It is common to see a herbalist reach into a huge, jumbled pile of roots and branches, pull out a root by sight, sniff it, throw it away, reach back into the pile, and pull out the correct one. In accompanying herbalists to the bush it is not uncommon to have eighty or more plants and their medical uses pointed out in the course of a virtually nonstop two- or three-hour lecture on the nature and practice of *maganin gargajiya*.

Medicines thus collected are treated in various ways. They may be sold by the bundle as raw ingredients, or they may be prepared as powders. In the latter case, once they are brought back to the village they are spread out on a mat to dry in the sun and are then placed in a mortar and pounded with a pestle until they have been reduced to a fine powder by the women of the household. This powder is then stored in a gourd bowl, wrapped in paper or placed in a plastic sack to be kept until such time as it is needed in treatment or is taken to the market to be sold.

Herbalists tend to be proud of their profession, which they view as a noble one in the sight of God. The idea is quite prominent that God has placed medicinal plants on the face of the earth for the use of man,

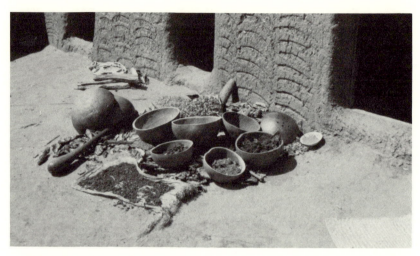

11. Herbal medicines drying in the sun.

and that by gathering and promoting the use of their medicines—which they often refer to as *maganin Allah*, "medicines from God"—they as medicine sellers are fulfilling a charitable, perhaps quasi-religious, role in life. Some even refuse to name a price for the medicines they sell, preferring to accept what the customer offers, regarding their work as a kind of *sadaka*, or "almsgiving," which while not gaining them much financial reward nonetheless gives them a sense of purpose and fulfillment that transcends the ordinary occupation (*sana'a*).

Garba the Kantankar is a case in point. He showed up in the village market one day carrying a big bundle of medicines and established himself under the shade of a large tree, where he spread out his wares and made himself at home. Clad in tatters and possessing literally only the clothes on his back, a few bowls, and a hoe, he nonetheless was a cheerful, happy man. He stayed in the village living under the shade of the tree in the market for nearly eight months, selling medicines on market days, going out to collect medicines at other times, doing a few odd jobs such as collecting firewood, teasing children, and gossiping with the people who passed by. His wife eventually came and joined him, and they lived together in the market for months, sleeping on the ground under the stars, before moving on. Many villagers who saw him only at a distance thought he was slightly crazy, but those who knew him well were impressed with his sense of dedication to his chosen occupation, his vast store of botanical knowledge, and his carefree personality. He was a man doing what he enjoyed, unconcerned for piling up material wealth and dedicated to what he saw as a somewhat higher purpose in life—herbal medicine—than that to which the average market trader clung.

Not all market medicine sellers are quite so dedicated or sincere, however, and the drugs available in the market are not always limited to traditional Hausa medicines. Nigerian drug regulation is virtually nonexistent and if one knows where to look and is willing to pay the price, nearly any drug may be obtained. *Magani* is *magani*, no matter what the source. Aspirin or A.P.C. tablets (aspirin, phenacetin, and caffeine) are ubiquitous, but amphetamines and similarly dangerous drugs are also easily obtained. Even in a rural village the lower social strata use *jan kafsu* ("red capsules") and combine them with alcohol to get high—a procedure regarded with disdain by the rest of village society.[5] Patent medicines and self-proclaimed "wonder drugs" do a brisk business, and the rural population is set upon by unscrupulous hucksters even as are their city brethren.

One market day a white Lada automobile, complete with loudspeaker pulled into the village four miles south advertising a cure-all for "toothache, headaches, stomach pains, internal ailments of all kinds" and many other disorders as well. For ten kobo one could buy this miracle cure from a handsomely dressed Hausa man standing in front of the automobile with an attaché case. Upon buying a small packet of this medicine and returning home, however, it was found to contain two well-wrapped aspirin tablets.

In another case one villager purchased a bottle of little yellow tablets to alleviate his coughing and chest pains. He had diagnosed his condition as *shawara* (extreme fatigue, usually associated with jaundice), a

5. The drug problem was considered severe enough by the state government to undertake some publicity on the matter. One day a loudspeaker van from the Ministry of Information pulled into the village for a film show. The showing of the film was preceded by a long exhortation to avoid drug use and to report those people who sold dangerous drugs. The film, oddly enough, was a twenty-five-year-old documentary on the visit of Queen Elizabeth II to Nigeria. Although the sound was inaudible and the reels were not shown in the proper order, it was enjoyed by all those present. Some aspects of the drug problem in northern Nigeria are discussed in Salamone (1973).

term he translated into English as "yellow fever." The bright yellow
color of the pills linked it with activity against the jaundice he feared
would result from his condition. The label on the bottle read:

> ALLIGOA GARLIC PILLS (EXTRA STRONG)
> combined with mistletoe and hawthorne,
> against senility, high blood pressure,
> arteriosclerosis and digestive troubles.
> Taken three times daily, two tablets before
> meals. E. Scheurich—Baden, Germany;
> Accra and Yaba—Pharmco, Ltd.

Such cure-alls are very popular and fit in with Hausa medical notions as
medicines ensuring bodily strength. Energizing tonics such as the omnipresent Maltona can be found in all towns of any size, often sold alongside Coca-Cola and Fanta. Guinness and Power Stout are felt by many
Nigerians to have similar health-giving (and aphrodisiac) properties.

■ *Wanzami:* The Hausa Barber-Surgeon

While medicine sellers function largely as pharmacists, the *wanzami* is
an important therapeutic practitioner who performs the functions of
both barber and surgeon. As a barber his principal occupation is shaving the heads of village men and boys at regular intervals.[6] (Women
take care of their own coiffures, plaiting their hair in braids close to the
head, a process known as *kitso.*) The procedure is simple. The customer
sits on the ground in the shade of a building or tree, and the barber sits
on the ground in front of him with his straight razor, a bar of soap,
and a cup a water. He wets the man's hair with water from the cup,
lathers it slightly with the bar of soap, and then proceeds to shave off
the hair, leaving the scalp completely bald. Nothing special is done with
the shavings; usually the customer will gather them up and give them

---

6. Among younger men, particularly secondary school students and those having
some exposure to the more cosmopolitan influences of the cities, this practice is
diminishing in favor of close-cropped or styled hair, which is often accompanied
by extravagant clothes, high platform shoes, and other forms of conspicuous con-
sumerism that mark the successful son of the village as thoroughly "modern" *'dan
gai,* a "son of pretentiousness" or a "dude."

to one of his sons to take inside and dispose of them, or the barber will accumulate a pile of them and dispose of them all at once. As a final touch the barber will often rub the pulp of a partially chewed kolanut over the shaved head. The price for this service is nominal—in 1976 it was generally ten kobo per head. In addition to his cosmetic functions as a barber, however, the *wanzami* performs a number of minor surgical operations.

Hausa surgery is rudimentary at best. There are no procedures that could compare, for example, with the delicate trephinations performed by the Arabs of Algeria described by Hilton-Simpson (1922).[7] The most common Hausa surgical procedure is cupping, known as *kaho* or "horn," in reference to the barber's cupping horn. As has been noted in chapter 5, in Hausa medical thought cold has the dual effects of killing the blood and causing an increase in the body's phlegm, which may likewise kill normal, healthy, red blood. Since the presence of "dead blood" in the body is a frequent cause of localized swellings, tiredness, and feeling out of sorts, in the Hausa view, cupping is the common remedy through which relief from these conditions is sought.

The procedure itself is simple and straightforward. First the part of the body to be cupped—usually the back, shoulder, neck, or chest—is washed. Then the cupping horn, a simple cow's horn with a small hole bored into the top to allow for suction, is placed over the area to be

7. In this regard the statement by Maclean in her book on Yoruba medical practices in Ibadan is puzzling. She writes, with reference to the Hausa quarter (*sabo*) of Ibadan (1971:65): "The Hausa community maintain their own customs in this part of Ibadan and their barbers are renowned for a knowledge of surgical procedures derived from the early days of Arabic medicine." It is unclear precisely what she means by this statement, for following it she describes the four major surgical procedures performed by Hausa barbers: cupping, uvulectomy, circumcision, and tattooing. This hardly constitutes renowned surgery from the early days of Arabic medicine, as a reading of Elgood's discussion of Safavid surgery in Persia (1970: 121–89) will demonstrate. Similarly, it is hard to believe that Hausa barbers have a renowned knowledge of Islamic literature, since the craft is one of relatively low social status and most barbers (at least in rural areas in the north) are illiterate. Then, too, Ismail Abdulla did not uncover any classical works of Arabic medicine and surgery in his researches on Arabic medical manuscripts in northern Nigeria (Abdalla 1979). The works of Rhazes and Avicenna appear to be virtually unknown in the Hausa heartland. Either Maclean means that the Yoruba perceive Hausa barbers as having access to the secrets of Islamic surgery, or she has overextended her prose.

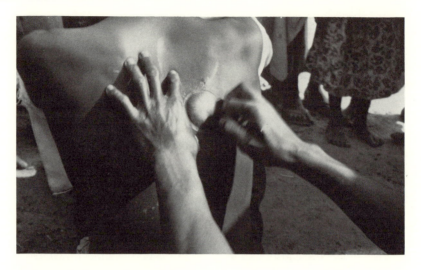

12. Cupping: Making the incisions.

treated and the air is sucked out, creating a partial vacuum inside.[8] The top of the horn is then capped with a small piece of tendon, slipped into place by the barber's tongue as he draws out the air. The horn is allowed to remain on the skin until it raises a welt, at which time it is removed. The welt is then washed with water and a series of cuts are made with the razor within the circle outlined by the horn—usually three rows of five vertical cuts each, although there is no special significance to the pattern of the cuts. The horn is then replaced over the welt, the air is removed, and the horn is again capped with a piece of tendon and allowed to set. Blood is gradually drawn out of the shallow cuts made by the barber and coagulates inside the horn. From time to time in the course of the treatment the barber will remove the horn, shake out the dark, congealed blood into a gourd filled with sand, and reapply suction to the horn. The dark blood thus obtained is regarded as the "dead blood" responsible for the area of swelling or the patient's lassitude and feeling of listlessness. Approximately one or two table-

8. An alternative, but less common method involves the use of a small, round gourd instead of a cow's horn. A hole is cut in the side of a dried gourd and a piece of cotton is placed inside. The cotton is then set alight and the gourd is placed over the area to be cupped. The flame inside the gourd uses up the oxygen, creating a partial vacuum sufficient to provide suction.

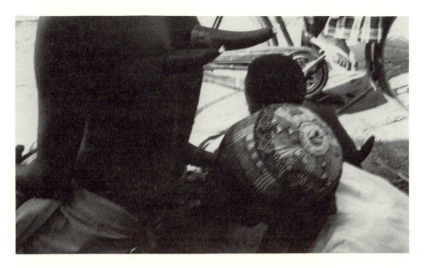

13. Cupping: Application of the horn over the incisions.

spoons of congealed blood is obtained from each cupping horn in the course of this procedure. The cost of treatment in 1976 was usually ten kobo per horn applied. The practice is very common and there is scarcely a single person in a Hausa village—man, woman, or child— who if examined will not bear the telltale series of small lines of scars somewhere where he or she has been cupped.

In addition to cupping, the barber performs a number of other surgical procedures: circumcision, uvulectomy, and tattooing. Circumcision was discussed in some detail in chapter 2. Uvulectomy takes place three or four days after the birth of the child. Using a long tool resembling a pair of pliers the barber excises the uvula (*beli*), it being feared that it will grow large over time and block the throat, leading to starvation or suffocation. The procedure may also be reperformed on adults.[9] Tattooing (*jarfa*) is done on the naming day to apply the familial dis-

9. Hospitals in northern Nigeria see numerous cases of this procedure gone awry, resulting in severe bleeding. When I showed villagers that I still had my uvula and insisted that it was not at all necessary to have it removed, they insisted that the reason mine had not grown to pathological proportions was the fact that I had drunk medicine to prevent this as a child, a medicine unknown to them. Clitoridectomy is not usually performed, there being no socially sanctioned ceremony of female circumcision equivalent to that performed on the male.

tinguishing marks, and is also performed on women and young girls for cosmetic purposes. (Aside from family markings men are not tattooed.) The procedure involves making a series of shallow cuts in the skin to form a pattern (stylized scorpions and lizards are popular, particularly on the forearms), then rubbing soot or ink into the incisions and allowing them to heal over. The area thus incised may be quite swollen and tender for several days, and the potential for infection is obviously high.[10]

Besides these surgical functions there are two ailments whose treatment is seen as the special domain of the barber: *ciwon saifa* and *balli-balli*. *Ciwon saifa* or "illness of the spleen," is a condition which primarily afflicts children. It is characterized by swelling in the left lower abdomen due to enlargement of the spleen. In an area where malaria is endemic and is a major cause of infant mortality, it is not surprising that this is a noticeable complaint. The condition is usually ascribed by the Hausa as either a creation of God (*halittar Allah*) which manifests itself in the early life of the child, or due to some disorder of the blood in the spleen. The treatment involves bleeding the child by making a number of incisions over the swollen area, after which the cuts are rubbed with a herbal medicine. *Balli-balli* refers to a disorder of the blood often found in children that causes palpitations of the heart. The treatment involves making a number of cuts over the heart and down the shoulder and arm on the left side of the body. Severe headache in the temporal area or over the eye—a condition called *jiri*—often accompanied by dizziness (*juwa*), is seen as due to "hot blood" or to the rushing and pounding of the blood in the afflicted region, and may also be treated by cupping or bleeding. Afflictions such as *balli-balli*, *ciwon saifa*, and *jiri* again point out the importance of the blood in Hausa medicine as an explanatory medium for illness, and in some respects the Hausa barber may be conveniently regarded as a kind of "ethno-hematologist."

Two other surgical procedures merit attention, at least in passing. The first of these is *sakiya*, or lancing. When inflammation develops in response to an infection the affected tissue begins to swell (*kumbura*). If the infection is contained by the body's defenses and remains local-

10. Hence the Hausa proverb *Wanzami ba ya son jarfa*, "The barber does not like to be tattooed," i.e., "The shoe is on the other foot."

ized, an accumulation of pus (*magunta* or "evil") forms in the center of the inflammation. When it becomes fluctuent the Hausa then say that the abscess "has made water" (*ya yi ruwa*), and it may be lanced to release the entrapped fluid. This is done by heating a metal arrow in a fire until it is very hot and then applying it to the wound as a cautery, a painful process that is not without its complications.[11] The other procedure, now rendered obsolete, was the traditional process of inoculation to prevent smallpox, a practice of considerable antiquity in West Africa, which was reported to exist in northern Nigeria by several early travelers through those regions. Denham, for example, wrote of his experiences with smallpox in Borno (1826, I:199–200):

> On my return I visited my patients, for Doctor Oudney could not move from his hut; and the small-pox raged amongst the slaves of two of our friends, added to the fever of the season. Out of twelve slaves who were seized, two had died; and the only child of Mo-hamed-el-Wordy had now taken it from his slave. They are not ignorant of inoculation, and it is performed nearly in the same manner as amongst ourselves, by inserting the sharp point of the dagger, charged with the disease; they never give any medicine but merely roll the invalid in a barracan, and lay him in a corner of the hut until the disorder takes a turn.

This procedure was reported in some detail and its effectiveness noted by a qualified medical observer at the beginning of this century (Foy 1915). Fortunately, government vaccination programs carried out in conjunction with the World Health Organization have now eliminated this disease completely and the traditional preventive measures (as well as their more scientific counterparts) are no longer needed.

11. One rather poignant example of this involved the son of one of my closest friends. This small boy, still a toddler, was sitting on the ground playing near the woodpile in his father's compound when he inadvertently knocked over a log. This large piece of wood fell over and landed on the boy's penis, resulting in an extremely painful injury. This wound became inflamed and swollen, and in an effort to alleviate the child's suffering his father applied a cautery to the child's penis some days later. As can be imagined, this made matters much worse, and it was only through his father's decision to seek more sophisticated medical care at a dispensary several miles away that an extremely serious situation was avoided. The application of antibiotics and dressings prevented further complications.

■ *Ma'dori:* The Bonesetter

Bonesetters are probably the indigenous medical practitioners most
highly regarded by the scientific medical community in Hausaland. By
and large they do a creditable job, in veterinary as well as in human
cases. Among the local population they have a very high reputation
indeed, and it is rare to find more than a few cases of broken bones
treated at government hospitals in rural areas in any given month. This
is partly due to the fact that indigenous bonesetters are far more accessible to the majority of the population than are hospitals; but even
among well-educated men and women the traditional bonesetter is often
preferred.[12] Following the setting of the bone a short splint, made of a
number of short sticks or cornstalks lashed together to form a flexible
mat, is applied around the broken limb, together with herbal potions.
Often (particularly among the Fulani) cattle dung is used as a poulticing agent. This indigenous splint is more "natural looking" and more
flexible than the unwieldy plaster casts applied at hospitals and is one
reason why local bonesetters are favored over hospital treatment. Additionally, local bonesetters tend to remove the splint earlier than would
an orthopedic surgeon, giving the impression of the bone having healed
faster under his care than under hospital supervision; but perhaps the
major reason why the *ma'dori* is favored in the treatment of broken
bones is, oddly enough, a consequence of the traditional treatment itself. Many of the orthopedic cases brought to the hospital for treatment
are complicated fracture cases which have first been treated in the local
setting. Given the poor sanitary conditions in which most of this treatment takes place, it is not surprising that sepsis sets in, and since hospitals are often "courts of last resort" for the sick from rural areas,
infection has often reached unmanageable proportions by the time the
patient arrives at the hospital. Often the only course of action is amputation of the limb, which alienates everyone concerned and serves to
enhance the reputation of traditional bonesetters, who do not perform
amputations. Once the view takes root that the hospital is a place where

12. For example, one friend of mine from southern Zaria, a respected laboratory
technician in a hospital in the north, told me incredible tales about the prowess
of a bonesetter in his home community. He told me how this man could manipu-
late the bones by his powers while away from the patient in another room, how
he had reattached limbs which had been severed from the body, even limbs which
had been chopped into pieces, and so on.

broken limbs are likely to be amputated, people are even more reluctant to go to them for treatment (see also Stock 1979:5).

■ *Ungozoma:* The Traditional Hausa Midwife

Undoubtedly the most common event in Hausaland requiring some kind of major medical intervention is childbirth (*haifuwa*). Children are greatly desired by the Hausa and the bearing of children is regarded as the principal usefulness (*amfani*) of women. The Koran (II:223) refers to women as the "tillage" of men, as fields wherein men grow crops of offspring, and children are frequently referred to by Hausa men as the profit (*riba*) of marriage which they obtain from the investment of their bridewealth. The notion of abortion is abhorrent and infanticide is unthinkable; both would be actions possible only for unbelievers (*kafirai*).[13] The only effective form of birth control available is abstention from sexual intercourse, particularly during the prolonged nursing period for each child which lasts two years before weaning.[14] If followed rigorously this would at least allow a regular spacing of births but, perhaps understandably, Hausa men regard this as an onerous imposition and many admit that they ignore it. Conversely, they also use this culturally sanctioned rule as a justification for patronizing prostitutes, as well as an explanation for the practice of having more than one wife.

During the course of the pregnancy the woman abstains from bitter foods and also from excessively sweet foods. The former is thought to "spoil" (*bace*) the child in the womb; the latter collects in the uterus and causes difficult childbirth by creating a film over the vagina, known in Hausa as *zaki* ("sweetness," also the term for the amniotic fluid) or *gishiri* ("salt"), this latter term also being used for the white exudations which appear on clay walls or the bottoms of pots as a result of dampness.

13. The Koran specifically prohibits infanticide (XVII:31–33) and says further (LXXXI:8) that on the day of judgment "the buried infant shall be asked for what sin she was slain." Prostitutes are widely reputed to know many abortifacient medicines.
14. This, too, is a practice enjoined by the Koran (II:233, XXXI:13–14, XLVI:14–15). Lactating women are, of course, relatively infertile (see Konner and Worthman 1980, Short 1984).

Women continue to work until the onset of labor, at which time they retire to their rooms to deliver, often alone and unassisted. When the child is delivered the midwife is sent for, usually an old woman who is a relative or friend of the family. Her task is to cut the umbilical cord and wash it until the bleeding stops; often considerable loss of blood attends this practice (Fleischer 1975). Following this she disposes of the umbilical cord and afterbirth (*mahaifa,* the same term as that for the uterus) by burying them behind the compound. In cases of difficult or prolonged labor surgical cutting is attempted on the vaginal wall to alleviate the condition of *gishiri.* This cutting is done with a small razor or sharp knife by a midwife or older woman with experience in the procedure and often results in hemorrhage, infection, and the formation of fistulas with long-term disability.[15]

Following the birth of a child the mother is regarded as weakened and in increased danger of becoming ill. She is thought to be particularly susceptible to the effects of damp cold (*sanyi*) and for this reason must undertake a long series of very hot baths. The effects of these baths are supplemented by a diet composed of hot, spicy foods and confinement in a hot room. These hot baths are regarded as mandatory for all births, but are thought especially necessary for the first. If the new mother has not delivered at the home of her parents on the occasion of her first birth, she will nonetheless return there for instruction and guidance (and possibly coercion) in the matter of these washings.[16]

The procedure is as follows. A large amount of water is heated over the fire, sometimes with the addition of herbal ingredients. The new mother is then forced to take a bundle of branches from a tree, dip it into the hot water, and beat herself with the steaming leaves to obtain the health-giving effects of the heat, which is said to make her body strong, build up the blood, and ward off *sanyi.* These baths must be undertaken twice a day for forty days, and thereafter once a day for several months. In women who have had more than one child, the length of the baths is usually reduced. In cases of miscarriage the cri-

15. Aspects of *gishiri* are considered in an interesting paper by Murray Last (1979) on the Maguzawa. Obstetrics and gynecology are the most dismal aspects of traditional Hausa medicine, and due to the practices of wife seclusion among the Muslim population are probably the areas least amenable to change.

16. An excellent discussion of Hausa pregnancy and childbirth practices is found in Trevitt (1973).

terion for taking hot therapeutic baths seems to be whether or not the fetus is recognizably human. If the age of the fetus is only three or four months it is thought that it is necessary to take only warm or cool baths. After about five months, however, the miscarriage is treated essentially as a normal birth for purposes of washing.[17]

Following this hot bath the mother is taken into her room and placed on a bed of dried mud. This bed has a cavity under it rather like a fireplace, and a small fire is kindled underneath while she rests on top, the object being to augment the effects of the heat. This is an ancient Hausa custom, remarked upon by the sixteenth-century traveler Leo Africanus, who observed (mistaking the reasons for the practice), as follows (L. Africanus 1896:831): "Some part of this kingdom is plane, and the residue mountainous, but the mountains are extremely cold, and the plains intolerably hot. And because they can hardly indure the sharpness of winter, they kindle great fires in the midst of their houses, laying the coles thereof under their high bedsteads, and so betaking themselves to sleepe." Should such a bed not be available, as in the case of a woman who sleeps on a modern metal-frame bed, hot coals are taken into the room to keep it appropriately sweltering.

In addition to these hot baths and the heat treatments in bed, the woman supplants her diet with large amounts of potash gruel (*kunun kanwa*). This is a food made from millet or guinea-corn heavily laden with pepper, spices, and potash (a type of salt consisting mainly of sodium carbonate), which is thought to be effective in helping fight off the effects of cold.

These practices seem to be related to the high incidence of peripartum cardiac failure found among Hausa women when compared with the women of surrounding areas in Nigeria (Davidson et al. 1974). It has been suggested that the massive sodium loading obtained from the medicinal potash gruel causes a marked increase in extracellular fluid and plasma volumes, with a resultant increase in cardiac work. The hot baths and lying on a hot bed in a hot room may then further increase cardiac output and cardiac work, ultimately resulting in heart failure if the myocardium for any reason is vulnerable, a condition to which Hausa women appear especially susceptible.

17. M. G. Smith (1954:26) reports that in the Zaria area these washings are not undertaken in cases of miscarriage.

■ *Mallam:* The Koranic Scholar

The Koranic scholar, or *mallam,* is a prominent figure in Hausa life and an important medical practitioner. The word *mallam* derives from the Arabic *mu'allim,* or "teacher," and refers to an educated person, particularly one who is literate in Arabic and knowledgeable about Islamic matters, although it is also used by polite extension as a respectful form of address for any man. In this extended sense the word has approximately the same meaning as the English "mister," e.g., Mallam Ibrahim, "Mister Ibrahim."

As an educated man the *mallam* has access to a body of information and ideas that remain closed to the illiterate village farmer. His ability to read Arabic allows him to penetrate the realms of Islamic thought and opens to him many secrets (*asirai*). As his knowledge (*ilimi*) of these things increases and he gains access to more secrets, his personal spiritual power increases. If he follows the path of Sufism and joins a Sufi *tarika,* his intellectual and spiritual quest may take him to the pinnacle of religious fulfillment, union with the godhead and the ultimate revelation of all spiritual secrets.

The *mallam* thus occupies a unique position as a keeper of the inner secrets and esoteric lore of Islam. Of course, the range of knowledge possessed by any one individual may vary greatly, and in general the more sophisticated and erudite Koranic scholars will gather in the large urban areas such as Zaria, Kano, and Katsina. Those living in rural villages possess a much rougher Islamic education. Depending upon what Arabic (or Hausa) materials he has at his disposal and his own personal inclinations, the *mallam* may function as a counselor, diviner, astrologer, fortune-teller, spiritual adviser, pharmacist, and physician. His books are the repositories of his secrets and he operates by "opening the papers" (*bu'de takarda*) or "peering into" (*duba*) his books to divine the causes and remedies for the illnesses that afflict his clients or to find the spells that will bring about the results they desire. The therapeutic strategies embraced by Koranic scholars lie within a tradition long established in Islam and known as the "medicine of the Prophet" (Arabic, *Tibb-ul-Nabbi*).

The core of classical Islamic medicine as it developed in the period from approximately 900 to 1200 A.D. was based upon the humoral theories of Galen, the great Greek physician of antiquity (ca. 131–201

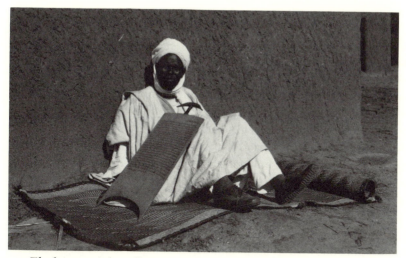

14. The limam *of the village mosque holding a slate covered with Koranic verses.*

A.D.), who modified the earlier traditions of Hippocratic medicine and built a complex medical system on their foundation.[18] The central theme of Galenic medicine was the interrelation of four humors as determinants of health and illness. Food was thought to arrive in the stomach, where it was transformed into other substances; the useful products of this "boiling" were carried to the liver while the extraneous material was expelled in the feces and urine. In the liver the remaining substances were transformed into four humors—blood, phlegm, yellow bile, and black bile—each having an appropriate quality: hot and damp, damp and cold, dry and hot, and cold and dry, respectively.

Health resulted from the proper balance of these humors and their qualities. This balance did not depend upon an equal contribution from each of the four humors. Rather, the composition of the balance varied slightly with each person according to his age, habits, complexion, and so on. The humor which predominated determined the individual's temperament: sanguine, phlegmatic, choleric, or melancholic. The function of medicine was to restore the balance of humors by countering

18. Galen's life and teachings are described in Sarton (1954) and Temkin (1973). The latter work contains a general discussion of the subsequent history of Galenism.

illness-producing imbalances; thus, "hot" remedies were used for "cold" illnesses, etc. A whole discipline became devoted to the classification of substances by their "qualities" in this system so that they could be used in the practice of medicine.

These theories could be used to explain nearly any morbid condition of the human body, and within the confines of the system they could hardly be refuted. This inner, logical symmetry appealed powerfully to medical minds, and the volume, clarity of exposition, and force of style of Galen's writings imbued the system with an authority that persisted for centuries. When the Arabs came into contact with the Hellenistic world they took this system of medicine and incorporated it into Islamic culture. Subsequent Muslim medical practitioners refined it to a high degree. The most notable of these practitioners was Avicenna (Ibn Sina), whose *Canon of Medicine,* a synthesis and synopsis of the Galenic system, became the authoritative textbook of Islamic medicine.[19]

For a variety of reasons this system of medicine did not progress. Slavish adherence to received authority and the lack of a critical experimental method resulted in a tendency to rearrange classical material and write commentaries upon it, rather than add to the body of knowledge. Medicine became a set corpus of material to be learned and gradually stagnated as a result. An important factor in this process was clerical opposition to the secular system of medicine. The Greeks had sought in their system to minister to the soul as well as the body, and the religious impetus of Islam to root all aspects of culture in the teachings of the Koran and the traditions of the Prophet Muhammed ran strongly counter to this. A body of medical belief and practice which could be thus sanctioned gradually grew up, fusing medical ideas taken from the Bedouin tribes of Arabia with holy writ and the traditions (frequently spurious) of the Prophet. The end result of this was a system of "Prophetic medicine" that included elements of folk practice, Galenic scientism, magical thought, and religious apotropaism. As

19. Surveys of Islamic medicine may be found in Browne (1921), Elgood (1970), and Ullmann (1978), and in a useful article by Burgel (1977). The first book of Avicenna's *Canon* has been translated into English by Gruner (1930). This book contains a number of useful charts and diagrams that compact the system into a shortened form and give some indication of the intellectual appeal it must have had to medical minds as a tool for organizing medical thinking.

Burgel has written (1977:59): "It was no longer a matter of discretion and reasoning whether a certain medicine should be administered or not, but primarily one of knowing whether the Prophet had approved it." As medicine became part of the general program of Muslim theology the orderly operation of the Galenic system fell into desuetude.

Nonetheless, the humoral theories promulgated by this system of medicine were transmitted in various forms to many parts of the world. The reentry of Galenic medicine to the Western world came about initially largely through the impetus of Arabic influences percolating through Spain and Sicily (Campbell 1926). The Spanish carried these humoral ideas to Latin America (Foster 1953; Madsen 1955; Simmons 1955; Ingham 1970; Suarez 1974) while the spread of Islam in the East carried them as far as the Philippines (Hart 1969). The humoral theories are well known in North Africa (e.g., Hilton-Simpson 1922:15–18; Greenwood 1980), and appear to have filtered down across the Sahara in diluted form. Remnants would appear to be found in Songhay (Bisilliat 1976) and among the Bambara of Mali (Zahan 1979), for example. Vague reflections of these humoral doctrines can also be seen in Hausa medical thought, as the functions of phlegm, blood, hot and cold, sweet, sour, bitter, and salty substances in the physiology and pathology of the body discussed in chapter 5 demonstrate. Hausa Arabic medical manuscripts contain dilute versions of humoralism as well, but the works of the great physicians of Islamic medicine such as Avicenna, Rhazes, and al-Majusi do not appear to have found their way to Hausaland (Abdalla 1979). The main thrust of classical Islamic medicine would therefore appear to have missed the Hausa.

Since the Galenic system of medicine as articulated by the great physicians of Islam is not found in Hausaland, the medical activities of the Hausa *mallam* focus on that melange of practices known in Arabic as *tibb-ul-nabbi* or "the medicine of the Prophet." The heart of this medicine is the utilization of remedies sanctioned by traditions concerning the Prophet Muhammed, and particularly the use of Koranic verses as medical remedies, a practice extremely widespread in Islamic Africa (e.g., I. M. Lewis 1966:23; Fisher 1973). Abdalla has described it as follows (1979:95–96):

> The Prophet Muhammed is believed to have recommended a few
> *aayat* or verses from the Quran for healing, but ever since that

time the Quran has increasingly become a major source of therapy among Muslims the world over. Various verses from the Quran are prescribed as remedies for different sicknesses, pathological or otherwise. The common feature of such verses is that they contain an explicit or implicit reference to the sicknesses for which they are prescribed. A person suffering from continuous vomiting, for example, will be treated with the *aaya:* "And We said, swallow up thy water, Oh Earth, Sky cease thy rain—And the water disappeared." And the *aaya* "To the fire We said: Be cold, and bring peace upon Abraham" is recommended to the person who complains of skin burns, while the *aaya* "I have bestowed love upon thee" is prescribed for the unsuccessful lover in order to remove all obstacles between him and the beloved. In the first of these three *aayat* the word *ma'* or water is mentioned, in the second, the word *nar* or fire, and in the third, *mahabba* or love. Thus there is an explicit sympathetic relationship between each *aaya* and the sickness or problem for which it is prescribed.

These remedies are administered in various ways. The most common way is as *rubutu* or "writing." *Rubutu* can refer to any kind of writing—in English, Hausa, or Arabic, for example—but used as medicine it refers to Koranic verses written in Arabic script. The verse specific for the complaint at hand is selected and written out several times on a wooden slate. The ink is allowed to dry and is then washed off and collected in a bowl. The resulting inky water is drunk as a tonic and washed over the affected part of the body as a cure or prophylactic. Koranic verses may also be written on small pieces of paper rolled or folded up into small bundles, wrapped tightly with string, and then sewn into a leather pouch (*laya*) to be worn around the neck, or into a leather belt (*guru*) to be worn around the waist. They may also be placed over a doorway, tied to the harness of a horse, or buried in some location as apotropaic devices to ward off evil and help bring good fortune.[20] If writing materials are not available the appropriate verses may be drawn in the dust. A popular remedy for headache recommends this practice at the onset of head pain. The verse thus written in the dust is gathered up and poured on the head at the location of the pain while reciting an appropriately pious exclamation such as *Alham-*

20. A good reproduction of such a charm is given in G. Nicolas (1975:404).

dulillahi, "Praise be to God." Occasionally, entire gowns may be covered with Koranic writing and worn for medical purposes (e.g., Heathcote 1974), and one sometimes sees men carrying small bottles of inky Koranic water with them to nip at during the course of their daily peregrinations.

Such practices have a long history in Islam and have been sanctioned by many popular medical writers. For example, Al-Suyuti, the popular Egyptian medical writer of the fifteenth century, wrote: "Know then that the recital of verses and the wearing of amulets are indeed useful if accepted by the patient and received with his consent as a method of cure. The recitation of charms and the wearing of amulets are a form of taking refuge with God for the purpose of securing health, just as is done in the case of medicine" (Elgood 1962:154). The use of Koranic verses for medical purposes can thus be seen merely as one kind of prayer, an act of piety or devotion aimed at providing succor or comfort for the sick, or as fervent expressions of the desire to avoid misfortune. There is, however, another important factor, firmly rooted in Islamic theology, that contributes to this practice.

The central place of the Koran as the Word of God in the religious life of Islam was described in chapter 3. The Arabic word *kalimah* ("word") is the substantive form of the verb *kallam,* meaning "he spoke to" or "he addressed." In theology this word is of great importance and is used to refer to God's word in its various forms. Arabic translations of the Old Testament, for example, use it to express meanings such as God's creative word, God's word of command in effecting the resurrection of the dead, God's decree, God's efficacious power, and God's divine revelation (O'Shaughnessy 1948:9). In its Islamic setting, but influenced by Christian theology, *kalimah* took on a meaning comparable to the *Logos* doctrine of the New Testament, a doctrine which was then applied to the Koran itself as being an eternal attribute and creative activity of God, as well as a revelation to the Prophet Muhammed. As O'Shaughnessy has written (1948:60):

> One of the earliest applications of *kalimah* in the primitive Moslem community was to the Koran. This latter had been announced by the Prophet as containing the very words of Allah but the piety of his followers went even further, making it uncreated and co-eternal with the Deity. Under Christian influence Islam evolved

the concept of an eternal "word," corresponding to the divine Word in the Christian dogma of the Trinity, but made tangible in the *revelation* sent down by God to his *Prophet*. Finally the orthodox theologians of Islam applied the notion to the Koran in its actual linguistic form.

After futile objections by the liberal Mu'tazilite school this opinion was imposed as obligatory under al-Mutawakkil (d. 861 A.D.) and definitely became the orthodox belief when the famous Islamic doctor al-Ash'ari (d. 936 A.D.) had publicly maintained that the Koranic revelation, written or recited, was identical with the eternal and uncreated word of God. Some indications can be gained of the possible conclusions from such a doctrine from the subsequent teaching that made "word" a synonym of the divine essence.

Thus, the Koran *itself* is a source of power that may be tapped for medicinal purposes. As such, it may be possible to use the verses or words medically without any real understanding of what they mean— a situation all too common in a culture where Arabic is a foreign language and literacy in Arabic is usually minimal at best. For example, a village tailor named Ibrahim had a pregnant wife. One day he was seen sitting outside his shop on the ground with a wooden slate, busily writing out a verse from the Koran over and over again. When asked what he was doing he replied that he was writing out a medicine for his wife to drink to ensure her having an easy labor when it came time for the child to be born. When asked what the verse that he was copying so assiduously meant, he replied, "Well, if you want to know what it means you'll have to go to a big scholar (*babban mallam*). I don't know that; but it doesn't matter because God knows what it means and that's that."

Because the *mallam* has access to the Koran and the mystically charged symbols of Islam, he is seen as a special custodian of charismatic power which can be tapped for healing purposes (I. M. Lewis 1966:29). It is but a short leap from this belief to the conclusion that all educated people possess access to similar secret powers and may likewise be approached to provide magical medical practices in a similar fashion. Nineteenth-century travelers in Hausaland were regularly accosted and begged to write out charms, remedies, and spells for one reason or another. Robinson (1900:143–44) reported several such requests, and at one point Clapperton's servants insisted on being paid for their work in such currency (Denham and Clapperton 1826, II:74). Richard Lander noted in his journal how he was detained by one importunate chief until he complied with such a request:

> 30th (August, 1827)—Having finished cleaning the muskets and pistols, asked the chief permission to leave Wowow. The old man, smiling, told me not half my business was done: he wanted six charms, which I alone could write. These charms were to be worn on his person, and to possess the following virtues: 1st charm. If his enemies thought of making war on him, it would cause them to forget to put it into practice. 2d. If they should be on their way to his city, for the purpose of warring, it would turn them back. 3d. If they should discharge their arrows at his people, when close to the city walls, it would cause them to rebound in their own faces, and wound them. 4th. It was the province of this charm to prevent his guns from bursting. 5th, was to preserve the person who might hold the gun from receiving any injury, should it unfortunately explode. The 6th and last charm was to make him the happiest and most successful of men.
>
> 31st—Carried the charms to the king, on which I had written scraps of old English ballads, which made him in the best humour in the world. (Lander in Clapperton 1829:280)

■ *Bori:* Illness, Therapy, and Vocation in Spirit Possession

Koranic scholars are not, however, the only persons who have access to a realm of knowledge not open to the common man or woman. Even as the *mallamai* have access to the mysteries of Arabic and Islamic esoterica, so the devotees of spirit possession (*'yam bori*) claim to have a special intercourse with the world of spirits, thereby having revealed to them secrets unknown to the ordinary villager. This claim to special knowledge is recognized by Hausa society, although springing as it apparently does from pagan roots it is given less respect and less prominence than that accorded to the *mallam* and his Islamic learning. The adepts of spirit possession use this special knowledge to give advice, perform medical consultations, and treat illness. In addition to these sober functions *bori* also displays varied aspects of masquerade, drama, and farce which serve as a lively source of amusement.

A variety of people are involved in *bori*, with differing levels of commitment to the cult. Because there is a strong element of theater and entertainment in *bori* ceremonies, particularly those which take place in the evenings on a regular basis in the compounds of prostitutes, many people attend such functions and take part in the dancing purely for the sake of participating in an amusing diversion. Many of these people do not perform *bori* falls, do not become possessed, and may even look upon such prospects with some fear or disdain. Others are serious devotees who sponsor these functions at their own compounds, venerate the spirits for their usefulness in treating illness, and have an active medical practice. People who attain prominence as dancers, regularly and easily attaining the trance of possession, or who are recognized for their deep knowledge of spirits and spirit-related medicines, are given the title of *Sarkin Bori*, "chief of *bori*," or *Sarauniyar Bori*, "queen of the *bori*," recognizing their preeminence.

Initiation into the cult through *girka* is the pathway to knowledge of the spirits as well as the most dramatic form of medical treatment provided by the *bori* adepts. As a verb form *girka* may refer to many acts, all of which are concerned with establishing some kind of order or with laying the foundations for a future action. Putting a cooking pot on the fire, erecting a granary on its platform, setting up the supports for a grindstone, establishing a school or market, laying the emplacements for a piece of artillery in the army, etc.—all of these constitute actions of *girka*. With reference to *bori*, *girka* refers to the ceremony of initiation through which the initiate establishes the foundations of a lifelong relationship with the spirit world in general and with a specific spirit in particular. Undergoing *girka* separates the casual spectator from the serious *bori* adept.

Girka is a form of medical therapy and is recognized as a last resort in cases of intractable illness. Not all cases of illness that do not respond to treatment will end in initiation into the *bori* cult—the individual personalities and social circumstances of each case are extremely important—but it is highly significant that the overwhelming majority of *bori* initiates are women. Politically powerless, socially restricted, often competing with other women for the attentions of a husband,

and faced with the necessity of being fertile in order to establish their position in the household as well as to ensure their future security in old age, women face social pressures which may be overwhelming. Many Hausa women adapt with only minor difficulties; many others, however, do not. The result may be a pattern of chronic insecurity which manifests itself in a variety of emotional and somatic complaints best described as hysteric.[21] The vague, chronic, poorly defined illnesses afflicting women that are recognized by Hausa medicine are one result of this. A prime example is *kwantacce*, the "lying down" of a pregnancy so that it becomes "dormant" for an indefinite period and the seat of innumerable complaints, excuses, and fears. Another example is *gishiri*, that constantly shifting, poorly defined complaint of the female reproductive system which figures so prominently in cases of difficult labor, but which also extends to many other aspects of female sexuality as well (Last 1976, 1979). In her study of *bori* among the Hausa of Niger, for example, Jacqueline Nicolas (1967) showed a high rate of divorce and a high incidence (60 percent) of *"troubles de la fonction maternelle"* among female *bori* initiates, as well as a childhood mortality of 57.3 percent among children born to such women—a figure nearly three times the officially established rate for the area.

Diagnosis of such complaints as due to harassment by a spirit allows a woman to assume the sick role, absolving her of blame for her condition. In addition it gives her added status. Involved with the spirits, she has now become an interface between the human and spirit worlds. In the state of illness, uncontrolled, this augments her social marginal-

21. Goodwin and Guze, in their book *Psychiatric Diagnosis*, describe hysteria (Briquet's Syndrome) as follows (1979:70):

> Hysteria is a *polysymptomatic* disorder that begins early in life (usually in the teens, rarely after the twenties), chiefly affects women, and is characterized by recurrent, multiple somatic complaints often described dramatically. Characteristic features, all unexplained by other known clinical disorders, are varied pains, anxiety symptoms, gastrointestinal disturbances, urinary symptoms, menstrual difficulties, sexual and marital maladjustment, nervousness, mood disturbances, and conversion symptoms. Repeated visits to physicians and clinics, the use of a large number of medications—often at the same time—prescribed by different physicians, and frequent hospitalizations and operations result in a florid medical history.

A fine historical study of hysteria has been published by Ilza Veith (1965).

ity; but through *bori* she is given the opportunity of establishing control over her condition and regulating her relations with the spirits. Performance of the possession dances and the hosting of *bori* functions allow her opportunities for self-expression and a chance to gain added prestige within the confines of her group. The possession dances, which involve a wide variety of spirits paralleling the human social hierarchy, give her an opportunity to mimic roles of power and authority not normally open to women in a society otherwise dominated by men. She may rest content with this or, taking full advantage of her unique position vis-à-vis the spirits and her access to the medical lore reposing in the older members of the cult, she may embark on a career as a healer, an occupation that allows considerable scope for a woman of insight, forceful personality, and determination. *Bori* would therefore appear to function in large part as a cult of female affliction similar to those found in other parts of Islamic Africa, particularly the *zar* of Ethiopia and Nubia (Messing 1958; Kennedy 1967; Gray 1969; I. M. Lewis 1969, 1971).

The process of *girka* has been described by various authors (Tremearne 1912:258–60; J. M. Nicolas 1967, 1972; Madauci et al. 1968: 77–84). It lasts at least seven days and during much of this time the prospective initiate is kept secluded and quiet, dressed in special garments, and is given medicines to make her body strong in order to withstand the violent falls characteristic of the *bori* dances, a toughening also designed to make her strong enough to tolerate the presence of the spirits. Essentially, *girka* is a rite of passage in which a person, usually a female, whose illness has been diagnosed as due to the unremitting harassment of a spirit, is initiated into a fellowship of sufferers and thereby ameliorates her condition.[22] By drinking herbal infusions and undergoing medicinal fumigations and washings, the offending spirit is tamed, made to reveal itself, and then propitiated by sacrifices, offerings, and invocations, after which a regulated relation-

22. This process would seem to have some interesting parallels with the formation of special interest medical groups in our own culture such as Alcoholics Anonymous, the Myasthenia Gravis Foundation, the Muscular Dystrophy Association, etc. One also thinks of those people who have suffered from a mental illness themselves and who subsequently elect to undertake a career in psychology or psychiatry.

ship between the sufferer and the spirit is established. The spirit ceases to harry her in return for her devotion.[23]

The adept may feel content merely to honor her patron spirit with periodic ceremonies, or may elect to embark on an active medical career, utilizing this special connection for therapeutic ends. Having suffered an attack by this spirit, she is now familiar with its manifestations and the herbal medicines necessary to treat it. In addition, the spirit now becomes a special source of information, revealing to the adept, through trances or dreams, medicines useful in the treatment of various illnesses. Such experiences—which one might label "medicine by intuition"—are combined with an apprenticeship under the watchful eye of an older, more experienced herbalist and devotee if the adept has serious aspirations to increase her knowledge. In cases such as this, where herbalism is to become a vocation, it appears that much of this specialist information is transmitted through family lines, and that possessing spirits as well as the herbal vocation are inherited. As the proverb says, *'Dan asali ya fi shigege,* "A son of the ancestors is better than a newcomer."[24]

23. "When a divine horseman rides, the behaviour of his medium generally includes an illustration of the ailment for which he may be held responsible. The possession-trance itself is evidence of a spiritual presence, and the medium's actions symbolic of the spirit's identity. These elements form the basis for symbolic healing. That is, when a person admits that his affliction is spirit-caused he may be relieved of its symptoms by dedicating his life to the possession-trance cult, demonstrating his commitment by serving as a medium. The medium is "cured" but in his altered state of consciousness he is hopelessly afflicted". (Besmer 1983: 114)

24. A good example of this was the herbalist Natakwibi, a village man who had migrated south from Katsina. Some years before he had been smitten by a severe mental illness which he called *haukar daji* or "bush-wandering madness." He had been taken in by a Katsina *'dan bori,* treated, and eventually underwent *girka,* establishing a special relationship with the spirit *Sarkin Rafi,* the "chief of the watercourse." Following his recovery he spent several months with this man learning about herbal medicines and the treatment of illnesses. He was not very successful as a herbalist, and remained poor, although he married and had a family and was widely known among the other *bori* devotees of the area. Other village herbalists, who came from family traditions of herbal medicine, had much more success and apparently knew much more about herbalism than did Natakwibi. Uwarture, a local female herbalist of considerable reputation, used to complain

One special aspect of the communication of the spirits with the human world is the *mai-Danko* or "owner of a *Danko*." *Danko* is a spirit who assumes the form of a snake and is generally reputed to be the son of the spirit *Inna*. In possession dances he causes the dancer whom he rides to writhe on the ground with her hands at her sides in imitation of the movements of a snake. He is known as a very chatty spirit who likes to hold conversations with others and *bori* adepts will attempt to summon him up to talk with him. A person who professes to have a relationship with *Danko* will often keep a model "spirit house" in a hut in his or her compound, surrounded with bottles of sweet-smelling perfumes and sugar—pleasant substances thought to attract spirits. In return for a small fee and an offering (usually of perfume, sugar, or some similar substance) to the spirit, the owner will arrange a séance at which *Danko* will manifest himself, answer questions, give advice, and so on. Unfortunately for the customer, the language spoken by the spirit is a tiny, high-pitched squeak not intelligible to the uninitiated. This sound is produced by the *mai-Danko*, who whistles softly through a small button held in the mouth. Following each whistling statement the *mai-Danko* interprets what the "spirit" has said. Such séances are generally recognized as being faked and are regarded as charlatanism by most people. Nonetheless, there are still those who seek out such advice in times of stress.[25]

■ *Boka:* The Consulting Herbalist

The heart of traditional Hausa medicine is herbalism, and the foremost specialist in herbal treatment is the *boka* (f. *bokaniya*, pl. *bokaye*). While this term may be loosely applied to anyone dealing in herbal

---

that Natakwibi was always coming around to her, trying to cadge medicines for his own use. As will be seen in the next chapter, Uwarture had a substantial family medical tradition behind her.

25. I witnessed several such séances and was unimpressed with the techniques used to produce the sounds. Most of the performers I saw were so bad that they made you sit facing the other direction, with your back to the *mai-Danko*, in order to prevent you from seeing their mouths. While using some of the same principles of performance—distraction and direction of attention elsewhere—this is not ventriloquism, which uses only the natural human voice modified in the nasopharynx to produce its effects.

medicines, most specifically it refers to a herbal *practitioner*, not just a salesman. The *boka* may make house calls or travel to other areas on request, but basically he or she is a settled resident of a community who accepts patients for treatment at his or her compound, either as out-patients who come for consultation and advice, or as in-patients who reside there with the healer for a prolonged period of treatment, as in the case of mental illness. Patients may come from considerable distances at substantial expense to see a *boka* whose reputation has spread beyond the local community, for in matters of sickness and health, word often travels remarkable distances. As the Hausa proverb says, *Ina amfanin ba'di ba rai?* "What good is next year without life?"

The absence of clans as functional social units in Hausa society and the presence of Islam as the dominant religion in Hausaland preclude herbalists from performing the priestly roles they might fill in other African societies. The art of the practicing herbalist (*bokanci*) is regarded simply as an occupation (*sana'a*), similar to those of farming, barbering, trading, leatherworking, and others. Although most of these occupations are closed to women, the occupation of herbal practitioner is open to them. While no respectable woman would be an itinerant medicine seller or hawk herbal wares in the marketplace, she may nonetheless operate a herbal medical practice from the settled confines of her home. Since this is the case, and since the sick role is open to anyone regardless of age or sex, the occupation of *boka* allows a woman much greater flexibility of movement and wider contact with human affairs than would normally be possible in a society that places such a high value on the seclusion of women. In this regard it is interesting to note that female herbalists tend to have strong personalities and seem to be as well known to the general population of the village as their husbands—an unusual situation among the Hausa.

Recruitment to the role of *boka* may take place through heredity or apprenticeship. *Bori* adepts who suffer from possession by a spirit and undergo the initiation process of *girka* may subsequently elect to become herbalists, learning the herbal craft from those who initiated them. Although all herbalists will claim to have knowledge of spirit-induced illnesses and their treatment, possession by a spirit is not a prerequisite for becoming a *boka*. An individual may grow up within a family tradition of herbal medicine and may take up the vocation as a consequence. In such cases the prospective healer is brought up with the craft, learning it both by observation of the daily practice and through formal teaching during medicine-collecting expeditions. Since herbalists may be of either sex, there are no restrictions on who may teach herbal knowledge and practice; females may teach males and vice-versa. It is also possible to find situations in which both family tradition and spirit possession play a role, the latter experience validating the choice of métier or being part of the tradition, as in a case where a special relationship with a particular spirit is handed down along with the fund of herbal knowledge.

The style of an individual practice may vary greatly. Some practitioners maintain heavily attended "open clinics" on market days; other herbalists live in bush homesteads, dabble in selling medicines in the market, and treat individual patients by request. Some are simple, humble healers who treat the sick on an essentially charitable basis; others are necromancers who indulge in chicanery and showmanship to bilk the unwary. Some have large numbers of patients, others only a few.

The village population showed variants of all these types. Alhaji Audu Boka and his younger brother, 'Dam Baba, devoted nearly all their time to the practice of traditional medicine. Although they were farmers they had no time themselves for agricultural work and hired laborers to tend their fields. They ran a lucrative herbal practice from their compound located on the edge of the market and on market days there was always a stream of patients going in and out for consultation and treatment. In addition, the two brothers also made trips—sometimes quite extended ones—to neighboring villages to fetch people for treatment at their compound, especially the mentally ill. Alhaji Audu went as far south as Jos on one occasion for several weeks at a patient's request. On the other hand, Uwarture, a female herbalist, confined herself mainly to dispensing medicines to such patients as came by her compound at irregular intervals. She accepted very little in return for her services, performing them *saboda Allah*, "for the sake of God." She treated children and small babies, infertile women, menstrual disorders, and the occasional case of more spectacular illness, such as paralysis. However, she too made frequent trips to other villages at the request of people desiring her services, and was often gone several days at a time. Uwale, another female herbalist, likewise worked from her compound and treated the occasional complaint without indulging in great fanfare. Dogo, a *boka* living out in an isolated compound in the bush rarely (if ever) treated patients at his compound, but confined himself mainly to selling aphrodisiacs (*yaji*) in the market and traveled to other isolated homesteads only at the request of the family of a sick person. 'Dam Mazadu lived in the village in a huge compound with four wives and numerous children, dressed richly, maintained an elaborate special room dedicated to his familiar spirits, and was reputedly well-known throughout the whole of Katsina (even to the emir); but he was also a cunning, artful man who took delight in sleight of hand and showmanship and projected a rather unsavory aura. Natakwibi, an impoverished ne'er-do-well, did odd jobs and dabbled in herbalism. An active *'dan bori,* he lived rather on the fringes of society and had a small, stagnant herbal practice.

Herbalism, it would seem, exhibits as wide a variety of personalities and styles of therapy as does scientific medicine. In order to understand these contrasting styles more fully and to provide a deeper insight into the dynamics of Hausa traditional medicine, the next chapter will describe the operations of two herbal practices in some detail: that of Uwarture, and that of Alhaji Audu Boka and his brother, 'Dam Baba.

VII

Two Styles in the Practice of Herbal Medicine

Daidai, majinyaci ba shi gode Allah sai ya ga wanda ya mutu.

(Truly, the sick man does not thank God until he sees the one who has died.)

HAUSA PROVERB

■ Uwarture: The Herbalist as Family Practitioner

Uwarture was a female herbalist and practicing midwife who lived with her husband in a modest compound surrounded by a delapidated guinea-corn fence near the edge of the village. A Fulani woman, she had been born in a cattle camp near Kaduna and had spent a goodly portion of her youth wandering with the herds and selling sour milk in the villages. Her family had been noted for their knowledge of medicines, and several of her relatives were active in the practice of traditional medicine. As is frequently the case with Fulani women, Uwarture married a Hausa man and settled down in the village to raise a family. When her children were grown and several grandchildren had been born to her daughters, her husband decided he wanted to move to another town some distance away. She refused and divorced him, later marrying her present husband, who had been married and divorced several times himself—a not uncommon phenomenon in Hausaland. The two of them lived together in his compound, each having a personal hut. Three other thatched huts were used for storage and for accommodating visitors and patients. A number of neighboring compounds had rear doors cut through to their compound and there was always a constant stream of women and children going in and out, for most of Uwarture's children, grandchildren, and great-grandchildren lived in the village. She was everybody's friend and "grandmother."

Uwarture gained her knowledge of medi-

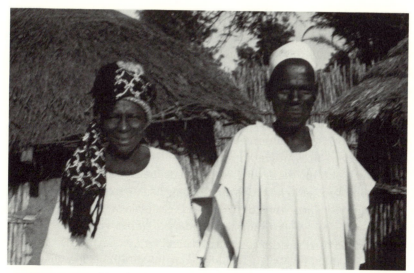

15. Uwarture and her husband, Damina.

cines from her family but this was reinforced—if not surpassed, in
her estimation—by an encounter with a spirit in the bush one day
many years ago. She had been out gathering shea nuts (*'kwara*) in
the bush with four other women and they were returning to the village when they stopped to rest in the shade of a large fig tree. Three
of the women passed on, but Uwarture and Ade remained behind.
Suddenly, they spied a female spirit with light red skin sitting in the
bush who demanded to know what they were doing there. Petrified
with fear, they told her they were gathering shea nuts for sale because they had no money and needed an income. They had not meant
to intrude, but they had not seen her there. Seemingly satisfied with
this answer, the spirit gave them leave to go. Uwarture and her companion caught up with the others and asked them if they had seen the
red woman in the bush, but they had not. Uwarture wanted to get rid
of all the shea nuts and collect them again the following day, but nobody else agreed.

On returning to the village all the women became ill except Uwarture, who remained in fine health until the same month in the following
year, when she was stricken down with an illness, lost her strength,
and was unable to get about without the aid of a walking stick. She
could not seem to recover. She called in a barber to cup her, but she

did not improve. She went to a government dispensary, but got no better. Then one night while she lay on her bed the female spirit reappeared to her and asked her what was the matter. She replied at some length, detailing her malady, and the spirit told her to get up in the night, go to the river, and collect three kinds of medicines, after using which she would recover. So she got up in the night, left the village, and went down to the river to collect medicines. Her husband discovered her absence and was afraid, thinking perhaps she had fallen in the well. She returned in the morning and told everyone what had happened. They thought she was crazy, but she persevered and began washing with the medicines given her by the spirit. In two days she had recovered, and from that time she actively pursued herbal medicine as her occupation.

The red-skinned Fulani spirit who had been instrumental in healing Uwarture's sickness struck a bargain with her prior to showing her the medicine necessary for her recovery. If she recovered she was obligated to practice herbalism for the benefit of others. Furthermore, she was not to engage in any kind of fortune-telling (*duba*), spirit worship or pagan sacrifice (*tsafi*), unless she wished the spirits to gather and return to plague her. The spirit also warned her not to wheedle money out of her patients, but to accept whatever they offered for their treatment. To all these warnings Uwarture scrupulously adhered. She avoided the disreputable aspects of *bokanci* and did not charge for her medical services, regarding them rather as a form of charity (*sadaka*) that she had been enjoined to observe by suprahuman agencies. She accepted "greeting money" (*ku'din gaisuwa*), as is normal Hausa practice, but took payment only when people offered it to her after their recovery, out of gratitude for what she had done for them.

It is to be doubted that this tale of spirit encounter has a solid basis in fact, but it is significant because it provides a spirit-sanctioned charter for the values, attitudes, and beliefs Uwarture expressed in her herbal practice. It forms a kind of personal theology reconciling certain tensions present in Hausa society, and as such its structure merits some discussion. In the first place, the initial encounter with the spirit took place out in the bush, away from human habitation. In Hausa thought the bush is always a liminal area, removed from human settlement and the world of normal human values. It is here that the gradual transition

begins. Similarly, her own position is mirrored in the fact that it was a
Fulani spirit that accosted her, speaking to her in *Filanci* instead of
Hausa. Uwarture frequently declared that *duk cikin duniya nan ba
abin da babu iska,* "in this world there is nothing that is without its
spirit." There are Nupe spirits, Gobir spirits, Kanuri spirits, European
spirits—there are spiritual counterparts for nearly every living thing,
human and animal. The female Fulani spirit is the logical outcome of
this system, an approach to the human world from its spiritual, metaphysical counterpart. The illness incurred by her four companions
points out the dangerous nature of such encounters, but the fact that
Uwarture did not succumb set her apart. A year after her companions'
recovery, however, Uwarture was suddenly stricken by an incurable
illness. Neither traditional practitioners such as the barber, nor scientifically trained practitioners like the dispensary attendant were of any
avail. Her status changed and, in assuming what seemed to be a permanent sick role, she moved from the world of normal, healthy life
into a liminal role, removed from it. In this uncomfortable and dis-
tressing state of affairs she was once again approached by the mys-
terious Fulani spirit, who struck an agreement with her. By showing
her the proper herbal medicines she returned her to a normal, healthy
state, and conferred upon her the new status of *bokaniya,* herbal healer.
She went out alone from the village, down to the river to collect medicines. This occurred at night under cover of darkness, and she returned
to the village as day was breaking—another indication of her immi-
nent change in status. Her announcement to her family and friends
that she had encountered a spirit and was now going to take up herbalism as her occupation was greeted skeptically, incredulously. It was
only with her rapid recovery under the influence of the medicines she
gathered with the assistance of the spirit that her claims were validated
in the eyes of others, and thereafter they began to flock to her for aid.

Morally, traffic with spirits as is described in this tale is disapproved
by orthodox Islam as setting up potential partners with God, splitting
His divine unity (Koran VI:100). Uwarture's tale avoids this difficulty
by having the spirit herself warn her against such paganism (*tsafi*)
and urge her to obey all the proper Islamic injunctions. The implication
is clear enough. The spirit, though herself the agency through which
a knowledge of the proper medicine is communicated, is in fact one of

the "believing djinn" of Sura LXXII of the Koran who accepted the message of Muhammed.[1] The spirit is thus plugged into the proper moral framework of the Muslim order and becomes an intermediary communicating moral truth as well as medical knowledge. Uwarture always maintained that she practiced *magani da ro'kon Allah*, "medicine with pleading to God," rather than *ro'kon iskoki*, "pleading with spirits," which would be *tsafi*, pagan abomination not to be tolerated in a believer.

Within this general framework, then, Uwarture practiced her medicine. In her general conceptions of the body, of its operation and proper functioning, she differed very little from the general paradigm set forth in chapter 5. She believed the interactions of hot and cold, of bitter, sweet, sour, and salt all to be important in causing illness. *Sanyi* (cold) she saw as the cause of coughing (*huka*), internal complaints (*ciwon ciki*), *amosani*, and the other common complaints previously discussed. All such illnesses she saw as caused by God (*ciwon Allah*), a part of the regular order of the world moving according to His guidance. Apart from this there were also those ailments caused by spirits: *ciwon iskoki, ciwon aljannu*. While she knew medicines for some of the illnesses of God, Uwarture maintained that her realm of specialty was *ciwon aljannu*. She claimed she was skilled at *karatun iskoki* and had *ilimin iskoki;* that is, she was able "to read spirits" and had "knowledge of spirits," establishing by the use of these terms an analogy with reading the Koran (*karatu*) and religious knowledge (*ilimi*). She was saying, in effect, that her knowledge of the spirit world was similar to the theological and religious knowledge of the Koranic teacher—a parallel

1. Scholars such as Watt (1953:104–9) have suggested that this was a political necessity for Muhammed, who needed some way of reconciling his monotheism with the political exigencies under which he operated. In order to obtain the support of certain tribes in his struggle for supremacy he was obliged to moderate his stance to accommodate, to some degree, the polytheist religious sentiments of some of his neighbors. This distinction as to "believing" and "unbelieving" djinn has its parallels in Hausaland, where the broad division into "white" and "black" spirits follows roughly this line. Some *bori* adepts maintain that the *iskoki* they are involved with in *bori* play (*wasa*) are qualitatively different from the evil *adjannu*, or "black spirits" who plague men. The existence of *Mallam Alhaji*, the Koranic pilgrim, as a prominent *bori* spirit supports this notion, and Uwarture told me that his normal abode was in the rafters of the village mosque, where he prayed his rosary without ceasing.

pathway to medical power. Of witchcraft and sorcery she professed to know nothing, being familiar only with medicines capable of warding off their evil effects.

Uwarture expressed the greatest admiration for hospital medicine (*maganin asibiti*). Indeed, in her view this was the best place to go for treatment of *ciwon Allah*. Surgery that was able to "take out the illness" ('*debo ciwo*) after which the patient was sewn back together was, in her mind, a miraculous capability. Similarly, the capability of replacing someone's blood through transfusions—which she regarded as a powerful cure for *shawara*—was equally marvellous. She was fond of saying *kowane ciwo da maganinshi,* "every illness has its own medicine," and she always maintained that if she saw a case of *ciwon asibiti,* "hospital illness," she refused to treat it and told the sufferer to hie himself there for treatment. In her view only a "false *boka*" (*bokar 'karya*) would do otherwise. The main difference between hospitals and herself was that they had no medicine at all for spirit-induced illness. That was her special domain.

The distinction between *ciwon Allah* and *ciwon iskoki* is not always very clear-cut, however. *Ciwon Allah* has other meanings as well. Since, in the Islamic view, all things ultimately come from God, any sickness for which there is no cure, any affliction for which there is no relief, is ultimately caused by God Himself:

> No affliction befalls in the earth
> or in yourselves, but it is in a
> Book, before We create it; that is
>   easy for God;
> that you may not grieve for what
> escapes you, nor rejoice in what has
> come to you; God loves not any man
>   proud and boastful.
> (Koran LVII:22–24)

> It is not given to any soul to die, save by the
> leave of God, at an appointed time.
> (Koran III:139)

This presents some problems for the practitioner, but it also provides a convenient explanation for failure. For example, while discussing leprosy (*kuturta*) and blindness (*makanta*), Uwarture said there are two kinds of each: the kind given by God, for which there is no cure, and the kind given by spirits. When pressed for a more precise distinction as to how one could tell the difference she replied that the outward manifestations of both are the same. That is, leprosy looks like leprosy and blindness looks like blindness, no matter what the cause. The only way to determine if the ailment is caused by spirits is to apply a course of treatment of herbal medicine. If the patient recovers, then the illness was due to spirits; if, on the other hand, no recovery is made, then it is obviously the will of God, and the only remedy is death! As the Hausa proverb expresses it: *Wanda zai mutu magani ba ya tsaishe shi*, "Medicine will not revive he who is doomed to die."

In actual practice Uwarture determined that most of the ailments brought to her were caused by spirits and made an attempt to treat them. In any case, since the amount of money involved was small unless treatment was successful, she felt a charitable obligation to try to bring relief to the suffering. Diagnosis was based on her knowledge (*ilimi*) of spirits and the effects of their activities. She used no elaborate procedures of divination. The cause, as well as the treatment, seemed obvious to one who knew. Several cases may be cited to give an indication of how such matters proceeded.

Case 1. A boy who had been suffering from a massive swelling of the throat and neck which caused severe constriction and choking was brought to Uwarture. He had been out in the bush away from his village chopping wood at the base of a tamarind tree when he suddenly became ill. Uwarture diagnosed the case as an attack of an *iskokin tsamiya*, "spirit of a tamarind tree," and treated him for such an attack. In this case it seems obvious that two factors entered into the formulation of this diagnosis: (1) the boy was out in the bush, a place where spirits are commonly thought to be numerous, and was chopping wood at the base of a tamarind tree—regarded as a favorite haunt of spirits due to the coolness and plenitude of its shade—and presumably the spirits were irritated by his noisy activity; (2) the illness came upon him suddenly while he was in the vicinity of the tree and grew worse during the night. Given that tamarind trees are favorite resting places of spirits and that sudden, paralyzing swellings of this kind are commonly thought to be the work of spirits, the link between the two is obvious. The two factors, channeled by Hausa presuppositions, com-

bine through their own situational logic to provide the obvious diagnosis: attack by a spirit living in a tamarind tree.

Case 2. In another case a woman came all the way from Funtua with
a boy of some fourteen years, tall and with a slight growth of beard.
His name was 'Dam Baba and he was suffering from an extremely
swollen face, very puffy cheeks, a swollen, distended jaw, and some
swelling of his neck. It was obviously quite painful for him to move his
head and neck in any direction. Uwarture only glanced at him very
briefly and pronounced her verdict, *ciwon daji,* or "bush sickness,"
caused by a spirit "shooting" his victim with a spirit arrow, causing
swelling and soreness of the body. The boy had been to the hospital in
Funtua, where he had been given an injection, but he felt he had gotten
no better; rather, his discomfort had increased, so he and his mother
set off to seek a herbalist's help. Uwarture's husband came in at this
point and said matter-of-factly, "Of course. You don't go to a hospital
for *ciwon iskoki.*"

This much decided, Uwarture collected some herbal powders for him
to mix with milk and drink, and then made up a pasty medicine from
butter and herbal powders and smeared it liberally around his face and
over the swellings. As she did so she spat slightly on her hand with the
medicine and addressed the spirits in Hausa as follows:

> Blessings of the spiritual power of Muhammed, may peace be
> upon him. Blessings of the spiritual power of Shehu 'Dan Fodio.
> Blessings of the spiritual power of [their] grandparents and par-
> ents. Blessings of the spiritual power of the Companions of God.
> Blessings of the spiritual power of the Children of the East, the
> Children of the South, the Children of the North and the Children
> of the West [all spirits]. Blessings of the power of the spirits who
> are in the water. Blessings of the power of those [spirits] who are
> on the high ground. May God relieve this suffering here. Blessings
> of the power of Tsoho Ubanku. Blessings of the power of Kembo,
> Gajere, Azabar Daji, Kerman Dawa, 'Dan Jigo, Abusa Kaho, and
> Auwale Dakanta [all hunter spirits of the bush]. All right. Leave
> this boy.

In this case the usual treatment with herbal salve applied externally
to the swollen area was accomplished by a long invocation to the

powers of the Prophet and his companions, the saintly Shehu 'Dan Fodio, leader of the Fulani *jihad*, and the powers of all the spiritual beings from all the cardinal points of the compass, above the earth in the high ground and down in the waters, as well as a succession of hunter spirits in the bush. The boy and his mother gave Uwarture a little money for her efforts and left. Uwarture told me that soon the water (*ruwa*) of the illness would come out, along with whatever had been shot into the boy by the spirit. She showed me some objects, including a black stone and some flakes of other substances, which she told me were the remains of other illnesses she had treated in similar fashion.

Case 3. A third example involves the case of a schoolteacher from Katsina who suffered from a paralyzed hand. About five months previously he had been sleeping in his mother's room at their home in Katsina, and when he awoke he found that he could not use his left hand, nor could he walk on his left foot and leg. His family, who were quite wealthy, took him to the hospital in Katsina, where he received some four months of treatment for his disability, but which seemingly did no good. Being referred to the Ahmadu Bello University Teaching Hospital in Zaria, he left Katsina and traveled south. He was admitted to the hospital and treated for two weeks, at which time he was discharged and sent back to Katsina to resume treatment there. Thoroughly disillusioned with his lack of progress, he heard about Uwarture from friends in Zaria and sought her out in her own village. She agreed to take him on for therapy, provided him with a hut to stay in, food to eat, and gave him daily treatments, which involved hot baths with medicinal solutions (rather like being bathed in hot tea), and daily massages with salves of butter and herbal compounds. He was also given a large stick of medicinal wood, which he was to grip continually in his left hand to allow the powers of the medicine to work on his arm. The cause of all this was *Inna*, one of the female spirits who is reputed to suck the blood out of arms and legs, causing paralysis and the withering of limbs. This fellow stayed for some weeks with Uwarture, and felt that he was making some progress, but it was slow, and he finally went back home to Katsina.

Uwarture provided a variety of medical services for a large number of people. Some were patients with chronic illnesses who, disillusioned with treatment at government hospitals, were attempting to keep their hopes alive by seeking out traditional herbal therapy. Others were women from other villages who had heard of her reputation and came because of infertility or for treatment of various menstrual disorders. Many of her patients were local women who came to her with sick children whom she treated by giving the mother herbal powders to use in bathing them. A great many were her relatives, either blood or affinal, who sought her help and advice as the family medical oracle before considering alternative treatments.

The style of these consultations was friendly and informal. Uwarture was a jolly and approachable woman who listened carefully and with interest to the complaints brought by her patients, or as was often the case, by their friends or relatives, who functioned as surrogates for the presentation of the chief complaint. Since Hausa concepts of illness are symptomatic rather than syndromic in nature, physical examination and history taking, if performed at all, tend to be cursory adjuncts to the business of handing out herbal remedies and listening to the patient's tale of woe. There is more sympathy than scrutiny and analysis in the process.

This done, she then prescribed her remedies based on her knowledge (*ilimi*), taking various medicinal compounds from the piles of powdered roots and wood chips she kept stacked in gourds, old plastic sacks, bottles, and empty bouillon cube tins, mixing and matching the ingredients as she saw fit, finally wrapping them in scraps of old paper and presenting them to her clients along with instructions as to their use. Thereupon she was presented with "greeting money" (*ku'din gaisuwa*) or "medicine money" (*ku'din debo magani*). Uwarture steadfastly refused to make demands for a specific amount of money, and never haggled over what was tendered to her. She handled the financial aspects of her herbal practice with much grace and modesty, consistently maintaining that she regarded herbal medicine as a vocation, a religious calling, not a business for making money. The money she was offered was based upon what her patients felt was polite and proper as a minimal payment for her trouble in collecting and preparing the medicines. If treatment was successful, often the grateful patients would return with some bolts of cloth or additional money as tokens of thanks for the renewal of their health. These payments may be properly regarded as acts of piety, religiously approved alms (*sadaka*) of gratitude.

■ Alhaji Audu Boka and 'Dam Baba: The Herbalist
as Consulting Specialist and Entrepreneur

Standing in sharp contrast to this simple, "at home" kind of therapeutic practice is the sort of herbal clinic run by Alhaji Audu Boka and
his younger brother, 'Dam Baba. Alhaji Audu and 'Dam Baba were
Zamfarawa men from Zuru in Sokoto. Alhaji Audu, who had only recently made the *hajj*, was a middle-aged *boka* with several wives who
lived in a big compound at the edge of the village market, detached
from the surrounding compounds and set off by itself. Afflicted with
wanderlust, Alhaji Audu stayed only a few years in any community,
then moved on, looking for new places and experiences. Even while living in the village he absented himself on numerous trips to other parts
of Nigeria—to Jos, Kainji, Sokoto, Kaduna, and Zaria. While off on
these travels he left his younger brother, 'Dam Baba, to mind the business, take care of patients, collect medicines, and see to the well-being
of the compound—a practice that was a source of irritation between
them.
    Herbal medicine was a tradition in this family going back as far as
anyone could remember, each generation being taught by the one preceding it and in turn passing its knowledge down to its successors.
Alhaji Boka learned his herbal craft from his father, with whom he
traveled in the bush collecting medicines. He claimed to have taken up
farming as a youth only to have people clamor so for his medical services that he was forced to take up herbalism as a full-time occupation.
'Dam Baba was an apprentice, living with and learning the trade from
his brother. Neither of them ever claimed to have had the kind of
spirit encounter so important to Uwarture—to them herbalism was a
gado, an inheritance from the past—*maganin gargajiya*, "traditional
medicine."
    Their compound had two entrances: a standard Hausa entry-hut
(*zaure*), which served as a waiting room, and another entry through a
pair of metal doors which swung open directly into the interior of the
compound from the outside wall. These doors were usually closed except when the entry-hut was in use for some other purpose, such as patient overflow. Upon entering the compound the visitor was confronted
with a large, rectangular courtyard with seven doorways debouching

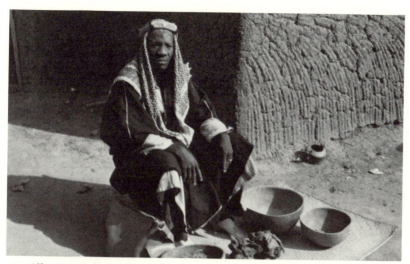

16. Alhaji Audu Boka dressed in his pilgrim's robe from Mecca and with a portion of his herbal pharmacopoeia.

onto it. Each doorway led to a separate room used for housing patients or as living quarters for members of the family. The compound eventually grew so large that two more rooms and an additional *zaure* were built. The outside entrance to the *zaure* was located near a large shade tree. Close by the doorway Alhaji Boka and 'Dam Baba had constructed a simple mud-brick prayer circle for use during the five daily prayers. This whole area, set off slightly from the main residential area of the village and located near a *gidan mata* (prostitutes' compound), the lorry-park, and the village market, was a perfect place for men to congregate and gossip, centrally located in the traffic of human affairs.

On market days (Tuesdays and Fridays) the compound was a welter of activity. These were the heaviest days for herbal consultation and the proximity of the compound to the market made it easy for people to stop off during the day while taking care of other market chores. There were always groups of people lounging in the shade of the tree, sitting in the entry hut, or standing around outside the doorway, waiting to come in for a bit of advice and some medicine. In contrast to Uwarture's practice, these people seemed to be outsiders coming in for medical services—Fulani herders, farmers from small settlements in the bush, people from other nearby or distant villages—rather than local residents. On a busy day forty or fifty people might pass through for medical advice.

The nature of these consultations was extremely interesting. Patients were seen individually, or in groups if more than one had come together. They were ushered into one of the rooms, either to wait or to be interviewed immediately. Alhaji Boka (or in his absence 'Dam Baba) would be seated on a mat on the ground or on a low cornstalk bed. There would be prolonged greetings as is the Hausa custom for any meeting, especially more formal ones. Kolanuts and cheap sugar candies were usually passed out to the patients, who often reciprocated with kolanuts of their own, or with a small amount of "greeting money" (ku'din gaisuwa). This was followed by a chat about family and general affairs, with Alhaji Boka asking leading questions about the health of the visitor's compound, obviously probing for clues and information that he might incorporate into his discussion. While talking to patients he kept a small mirror in front of him into which he gazed continuously, glancing only occasionally at the patients and talking in a low, prescient voice. He said that this was because "every illness has its shadow" (inuwa) and through the mirror he was able to see these shadows and discern the ailment troubling the patient.[2] Once the ailment was described Alhaji Boka would arrive at a diagnosis based on his knowledge (ilimi) of illness, its causation, and treatment. Often the patient himself would not need to be present. A simple description of the sickness, perhaps drawn out with leading questions, was sufficient. As with Uwarture, physical examinations were not performed unless the malady was one perfectly obvious to the sight, in which case it was only a casual observation of the problem—almost like a polite expression of interest—rather than an examination in detail. A diagnosis arrived at, he would then state the sum that would be required as ku'din magani, "money for medicine"—usually quite a large amount. The patient would invariably counter this demand with a much lower offer, presenting him with a modest amount of money rarely exceeding two or three naira. This money Alhaji Audu would gratefully accept, assur-

2. In Hausa the common word for mirror is madubi, "place for looking," which with a change of tone and stress also means "fortune-teller." Duba, the verbal root, means "looking, seeing, inspecting, fortune-telling, prophesying." Boka, the term for a herbalist, is also an alternative word for "mirror."

ing the patient that he or she would recover completely, God willing.[3] Following this business transaction, he would reach behind him into one of a number of gourd calabashes, pull out some herbal powders, wrap them up in paper, and give instructions for their use—to drink, to wash with, to put on a fire as medicinal smoke, to inhale up the nose like snuff, to boil in water creating medicinal vapors, or whatever— sending the patients away while ushering in the next, a process that went on hour after hour.

To understand the nature of this practice more fully, let us consider a number of cases Alhaji Boka saw in the course of one afternoon on a Tuesday in August.

Case 1. I arrived at the compound about 1:30 in the afternoon. Alhaji Boka was found in conversation with two Fulani women, one of whom was suckling a baby. The other woman was a young girl just reaching sexual maturity. They engaged in conversation with Alhaji Boka for some time and then left about 1:45, returning again at 2:15, at which time they were given several medicines for their complaints—dizziness and disturbing dreams at night about men, known in Hausa as *namijin 'dare.* As mentioned previously, these dreams in which a woman has sexual relations with a strange man (or incestuous intercourse) are thought to be caused by spirits, and can result in obstetrical difficulties, gynecological complaints, or be the harbingers of other impending physical ailments. The women were given medicinal incense (*turare*) for use against the dizziness and evil dreams, made up of *kauci*, a parasitic shrub (*Loranthus pentagona*) which grows on various trees and shrubs in the bush and is thought to be efficacious against spirits due to its relationship with high places. *Kauci* is especially useful when taken from certain trees (it has different medicinal qualities depending on where it is found), and the incense in this case was made up of *kauci* taken from *tsamiya* (the tamarind tree, *Tamarindus indica*),

3. After the patient's recovery the remainder of the money—or at least an additional amount of some kind—would be paid, this taking the form of *sadaka*, a charitable gift. In practice, of course, this is somewhat uncertain, depending as it does on one's conception of the word "recovery" (*warkewa*). Since the patient is the one who determines when he is well, payment of such moral (though not legal) debts is frequently irregular. Nonetheless, that this was a rather lucrative business cannot be doubted, since Alhaji Audu Boka was able to save up enough money to perform the pilgrimage to Mecca, which entailed a minimum amount of one thousand naira ($1,600) at the time of my fieldwork.

katsari (an acacia-like tree, *Albizzia chevalieri*), and *gamji* (the gutta-percha rubber tree, *Ficus platyphylla*). In addition, Alhaji Audu gave them powdered *katsari* to ward off the effects of sorcery (*sammu*), and *kadanya* bark (*Butyrospermum parkii*, the shea butter tree) to be used as a tonic against *ciwon ciki*, internal disorders. These two women had traveled fourteen miles to consult him.

Case 2. At 1:45 P.M., when the Fulani women went out the first time, a woman named Hajiya arrived. She was a middle-aged woman and a good friend of Alhaji Audu, having made the pilgrimage to Mecca at the same time he had the previous year. She was complaining of dizziness (*juwa*) and dreams about men, itching (*kaikai*) on the arms, headaches, and general lassitude. He talked with her for some time and later said that she had been having marital difficulties and was considering divorce from her current husband, having previously been widowed. She had, however, decided to try to make the best of it, only to be beset with these ailments. Alhaji Boka gave her several medicinal preparations: *kadanya* bark to be put into solution and washed with as *maganin ciwon jiki*, to take care of her general bodily tiredness; *gawo* (*Acacia albida*) to be used as a powder against sorcery; and some incense identical to that mentioned in case 1 above to ward off spirits. He explained after she had left that she was suffering from a combination of sorcery and spirits, the internal pains and itching being caused by sorcery from some unspecified rival, and the dizziness and bad dreams from spirits. This woman had come from a village seven miles away.

Case 3. After the two Fulani women had again left, about 2:20 P.M., a man came in who had been seen that morning outside the compound cupped by a barber with five different cupping horns. He was complaining of chest, hip, and back pains, as well as general tiredness and lack of energy. After he had been cupped by the barber that morning, Alhaji Audu had applied herbal medicines to the cuts and had told the man to return later.[4] When he came in again, Alhaji Audu gave him two medicines: powdered *gawo* to be taken in *fura* (sour milk with pounded millet) as a preventive against sorcery attacks, as well as powdered *kadanya* bark as a tonic to restore his energy. This latter herbal

---

4. The application of medicines to the cuts made in cupping is rather unusual among the Hausa.

medicine was the same as what had been rubbed into the cupping cuts earlier in the day. Alhaji Boka said that this particular man had been struck down with his illness while working in his fields and was suffering very definitely from sorcery. Someone had made a sorcery poison (*sammu*) and had buried it on his farm. Coming across it unaware in the course of his work, he had been laid low through this treachery. Later in the day this patient came back again and was given some *katsari* powder (*Albizzia chevalieri*) as a medicine against spirits, as well as some more *kadanya*. A local Maguzawa man, he had come about four miles for treatment.

Case 4. About 2:35 P.M. two old Fulani women came in from a camp some seven miles away. They presented three different complaints. One of them had a girl at home who had just given birth but was suffering from general swelling (*kumburi*) of the body, lassitude, vomiting (*amai*) and small, dry feces (*bushin kashi ka'dan-ka'dan*). Alhaji Audu immediately diagnosed this as due to spirits (*iskoki*). The second case was one of a man at home suffering from *ciwon 'kafa da baya,* "leg and back pain," which they described as severe and disabling. Alhaji Boka said this was due to *amosanin 'kashi,* "rheumatism of the bones," due to the actions of spirits.[5] The third complaint was presented by one of the women herself—foot and leg pain, *ciwon 'kafa.* Alhaji Boka told her that this was due to *amosanin ciki,* "disruption of her internal organs due to the penetration of cold" (*sanyi*), which had then spread down her leg causing her discomfort. He gave them *turare* for use as medicinal incense as mentioned above, and *kadanya,* to take care of their needs.

Case 5. While the two Fulani women just mentioned were present, Alhaji Boka left to give some medicine to a woman who was waiting outside. After the Fulanis had left he said that he had given this unseen woman *kadanya* for *ciwon jiki* (generally bodily illness), and *cindazugu* (the physic nut, *Jatropha curcas*) for *ciwon ciki,* "belly complaints." Her general problem, he said, was *amosanin ciki* caused by spirits. He made a special effort to see her because she had come about fifty miles and had to catch a lorry back to her village. It should be noted in this

---

5. Note here the mingling of two medical concepts. *Amosani,* an internal complaint usually said to be caused by cold, is here attributed to spirits. Many Hausa notions about illness are similarly flexible. In this case *amosani* is used as a semantic label to cover the affliction, while its cause is determined to be *iskoki,* spirits.

case that although he said her *amosani* was due to spirits, he made no effort to give her a spirit-related medicine.

Case 6. This woman, who arrived about 3:20 P.M., was not really a case for treatment, but rather a former, satisfied patient who was coming by to pay her respects. A Fulani woman from some distance away, she had been married for many years without ever having given birth to a child. The previous year about the time Alhaji Boka was leaving on his pilgrimage to Mecca, she had come to him for help. He had given her some medicine to induce fertility, and now she was seven months pregnant, thoroughly pleased with his treatment.

Case 7. After the pregnant woman had gone a Fulani herder came in and got two medicinal charms (*layu*) which he had requested to help him ward off attacks from evil spirits. These were small leather pouches with herbal medicines inside, consisting of *kaucin tsamiya* (the parasite from the tamarind tree) and *kaucin tumfafiya* (the same parasitic growth taken from the milkweed shrub *Calotropis procera*). And so it went, on into the later afternoon.

The variety of Alhaji Audu Boka's herbal practice can be clearly seen from these brief case descriptions, and yet certain patterns run throughout. Most of the patients came from outside the village: from rural homesteads or farms, from Fulani cattle camps, or from villages and towns some distance away. A large portion of time was spent on general conversations about life, on greetings, exchanging small gifts of one kind or another, and in intimate personal interaction during the course of each consultation. In all cases Alhaji Audu assured the patient or his friends that he or she would recover. Assurance held a major role in his bedside manner. The fact that absent patients were also treated indicates that diagnosis was not based as much on physical examination as on a general perception of the nature of the patient's illness. *Ilimi*, "knowledge," of herbal remedies, is the major factor involved, not an elaborate etiology of disease. It matters foremost that one knows how to *cure* the sick; how the illness came about is of secondary importance.

Adhaji Boka attributed most illness to malign influences, but wasted little time on which witch, which sorcerer, or which particular spirit was causing the problem in question. Most of the medicines used were general in nature rather than specifics against very narrowly defined ailments. Medicines for *ciwon jiki*, "body pain," or medicines for *iskoki,* "spirits," loomed large in his pharmacopoeia. If only a few medicines were on hand, those were given out, much as a dispenser at a hospital or clinic might give out broad-spectrum antibiotics. Patients never went away empty-handed if they had come for medicine. Since the patients were not told the names of the herbal powders they were given, only that they were *magani* for the malady under consideration, it mattered little to them which specific ingredients were present. If several different kinds of medicine were dispensed in liberal amounts, they went away happy.[6] When one observed a healer such as Alhaji Audu at work over a period of time, it became obvious that he had relatively few kinds of herbal powders, the precise types depending on what had been collected recently in the bush, and those medicines were then the ones utilized. Preferences for particular plants varied over the course of time, depending on their availability and the ailments under treatment, but the specificity of herbal remedies frequently was not very great. Since Hausa medicine tends to view *symptoms* themselves as individual entities or as manifestations of very broad underlying causes such as cold, heat, spirits, witches, or sorcery, specificity of diagnosis is not of great concern. As long as the plants are good *magani*, as long as the herbalist has a good knowledge of herbal practice, things will proceed smoothly. This ad hoc use of plants corresponds nicely with the ad hoc kind of diagnosis practiced, as well as with the sporadic nature of illnesses and the irregular patterns of consultation found in Alhaji Boka's out-patient practice.

It should not be assumed, however, that this sporadic out-patient medicine, this "office consultation," marks the limits of herbal practice. In addition to this short-term therapy, Alhaji Boka and 'Dam Baba engaged in long-term treatment of illness, particularly mental disorders. These in-patients were severely disturbed people brought to them from other locations for prolonged treatment, who stayed several weeks or

---

6. Hausa patients at hospital out-patient clinics are sometimes upset if they are only given a few pills, considering such a small amount of medicine hardly worth the bother of taking. In this regard it is interesting to recall Barth's unfortunate tale (1859:177–78) of the man who pestered him for medicine at Kukawa. Barth gave him two strong doses of Epsom salts, and later three doses of a vermifuge, with instructions to use these medicines on successive days. Unimpressed with such small doses, he preferred to take them as a bolus to enhance their effects, and killed himself as a result.

even months. They would be given a room in the compound, watched, fed, and treated with herbal remedies until such time as they were pronounced "well" and ready to return to their home communities. Consequently, these long-term cases provide interesting material for studying another facet of the herbalists' craft.

As was noted in chapter 5, there are many causes and kinds of madness (hauka), ranging from unacceptable social behavior (drunkenness, drug taking) to neurological diseases (epilepsy, palsy) to complete dementia. Total derangement is almost always regarded as the work of evil forces and those pathetic creatures who wander around stark naked, going from village to village and sleeping in the empty markets; those who sit and drool, the mentally retarded, spastics; those who laugh insanely; those who sit in total silence, autistic and oblivious to the world; or those who erupt in uncontrolled violence against their fellows are put beyond the pale of normal human society and consigned to a hellish world of their own. For them the only hope is in God's mercy or in the skills of the boka, and the prospects for recovery are rather slim. As the Hausa proverb says: Mahaukaci ba ya warkewa, sai rangwame, "The madman does not recover, he only gets a trifle better." 'Dam Baba, in a moment of pessimistic insight, remarked "Medicine for madness is extremely difficult." Nonetheless, when mental illness strikes, the boka is summoned to try his skills against this fearful adversary.

Case 8. One Sunday evening as I was out walking in the village I met Alhaji Audu, who told me he had just returned from Kankara, where he had been summoned to take charge of a madman. This man had a past history of mental problems and suddenly went berserk, attacking people with a hoe. The authorities decided that the man was not a criminal, but rather was insane and so they sent for Alhaji Audu to get him and try to treat his disorder. It took several men to subdue the patient and transport him back to the village. Once there, the poor fellow was taken inside the compound and locked inside the entry-hut. When the door was opened, the man could be seen sitting in the dark. There was a heavy log in the center of the room. He was fixed to the log with a long, thick, metal staple called a gam, which had been fitted over his ankle and pounded into the wood, immobilizing him. He was quiet and docile, but had a wild, fierce look in his eyes, made all the more unnerving by the flickering light of the kerosene lamp. He did not reply when addressed.

The following morning his treatment began. Just before eight o'clock Alhaji Audu prepared the medicine, called *sha'ke*, a generic term for medicines inhaled up through the nose like snuff, penetrating to the brain (so it is said)—a useful treatment both for headache and for madness. This was a reddish-brown powder of an extremely pungent nature. Upon entering the room the sight presented was far different from that of the day before. The patient was sitting on the floor stark naked, having ripped off his clothes, his body ghostly white from his wallowing in the dust. He had a look of fear, anger, and suspicion in his eyes, and motioned everyone out of the room in violent gestures. He was belligerent, totally unamenable to taking anybody's medicines. In no uncertain terms Alhaji Boka told him he had to take it. It was for his own good. Alhaji Audu took the medicine in his hand and tried to get the deranged man to inhale it, but he refused, pushing it away. Alhaji went behind him, took a pinch of medicine in his hand, inserted it in the madman's nostril, and pushed it inside. Immediately he blew it back out and started to fight, constrained though he was by his leg stapled to the log. Alhaji Boka slapped him about the head and shoulders until he finally submitted, then took the medicinal powder in his hands, shoved it up the man's nostrils, and blew it into his nose. This he repeated several times, amid loud protestations from the patient. Finally, the poor man was left alone, sitting quietly, his eyes filling up with tears from the effects of the medicine, mucus and saliva running down his face.

Later in the afternoon the deranged man became violent again and succeeded in creating a terrible commotion inside the *zaure*, tearing the entire door out of the wall in the process. There was a large crowd of onlookers gathered outside, and it was difficult to see what was going on. Pushing through the crowd one could see the deranged man sitting on the floor, covered with his own feces. Bawa, Alhaji's Audu's little boy, was coming in with piles of dirt to cover up the mess, and Alhaji Audu himself was angry, slapping the suffering madman about, browbeating him into submission. Alhaji Audu finally pinned the poor fellow's neck to the ground with his foot—he himself was a big, burly man—and admonished him roughly about his behavior. Other men went off for some rope and bound the patient's hands behind him, while a local carpenter came by to repair the door. When all was done the fellow was locked in a dark room and left muttering to himself, while Alhaji Boka came away muttering, "Madmen are no good."

Two days later the scene was completely different. The madman was sitting peacefully in his room, washing himself with a basin of water. His two wives had come down to see him. He seemed much improved. Several days later the man was barely recognizable. He was sitting outside the compound on a grass mat, dressed neatly in clean clothes, eating a bowl of *tuwo* by himself, unrestrained in any fashion. He greeted people quietly and deferentially when spoken to and seemed like any other shy, normal person. Alhaji Audu said that the man was almost recovered and would be returning to Kankara in a few days. The contrast in behavior in such a short time was truly remarkable. Several days later the man was taken home, riding on the back of a motorcycle. Alhaji Audu was promised fifty naira ($80) for treating him.

Case 9. Not all such long-term cases were as financially profitable or as successful as the case of the man from Kankara. The madwoman of the village market, Dala, provides an extremely interesting contrast. Dala was a girl from a homestead in the bush a few miles from the village. She grew up as a reasonably normal girl, insofar as one could discover, and once was married; but shortly afterward she went mad and took to wandering around in a crazy stupor, and her husband eventually divorced her. Then, for several years she lived in the village market. She wore nothing but a tattered body cloth which she actually kept wrapped around her only occasionally, the rest of the time waving it in the air, strutting about completely naked, exposing herself to the world, and laughing insanely while she talked to the dogs. When thirsty she would drink water from the borrow pit near the market, a slime-covered swamp of muck into which urine from the prostitutes' compound ran in a muddy stream. Ducks slopped about in it. Nothing could have been more repulsive to any human being than to drink from such a mess. At night she slept in empty market stalls, covered or uncovered. Numerous times her family came and caught her, taking her back home, but each time she ran away again until finally they gave up, content to let her live as she seemed to think fit.

After such a long time it seemed that Dala was hopeless. Common Hausa belief holds that such "market madness" is incurable. Finally

her father, Mallam Usuman, came to Alhaji Audu and persuaded him
to attempt to undertake to cure her. As a poor farmer, he said, he had
no money to pay for treatment. Finally Alhaji Audu agreed to treat her
saboda Allah, "for the sake of God," that is, as a charity case. Alhaji
Audu and 'Dam Baba caught her and took her to their compound,
where they locked her up in a room filled with medicinal smoke
(*turare*). At first they had problems with her, but with a place to stay
and someone to feed her and look after her, Dala finally decided to remain with them. They gave her *sha'ke* up her nose, to which she ob-
jected violently, and other similar treatments. Nonetheless, she stayed.
Aside from this she was treated well and not abused and after a few
months her condition improved. Whereas before she was a filthy, half-
naked wretch, living with dogs and drinking slimy water, she was now
clean, bathed regularly, greeted people in a quiet, subdued voice, and
managed to speak a few words of conversation where before she only
laughed or talked incoherently to herself. She also performed simple
chores for the compound such as fetching water from the well. Still
severely ill, she was nevertheless improved in her condition and living
a much better life, and although it was doubtful that she could ever
return to a completely normal state of mind or adjust to life outside the
structured living of the herbalists' compound, there was no question
that she did make some progress as the months went by.

Case 10. A final case gives some insight into what happens to the
family when mental illness strikes, demonstrates the relationship between the *boka*, his patient, and the family, and also sheds additional
light on the general treatment of the mentally ill. One Sunday morning
Alhaji Boka was found going to the blacksmith to get three leg staples
(*gam*) made for the purpose of subduing violent madmen. He said that
a man had come to him from a hamlet several miles away to ask for
help in treating a madwoman. 'Dam Baba was sent to fetch her.

We left the village at noon by motorcycle, making tortuous, slow
progress over the miserable bush paths, which were buried in several
inches of fine, dry dust. Cindo, a ne'er-do-well and sometime drunkard
who was occasionally employed for the purpose of herding madmen
around, had left for the hamlet sometime earlier by bicycle, and was to
meet him there to help restrain the patient and bring her back for treatment. It took nearly two hours to travel the seven miles out to the
hamlet.

Numerous people were there to meet 'Dam Baba when he arrived. As is customary, the greetings of arrival were profuse, and as it was a hot day, cool water mixed liberally with leftover *fura* was provided for refreshment. The initial ceremony concluded, 'Dam Baba entered the compound in question. It was a large compound packed with people— men, women, and children—standing and watching. Several women in the background were weeping, wailing and crying as if somebody had died. Cindo was there, standing between two thatched compounds with the stricken woman, who was chattering away incoherently in a disoriented voice. She was dripping wet with water, which had been thrown on her in an attempt to calm her down. Cindo was remonstrating with her, a rawhide whip in one hand. The woman was taken over to the shade of a third hut and made to sit down, but with difficulty. She did not cooperate. 'Dam Baba went over to the compound head to discuss the situation with him. A small mirror was brought, which 'Dam Baba took and glanced into as he and Alhaji Audu were accustomed to do when diagnosing illness. Finally, he pronounced his verdict: she was stricken by evil spirits (*bakin aljannu*), but would recover with his help. The people seemed relieved to hear this. 'Dam Baba later declared that he had seen in the mirror all sorts of evil spirits which were disrupting her mind, causing her to go mad. 'Dam Baba and a number of senior men from the compound retired to discuss the details of her treatment and the financial arrangements that would be necessary.

The deranged woman was middle-aged, covered in a blue-and-white striped body cloth of the sort made locally. She was naked down to the waist and was without head covering of any kind. She seemed very disoriented and talked in a continuous stream of unrelated sentences, switching topics, speaking of somebody and then asking for somebody else. She wanted to get up and wander around, but everybody urged her to remain seated. She had a bewildered, perplexed look on her face; her eyes in particular seemed troubled. Her conversation wandered in random directions. Her movements were disconnected, all to no apparent purpose.

She kept asking for somebody named 'Dan Juma. A little later she started talking about cattle and laughing, then stopped and lit a cigarette. She began asking in plaintive tones to be given her baby. Finally, a baby was brought out for her to carry around. She gave it a breast to suck, held it, and looked bewilderedly about, asking strange questions, talking about Fulani milk, singing, staring, asking about 'Dan Juma, grabbing at things people were holding. 'Dam Baba gave her some water to drink. She started a conversation asking about her rooms, tried to grab a box of matches, and kept asking about 'Dan Juma. They tried to keep her seated, but she kept getting up to wander around with the baby strapped to her back, and people kept forcing her back into a sitting position.

During this time forty or so people were standing about, staring at her. Women were crying in the background, distraught by the entire situation. It was quite a dramatic scene. She was completely isolated and set off from the rest of the community, surrounded by puzzled, grief-stricken friends and relatives who were at a total loss as to what to do.

She babbled on, finally deciding she needed to go down to the river to wash, asking about her *kabila* (tribe) and its location. Her speech was a constant stream of nervous, disjointed talking, with a very short attention span and no presence of mind or sense of where she was or what was going on around her. She wanted to dance, then to sit down, kept asking for the baby (who had been taken from her), asked for God's help and said *"Hankalina ya dawo kaina,"* "My sense has returned to my head." She kept grabbing at men's clothes when they walked by. In turn they brushed her off roughly. Clearly everybody in the compound was under great emotional stress. The senior men showed it deeply etched on their faces. One younger woman in particular had to be helped into a hut, where she broke out in a most fearful sobbing.

Finally, 'Dam Baba came back from his conference, bringing a pouch full of *sha'ke*, medicinal snuff. He approached her with it. She put up a stiff resistance, fighting him off with her arms. It finally took four men to administer the medicine to her. Three men held her down while Cindo placed the powder in her nostrils and blew it up into her nasal passages. It was obviously very unpleasant for her, but she sat quietly and submissively after having received it, with watery eyes and tears streaming down her face. She was given some water to drink and sat quietly, wiping her face and trying to recover from the shock.

'Dam Baba said that this confirmed his opinion that she had definitely been seized by an evil black spirit, but that it would be possible to treat her. He said the family had agreed to pay him twenty naira ($32) now, of which he had already received seventeen, the three remaining to be paid a little later. After she had recovered they would pay an additional eighty naira ($128), bringing the total up to one hundred naira. This was an enormous amount of money for Hausa villagers to get together.

The compound head was asked when this illness had struck. He said she had been perfectly well until two days previously, when she had suddenly been smitten about noon. She had been incoherent and disoriented ever since. The sudden onset of this illness certainly must have contributed to the great emotional disturbance this misfortune had caused, and it was easy to see how such an occurrence could be attributed to the intrusion of a malevolent evil spirit.

Cindo was of very little help throughout all this, occupying himself mainly by threatening the poor woman with his whip if she did not remain seated; but his activities did not seem to bother anyone.[7] A number of the men in the compound were very agitated with the woman and 'Dam Baba frequently reprimanded her in a loud, stern voice, telling her to behave herself. Cindo appeared just to be waiting for a chance to lay about her head and shoulders with his whip.

The activities in the compound took about an hour, and when the party was ready to leave they were escorted out to the road by the members of the compound. The woman followed 'Dam Baba, holding onto his gown. She was not eager to go anywhere, but was not really aware enough of what was happening to follow the proceedings. She

7. Cindo, being one of the town drunks, was often a cause for concern in the village. On one occasion I helped 'Dam Baba and Alhaji Boka catch him, throw him to the ground, and staple his leg to a log when he got drunk and started throwing ax handles at a group of village children who were taunting him. He was so drunk he didn't even remember it the following morning, even though he was still pinned to the log when he recovered.

The fact that 'Dam Baba and Alhaji Boka were forced to employ somebody like Cindo to fetch back a mentally disturbed person seems to me to have parallels in the staffing of many mental institutions in European and American society, particularly in the past. As people on the margins of society, the mentally ill are set aside and often are dealt with only by people who also have a marginal status but who can gain a feeling of superiority by ordering such others around. This was clearly the case with Cindo. His use of violence and the whip was a clear indication of such an urge.

went along simply because she could not think of anything better to do at the moment. If another idea had entered her mind she would have wandered off someplace else.

The question of how she was going to be taken back to the village was intriguing. There were already two passengers on the motorcycle. Cindo had ridden over on a bicycle. The proposal was to carry her back to 'Dam Baba's compound on the bicycle. Cindo would balance her on the handlebars and take her back that way—a common practice all over Nigeria, provided of course that the person on the handlebars is willing to go. This was the problem. She did not want to go anywhere. What followed was a magnificent comedy routine.

First, the bicycle was brought out and she was told to get on it so she could be taken back to the village. She did not seem to understand, but just stood there, oblivious to the whole proceeding, a small smile on her face, staring wide-eyed at everybody. Not getting anywhere, they picked her up and put her sidesaddle on the bicycle frame in front of the seat. She kept sticking her feet onto the pedals, however, or onto the chain, knocking off the pump for the tires, getting tangled up, moving on and off the seat. All this time, of course, people were trying to hold the bicycle upright. She kept trying to climb off; they kept trying to balance her on the frame. Finally, it looked as if she was on and holding onto the handlebars, so Cindo gave the bicycle a little push to start it rolling, and began weaving an unsteady course down the bumpy, dusty path, clambering onto the seat just as she got off, dumping them all in a heap. After ten minutes of trying to get her on the bicycle they had traveled fifteen feet.

Finally, in anger, they decided she would have to be tied to the bicycle frame to prevent this from happening again—as if anybody could ride a bicycle over a footpath in the bush with a woman tied to the handlebars, struggling to get off, bearing in mind that most Hausa bicycles have no brakes and that a goodly portion of the trip back would be downhill and over several dry watercourses. Nonetheless, a number of villagers held her down while the rest held up the bicycle. They put her legs down on either side, tied them to the frame, and then tied her hands and arms securely to the handlebars. This done, they held the bicycle upright and Cindo started it rolling again—balancing precariously—and wobbled unsteadily down the road, around a bend at the edge of the village, behind some shrubs, and out of sight.

'Dam Baba said goodbye, hopped on the motorcycle and slowly set off down the same path. As he reached the edge of the village and rounded the turn, there, behind the shrubbery, lying in a heap, were Cindo and the woman. She was angry, struggling to get loose and un-tangle herself from the bicycle, the rope, and Cindo. 'Dam Baba got off the motorcycle, untied her, and went through the whole ludicrous business of setting the bicycle back up, putting her on the handlebars, and trying to set off down the road again. They seemed to have suc-ceeded, bouncing uncertainly along the path until they were almost out of sight. 'Dam Baba and I followed on the motorcycle, with a number of villagers on bicycles escorting us out into the countryside.

About a quarter of a mile from the village the bicycle tipped over again. This time the patient got up and ran away. Cindo, extremely angry at this point, followed her with the whip, flailing away at her, finally grabbing her arms and flinging her to the ground. It was finally obvious to everyone that they would not get her back to the village by carrying her on the bicycle, so a boy was sent to ride the bicycle back to the village, followed by a man on another bicycle to take him home again. The poor woman was bound with her hands tied together in front, still oblivious to everything and chattering away disconnectedly with that smug little smile on her face. She trudged along in front of Cindo, who held the other end of the six feet of rope tied to the two strips of cloth which immobilized her hands. The rope in one hand, his whip in the other, he followed her down the dusty path, preceded by two bicycles, the motorcycle bringing up the rear—an extraordinary cavalcade in the late afternoon sun. Eventually, the motorcycle pulled on ahead, arriving back in the village about six o'clock. Just over an hour later Cindo and the patient came trooping in. She was placed in a room with another madwoman, where a wood fire billowed out smoke from the medicinal incense that was burning to drive out the evil spirits. Her course of treatment had begun.

" 'Dan Juma," for that was the nickname given her after her inco-herent ramblings about the unknown man of that name, stayed with 'Dam Baba and Alhaji Boka for a long time. Each day she was given medicine—either *sha'ke*, fluids poured up her nose, or medicinal smoke—and was given simple tasks to perform. Somebody from her home village brought her baby to her, and she carried it around with her. It was not very long after her arrival that she reoriented herself and began to realize that she was living in a herbalist's compound. She gained intelligibility in her conversation and returned to normal fairly quickly. Although she still seemed rather a strange women, nonetheless she was a functional member of society. She became an accepted part of the compound and got along well with everybody.

Weeks passed and turned into months. 'Dam Baba sent word back to her hamlet that she had been cured, and that they should come get her and pay him his money. They ignored him. He sent again, and was told that somebody would soon come to get her; but nobody came. After this had gone on for several months it became apparent that no one would come for her. Originally it had seemed like 'Dam Baba was attempting to extort a great deal of money from a bereaved family. As matters progressed, however, it became obvious that what he had done was necessary, for he was stuck with feeding and taking care of a sick woman for months. The amount of money he had been paid initially for treating her seemed small indeed as time stretched on. It was also clear that the herbalist's compound served as a convenient place for dumping an embarrassing and mentally disturbed person, much as mental hospitals and nursing homes in the West are frequently little more than places for disposing of the mentally ill. Once they had accepted her for treatment they were stuck with her indefinitely.

In all three cases of mental illness mentioned above, however, it appeared that the treatment given by the *boka* had a positive effect. The medicinal smoke and the *sha'ke* forced up the nose to drive the spirits out of the brain through violent sneezing, especially in the initial stages of treatment, where a conflict of wills between the healer and the patient was often encountered, served to break the patient and force him or her into a dependency on the healer. This done, the healer then asssumed a supportive role. Patients were not mistreated, only forced to conform to a rather unpleasant therapeutic regimen. Their integration into the life of the compound and their acceptance by the people with whom they lived must have worked toward building in the patients a more positive view of the world and their surroundings.[8] It would be overstating the case to say that all these patients were

8. In *bori* spirit possession the final sign that the possessed person is returning to normal is a series of three violent sneezes, signaling the departure of the spirit which has been "riding" the dancer. The relationship between *sha'ke*, sneezing, and the cure of spirit-induced mental disorders should be apparent.

"cured." The Hausa proverb mentioned earlier recognizes the fact that mental illness is a difficult thing to correct, but in these three cases the patients all seemed to make some kind of adjustment, to regain some stability, or at least to accept their environment to a greater degree than they had before.

In their style of practice and clientele Alhaji Audu Boka and 'Dam Baba differed sharply from Uwarture. Much of this difference stems from the different opportunities open to them as a result of the differing Hausa sex roles. As a woman, Uwarture was essentially a family practitioner, operating within the scope of her friends and relatives, who formed a large group of potential clients due to her long residence in the village and her large family. The two brothers, on the other hand, were outsiders, strangers who had been resident in the village only a short time. As men, they were allowed greater freedom of movement and more forceful expressions of behavior than those appropriate to women. These things they exploited energetically, making herbalism an occupation which paid them rather well. Building their compound immediately adjacent to the village market and lorry-park showed shrewd business judgment and gave them both easy access to passers-by and high visibility, with resultant good advertising. Having made the pilgrimage, Alhaji Audu Boka was able to combine aspects of Islamic piety with his knowledge of herbalism, and the presence of his younger brother, also a herbalist, allowed them to undertake independent trips to other parts of the country to augment their herbal practice, as well as to undertake the treatment of violent mental patients who might need the full attentions of two strong and skilled men. In spite of these differences, however, the core of both practices was herbalism: the modes of administration and the medicines given were very similar.

■ Rivalry and Therapeutic Options

Herbalists are individuals, each practicing his or her chosen occupation. They are a category of people, but not a corporate entity. There are no guilds of herbalists (with the possible exception of the *bori* network), even though an incipient Nigerian Herbalists' Association is being created. The *bokaye* deal with individual matters, not with relations between larger social units, as might be the case elsewhere in

Africa. It is a matter of some interest, therefore, how herbalists inter-act with each other. The nature of the relationship depends mainly upon the personalities of the individuals involved. Some healers have noth-ing to do with each other; others have continuing relationships of vary-ing cordiality. Alhaji Boka and 'Dam Baba, for example, utilized other herbalists and medicine sellers as suppliers, asking them to collect cer-tain herbal ingredients out in the bush, for which they were paid. In general, however, herbalists tend to be competitors with each other, downgrading their rivals in order to increase their own reputations.

The distinction between *maganin gaskiya* ("true medicine" or "real medicine") as opposed to *maganin 'karya* ("false medicine" or "fake medicine") is a significant one in the minds of both herbalists and pa-tients. There is a plethora of potential herbal ingredients, and these can be combined in almost infinite permutations. Every herbalist has some kind of *ilimi*, knowledge, of herbal remedies, but the extent and quality of this knowledge is subject to variation. The notion that one's own knowledge of these medicines is superior to that of one's rivals is strong, and if the matter is discussed the opinion will often be ad-vanced that "so-and-so's medicine is 'false,' " that he is a deceiver and a scoundrel, not fit for treating those who are sick. Where money is involved such rivalries may become heated. One such instance arose between Uwarture and Alhaji Boka. It went so far as to be brought before the village headman, something clearly beyond the normal limits of such rivalry.

According to Alhaji Audu, a patient with partial paralysis of his arm came to him for treatment, moved into the compound, and began tak-ing medicine, promising to pay him some thirty naira. Several days later Alhaji Audu went to market in another village and discovered upon his return that the man had run off without paying. Sometime later he found out that this man, rather than returning to Funtua as he had thought, had actually gone over to Uwarture and, being dissatisfied with the treatment he had received from Alhaji Boka, refused to pay him anything at all. Alhaji Boka became angry, confronted him, called him a "worthless, lying bastard," and threatened to afflict him with a disease so terrible that he would come crawling back for treatment and pay him two hundred naira to cure it rather than the paltry sum he owed him. Then he stormed off in an angry temper.

Uwarture's version of the story (confirmed by the patient who was still resident in her compound) was rather different. This particular patient had been plagued with weakness and paralysis of his entire left side for some time. Hearing of Uwarture in Funtua, he made the trip to the village in search of her, hoping that he could be cured. After arriving at the lorry-park on the edge of the market he inquired about her, only to run into Alhaji Boka, who told him that she was no good and that her medicines were a pack of lies. Alhaji Audu told him that he was perfectly capable of curing his condition. With help so near to hand, the man consented to go with him and moved into his compound, paying him the sum of three naira for treatment, which was most of the money he had. He stayed in the compound for five days, but was very short of money and had little to pay for food. He even claimed that he had tried to sell his gown to obtain money to buy food. Alhaji Audu, he said, did not provide him with anything to eat, or at most a bare subsistence, and after five days of rather intense discomfort he took the opportunity of Alhaji Audu's absence to leave, going in search of Uwarture.

When he arrived at her compound he explained the situation to her and moved in to begin a course of treatment. Shortly afterward Uwarture and her husband left on a one-day trip. From the lorry-park near his compound Alhaji Boka saw them leave and decided this would be a good time to get his revenge. He went over to her compound and walked right in, an egregious violation of Hausa etiquette. One of Uwarture's neighbors, an old woman, told Alhaji Audu that nobody was home, but he ignored her, went in, and began poking around among her possessions and looking through her medicines. He had a violent confrontation with the patient and then stormed out. The following day, when Uwarture and Damina returned and discovered what had happened they were livid with rage. They went straight to the village headman and told him what had occurred. Alhaji Audu was summoned and thoroughly chastised. Nothing else was done, but Alhaji Audu was very subdued for a number of days thereafter, keeping a distinctly low profile around the village. The patient remained with Uwarture, who treated his condition by rubbing him with herbal medicines mixed in butter, massaging his left side, starting with the head and working down to the limbs, then bathing him with a hot medicinal tea composed of ten different ingredients, which was designed to rid him of the spirit plaguing him: *Inna, mai-shan jini; "Inna*, the drinker of blood."

The American cynic Ambrose Bierce once defined a physician as "one upon whom we set our hopes when ill, and our dogs when well" (Bierce 1958:99). Physicians are frequently maligned until someone becomes sick, at which point everything is forgotten except the desire to recover. Several Hausa proverbs express these sentiments: *Rai ya fi dukiya*, "Life is worth more than wealth." *Ina amfanin ba'di ba rai?,* "What good is next year without life?" When someone becomes ill, hope of recovery is a great sustainer, staving off the hidden fear of death which always lurks in the uncertainty of illness. The proverbs say *Rama ba mutuwa ba ne*, "Being thin is not being dead"; and *Daidai, majinyaci ba shi gode Allah sai ya ga wanda ya mutu*, "Truly, the sick man does not thank God until he sees the one who has died." Hope reposes in the medical practitioner: *Abin majinyaci na mai-magani ne*, "The possessions of the sick man belong to he who has the medicine." Nonetheless, the costs of illness are difficult to bear: *Magani da ku'di, shi ne da wuyar sha*, "Expensive medicine is difficult to drink." More pointed, perhaps, is that proverb which raises doubts about the efficacy of treatment: *Yau da gobe, 'karya ta boka,* " 'Slowly but surely' [you'll recover] is the herbalist's lie."

The interplay of these emotions helps explain many aspects of Hausa illness behavior. The sick Hausa villager is not particularly concerned with who or what brings recovery, as long as he gets well again. The case involving Uwarture and Alhaji Audu Boka described above is indicative of this not uncommon phenomenon. The patient goes for treatment to one healer, stays for a while, but then becomes dissatisfied and changes to another herbalist, or indeed switches to another mode of therapy altogether. A number of therapeutic options are open to the sick, both in the traditional culture as well as in the modernizing one. All are regarded as sources of *magani*. They are not mutually exclusive systems of medicine, but are perceived as different modes of therapy which may have varying effectiveness in different circumstances and different illnesses. As such they are utilized in combination with each other by the local population. Hospitals, dispensaries, and scientifically prepared drugs are utilized alongside the traditional modes of healing.

One of the most common areas where the two cultures of traditional and scientific medicine mingle is the injection. *Allura*, the Hausa word for needle, is the common word for a medical injection. To say of somebody that *an ba shi allura*, "They gave him the needle," is to say that the person was given an injection of some kind. This practice has no real counterpart in Hausa traditional medicine[9] and the idea of putting medicine directly into the body in this manner has been heartily accepted—so enthusiastically accepted, in fact, that patients going to a hospital for treatment are often greatly disappointed, if not angry, when they are not given an injection. Dispensers in rural areas may take advantage of this fact by charging patients for injections and pocketing the illicit fee. In addition, there are growing numbers of people in towns and rural areas who have gained possession of syringes and needles and who give injections on demand (see chapter 4). The rural villager may not distinguish properly among these practitioners, viewing all injections as approximately equal in value whether given by a doctor, a nurse, a dispenser, or a local entrepreneur. If the patient feels he needs an injection he will seek someone who will give him one, and since an enterprising local enthusiast is often more willing than are hospital personnel, it is to the market source that he will go.

Uwarture herself was an interesting example of the utilization of therapeutic options of this kind. An accomplished herbalist, she nonetheless had great respect for the abilities of doctors. Suturing and surgery in particular impressed her. Although she did not give injections herself, she felt no aversion to receiving them. On one occasion in particular she felt ill and had a local man come around to inject her. Rather than recovering, however, she got much worse. The injection was given in her left arm and an infection developed. Her entire left arm, shoulder, armpit, and breast became swollen and painful. She was unable to lift her arm or even grasp anything with her left hand. The experience left her prostrate for several days, during which time there was much concern for her recovery. A steady stream of sympathetic visitors came by to see her, and a number of women were always

9. Some village friends explained cupping to me by analogy with injections, calling this practice *allura irin namu* or "our kind of injections," or *allura ta gargajiya*, "traditional injections." The practices are not really comparable, however, especially since medicines are rarely rubbed into the cupping cuts.

present with her in her hut. Fortunately, the swelling and pain subsided after a few days and she recovered.[10]

In a setting of such demand it is easy to understand how the principal usefulness of dispensaries is seen as a place to get injections. A dispenser who is ready with his needle is always more highly respected than one who is not. The closest dispensary to the village was four miles away. It was manned by a young, arrogant dispensary attendant only recently graduated from the Medical Auxiliary Training School. He showed little interest in treating patients and was poorly regarded locally. The common opinion was that *ba shi da magani, sai episi*, "He has no medicine, only A.P.C." (Aspirin-phenacetin-caffeine tablets). The other dispensary, some eight miles away, was much more heavily used, for the attendant was an older man, intent on helping people, who was interested and well trained. He took a personal interest in his patients, bounced babies on his knees and chucked them under the chin. He treated people as individuals, which they appreciated.

As with most human beings, convenience plays an important role in the utilization of health services by the Hausa (Stock 1979). The dispensaries were used only sporadically, and then only for serious ailments such as a deep gash on the leg, a severely infected wound, or some other ailment where scientific clinical medicine was reputed to be of especial usefulness. Hospitals were used very infrequently, due largely to the cost of travel and the time spent waiting. The nearest hospital was well over twenty miles away, and for a rural person to make the trip it was necessary for him to have a severe ailment, time and money enough to spend in transit, and faith in the effectiveness of treatment.

For the villager hospitals are large, unfamiliar places. In Hausaland they are frequently staffed with southerners—Ibos, Yorubas, or Tiv—due to the poor educational system in the north. The attendants are fairly sophisticated people (by rural terms), used to big cities and their ways. Frequently they have little patience with uneasy, nervous people from the countryside and treat them curtly, if not rudely. The lines are long and, for outpatient treatment, the rewards are frequently no

10. Others are not so lucky. One "modern" schoolteacher in another village decided he knew enough to set up an injection practice for the fee of one naira per injection. Shortly thereafter a small boy he had treated died as a result.

more than a few quick questions and a small packet of pills. It is a regimented, impersonal business—a major reason why the *boka* will likely be around for many years to come, for in dealing with a traditional herbalist the patient is treated attentively and individually, in surroundings with which he is familiar, and in terms he can understand. Hospitals frequently are sources of bewilderment, with people marching to and fro from room to building to room for no apparent reason. In cases of deep wounds, severe bleeding, and illnesses where antibiotics or sophisticated technology (such as surgery) can produce immediate, dramatic results, the hospitals' reputations are high indeed; but in those cases where the ailment is unusual, difficult to diagnose or treat, or of an unspecific nature, the failure of scientific medicine to provide a cure often pushes the patient back into the world of traditional practice.

Uwarture and others frequently said that hospitals had no medicines for spirit-induced illnesses, for sorcery, for witch attacks, or for other ailments caused by the intrusion of malevolent spiritual forces. In these cases the *boka* was the only recourse for treatment. One such case, a sad one, was that of Mai Ku'di, a small boy who had a permanent neurological defect. This child had severely crippled hands and feet, which appeared to be congenital defects, accompanied by poor motor control and severe retardation. This child and his mother came to stay with Alhaji Audu, where the boy underwent treatment for spirit-induced illnesses (as well as for intestinal roundworms). He just sat and stared, moving his arms around in uncontrolled movements, sucking the backs of his crippled hands, with no control over his excretory functions. Alhaji Audu said the child would eat anything left lying around, plastic bags, feces, anything he could get into his mouth. His mother said that he had been normal up until the time he was weaned, but then was stricken with this horrible affliction. She had taken him to the hospital in Kaduna where they treated him for some months. He did not improve, so she took him to a herbalist in Kaduna, who also treated him. Again, he did not improve. From Kaduna she took him to the Ahmadu Bello University hospital in Zaria, where again no help was obtained. Hearing about Alhaji Boka in Zaria, she traveled to his village to seek help from him, and remained there for five months, always hoping to see some improvement in her boy. When this, too, failed, she went to see Uwarture, who turned her away saying it was *ciwon Allah,* "God's sickness," and that there was no cure for it. Still seeking hope anywhere she could find it, the distraught mother spent most of her time and money traveling the countryside from herbalist to hospital and back, looking for a ray of hope.

In circumstances such as this, countless daily dramas of illness and treatment are played out in Hausaland. The task now remaining before us is to explore something of the internal logic of the system and its metaphysical assumptions in order to grasp the interrelationships of illness, its explanation, and the design of therapy.

VIII

Allah, Herbs, and Spirits: The Logic of Hausa Medicine

What we are to seek . . . is not when superstition in medicine was replaced by science (has it been?), but how the diverse elements of human imagination have operated to bring about the contemporary rationale of medicine that has everywhere and in diverse ways, not all desirable, transformed the conditions of human existence.

W. P. D. WIGHTMAN, *The Emergence of Scientific Medicine*

Wanda zai mutu magani ba ya tsaishe shi ba.

(*Medicine will not revive one who is doomed to die.*)

HAUSA PROVERB

■ The Metaphysical Foundations of Hausa Traditional Medicine

To this point a broad range of topics pertaining to rural Hausa life has been discussed. We have seen something of the nature of rural living and the ways in which the span of human life is divided and marked in Hausa rites of passage. Muslim Hausa views of the moral order and the nature of virtue have been discussed, as have the contrary values of evil and their social setting. The central concept of *lafiya*, or "moral and physical balance," has been emphasized, as well as those things which upset that balance, especially within the human body, and cause illness. The Hausa idea of *magani* or "medicine"— "that which brings about or restores *lafiya*"— has been described, and we have surveyed the various medical practitioners who offer these remedies to those in ill health. Finally, we have followed two such practitioners in some detail to gain a better understanding of the social setting of traditional herbal practice. In this chapter our purpose is to focus more closely on the logical structure of Hausa medicine, especially in regard to therapeutic practice, and to elucidate some fundamental principles under which this system operates; in short, to examine the metaphysical foundations of Hausa medicine and to discuss some of the implications that result from these starting points.

Metaphysics deals with the largely unarticulated foundations of thought, the assumptions that form the background for thinking. As R. G. Collingwood stated in his highly stimulating work *An Essay on Meta-*

physics (1940:21): "Whenever anybody states a thought in words, there are a great many more thoughts in his mind than are expressed in his statement. Among these are some which stand in a peculiar relation to the thought he has stated: they are not merely its context, they are its presuppositions."[1] These presuppositions are the foundations on which every thought that follows is based; they are assumptions about the nature of the world, a view of what composes "reality." They are logically prior to everything else in that system of thought, and as long as one operates within that system of thought it is impossible to get around them; because they are the determinants of "sense," any attempt to do so would result in "non-sense." These "absolute presuppositions" form the categories of thought through which human observations are channeled, defining the structure of thinking and giving it meaning.

In short, these presuppositions form the tools by which experience and reality are gauged. Collingwood drove this point home with a hypothetical anthropological example: a tribe of people who supposed that everything in the world happened because of magic (1940:193–94):

> An absolute presupposition cannot be undermined by the yardstick of "experience," because it is the yardstick by which "experience" is judged. To suggest that "experience" might teach my hypothetical savages that some events are not due to magic is like suggesting that experience might teach a civilized people that there are not twelve inches in a foot and thus cause them to adopt the metric system. As long as you measure in feet and inches, everything you measure has dimensions composed of those units. As long as you believe in a world of magic, that is the kind of world in which you live. If any group or community of human beings ever held a pan-magical belief about the world, it is certainly not "experience" that could shake it.

The end result of such beliefs may be medical error and ineffective treatment, but these results stem from the faulty presuppositions with which they began. The process by which conclusions are reached may be very logical. The anthropologist and physician W. H. R. Rivers

---

1. This entire section owes much to Collingwood's discussion of metaphysics.

pointed this out long ago in his remarks on indigenous medical practices in Melanesia (1924:51–52):

> The practices of these peoples in relation to disease are not a medley of disconnected and meaningless customs, but are inspired by definite ideas concerning the causation of disease. Their modes of treatment follow directly from their ideas concerning etiology and pathology. From our modern standpoint we are able to see that these ideas are wrong. But the important point is that, however wrong may be the beliefs of the Papuan and Melanesian concerning the causation of disease, their practices are the logical consequences of those beliefs. We may say even that these peoples practice an art of medicine which is in some respects more rational than our own, in that its modes of diagnosis and treatment follow more directly from their ideas concerning the causation of disease. According to the opinion of the civilized world, these ideas of causation are wrong, or contain but grains of truth here and there; but once grant these ideas and the body of medical practice follows therefrom with a logical consistency which it may take us long to emulate in our pursuit of a medicine founded upon the sciences of physiology and psychology.

Other cultural and social systems can thus be seen as differing in the metaphysical presuppositions they make about the world, the assumptions which undergird the rest of their social thought. The purpose of metaphysical analysis, in Collingwood's view, is thus to elucidate and analyze the myriad clusterings of absolute presuppositions made by various people at various times in history and in other cultural settings.[2] Such clusters he termed "constellations of absolute presuppositions," the analysis of which gives the metaphysician "a hint of the way in which different sets of absolute presuppositions correspond not

2. "To sum up: Metaphysics is the attempt to find out what absolute presuppositions have been made by this or that person or group of persons, on this or that occasion or group of occasions, in the course of this or that piece of thinking. Arising out of this, it will consider (for example) whether absolute presuppositions are made singly or in groups, and if the latter, how the groups are organized; whether different absolute presuppositions are made by different individuals or races or nations or classes; or on occasions when different things are being thought about; or whether the same have been made *semper, ubique, ab omnibus*. And so on" (Collingwood 1940:47).

only with differences in the structure of what is generally called scientific thoughts but with differences in the entire fabric of civilization" (Collingwood 1940:72). From our viewpoint it is obvious that this is one way of describing the anthropological endeavor. Theoretically, at least, it should be possible to describe and analyze the various constellations of presuppositions that form the foundation for any given cultural system. In practical terms, to do this for an entire society would be a formidable undertaking indeed; but an analysis of the foundations of some small, selected aspect of thought should be much easier to accomplish.

Fruitful areas in which to pursue this type of analysis are those aspects of a culture that involve active problem solving, such as its medical system. Metaphysical assumptions about the world are crucial in defining the nature of the perceived "reality" that generates problems, and hence are also crucial in defining possible pathways to their solution—and no system of thought is without such assumptions.[3] The resultant mode of thinking, which is adopted to produce explanations of and solutions to problems in such a setting, may be called an explanatory or problem-solving "paradigm," borrowing the phrase so usefully coined by Kuhn in his book *The Structure of Scientific Revolutions* (1970). In this chapter an attempt will be made to describe the essential presuppositions that form the metaphysical foundations of Hausa traditional medicine. It is these basic beliefs that determine the

3. See, for example, E. A. Burtt (1932), *The Metaphysical Foundations of Modern Physical Science*. In this regard Collingwood noted (1940:179–80):

> In point of fact the Kantian "principles" are nothing more permanent than the presuppositions of eighteenth-century physics, as Kant discovered them by analysis. If you analyse the physics of to-day, or that of the Renaissance, or that of Aristotle, you get a different set. . . . When once it is realized that the absolute presuppositions of eighteenth-century science, far from being accepted *semper, ubique, ab omnibus*, had only a quite short historical life, as we nowadays think of history, in only a quite limited part of the world, and that even inside Europe other systems of science worked before then and since then on different presuppositions, it becomes impossible for any one except for the most irresponsible kind of thinker to maintain that out of all these and all the other possible sets of presuppositions there is one set and only one which consists of propositions accurately describing observable characteristics everywhere present in the world, while all the other sets represent more or less systematic hallucinations as to what these characteristics are.

structure of the Hausa medical paradigm and constrain their attempts at dealing with any given situation of illness. It should also be stressed that these formulations are *not* "propositions" advanced by the Hausa for proof or disproof, but rather are "suppositions" taken for granted as inherent parts of the reality in which they live. By making these principles clear, the nature of the system and its limitations becomes clearer and the actions of traditional medical practitioners become more readily understandable.

Six Presuppositions of Hausa Traditional Medicine

1. Allah is the one, the only, supreme God, the creator and ruler of the universe. He is the ultimate cause of everything that happens, and nothing happens that is not ultimately His will.

2. Allah has made Himself known to mankind through the prophets. The last and greatest of the prophets is Muhammed, through whom Allah transmitted his final revelation in the form of the Holy Koran.

3. Subordinate to Allah there also exists a body of sentient (but capricious) beings with lesser but still substantial powers who may establish relationships with men. Such relationships may occasionally be beneficial, but most often they are not, and result in sickness, disablement, or death. These beings include a wide variety of spirits (*aljannu, iskoki,* the *dodo,* etc.), the souls (*kurwa*) of the recently departed dead, and witches *(mayu),* whose evil intentions are carried out through the unique powers of their souls.

4. Proper well-being (*lafiya*) depends upon an individual's ability to live in harmonious balance with his surroundings, which include the moral, physical, and spiritual realms. Illness results from the disruption of this balance within the body by the intrusion of environmental factors (especially cold) or through the actions of spiritual powers.

5. For each illness Allah has ordained a remedy, according to His will. Success in the treatment of illness comes from proper knowledge (*ilimi*) of these medicines. Some illnesses are of minor concern and can be treated with weak remedies, but more serious illnesses are more difficult to treat and require more powerful medicines. Such knowledge is not easy to obtain. In cases of more severe illness, knowledge of the proper medicines becomes harder and harder to attain, and consequently it will be known to fewer and fewer people.

6. The ingredients of successful medicines are to be found in the trees, shrubs, plants, and animals created by God; in His Holy Koran;

and in the traditions (*hadisi*) of the Prophet Muhammed, who transmitted God's revelations to mankind. The essence of medicine is the
knowledge of the correspondences among these things and the ailments
of the patient. Such knowledge may be obtained by (a) studying the
direct revelations of God as recorded in the Koran, the traditions of the
Prophet, and the commentaries of the learned men of the past; (b) direct revelation from the spirits, who reveal useful medicines to their
followers; (c) gaining access to the secrets of other traditions such as
through the inheritance of medicinal recipes within a family line, or by
apprenticeship to the owner of such secrets as, for example, in the
course of initiation into the *bori* cult; and by (d) judiciously combining
intuition, speculation, and crude empiricism with the information obtained from the first three sources.

Of all these unquestioned axioms of Hausa medical thought, the first
has the most profound implications. As has been noted earlier, *Islam*
in Arabic means "submission" to the will of God. The believer acknowledges God's supreme power and agrees to live according to His
will, thereby finding peace and gaining salvation. As in the physical
world where the power of God is seen as controlling, ruling, motivat-
ing, and restraining the forces of nature, so His will also ultimately
determines what happens in the lives of men. All success and all misfortune alike is sent ultimately by God. In medical thinking this means
that all illness ultimately comes from God for unknown and unfathomable reasons, and that all recovery also comes because of God's
will. In the last analysis, God is unreachable and transcendent, the final
cause of all events. In some non-Muslim African societies, this ultimate
"why" is answered by witchcraft: in Hausaland the final explanation
is the will of Allah.

Consider, for example, the famous case of the Zande granary, detailed in Evans-Pritchard's *Witchcraft, Oracles and Magic Among the
Azande* (1937:69–70). In Zandeland old granaries occasionally collapse because termites have eaten their supports or the wood has de-
cayed. There is nothing unusual in this; but sometimes—because granaries provide shade and thus are convenient places to chat or play the
African hole-game—it happens that somebody is sitting under one
when it does collapse, and sustains serious injury as a result. The Zande
do not question why the granary should have collapsed—everybody
knows that old, broken-down granaries *may* collapse; nor do they ques-

tion why people should sit under them in the shade, for these reasons, too, are obvious. The grave question for the Azande in such a case is why *that* particular granary should have collapsed at *that* particular time when *those* particular people were sitting under it. What to our notions is merely coincidence is for the Azande an instance of witch-craft. Without witchcraft either the granary would not have collapsed, or there would not have been people sitting under it when the collapse occurred.

Among the Hausa the interaction of such chains of events is ex-plained by the will of God. For example, in the village that formed the locus for most of this fieldwork it was not uncommon for old buildings to be in rather shabby states of repair. The entry-huts of several vil-lagers were in terrible shape, but nonetheless formed the social centers of their households when friends came by to chat with the compound head. One villager, Muhammadu Mai-Shanu, had such an entry-hut. It was incredibly dilapidated and was kept standing only by propping up all four sides with large logs. Even so, the walls sagged away from the perpendicular by an alarming number of degrees. In the course of several discussions the subject of his entry-hut arose; I pointed out that he should repair it before it collapsed and killed somebody. Wouldn't he be liable for such an injury? In response he noted that he had propped up the walls and had also taken chalk and written a long Koranic charm around the inside of all four walls—the idea being that the power of the words would act like steel bands around a box, hold-ing the sides together. The walls would not collapse and injure someone unless it was the will of God. Preventive maintenance is not a notion that takes hold easily in such a setting, for who can anticipate the will of God?

In the final analysis God is thus responsible for all illness. As the ulti-mate mover of the entire universe, He sets in play the environmental forces (such as damp coldness) that penetrate the body and cause sick-ness. Other sentient powers, such as the spirits, cause illness ultimately because of the will of God. As one herbalist exclaimed in exasperation when pressed to answer the (to him) elementary question of why the spirits attack people: *Allah bai aike su ba!?* "Doesn't God send them!?" There is, however, a certain latitude in this process. One can imagine that as a chief (and God is frequently envisioned as the supreme chief of the world),[4] He has many things demanding His attention. As with the subordinates of any chief, the spirits may decide to act on their own without informing their master precisely what they are doing. God may be unaware of such doings temporarily, but ultimately He will find out and take action, either granting His permission or causing the illness to go away. Thus, because God ultimately controls everything, recovery also occurs because it is God's will. One often hears expressions such as *Allah ya sallame ni, na warke,* "God released me; I recovered from my illness," —the verb *sallame* meaning "to dismiss from one's presence" or "to grant permission to depart," etc. God thus dismisses the illness and the patient is allowed to resume his or her normal life.

The omnipotence of God is a very important concept in Hausa thought, and nobody elaborated it better than the herbalist Uwarture. According to her all illnesses may be grouped into two categories, *ciwon Allah,* "illnesses from God," and *ciwon iskoki,* "diseases of the spirits." All sickness results from one of these two causes, but the outward appearance of both is the same. Thus, for example, there could be leprosy sent from God or caused by the leper spirit, *Kuturu;* or there could be madness caused by God or caused by the attack of a spirit; and so on for any ailment one would care to name. Only through the application of the proper medicines can they be distinguished. If spirits cause the illness, it vanishes when confronted by the medicine and the patient recovers; if, however, the affliction is caused by the will of God, medicine is of no avail. In such a scheme medicines are almost diagnostic tools more than therapeutic regimens: if no response is obtained it is because God is counteracting (or countermanding) the effects of the medicines, not because the medicines are powerless—a very convenient way of avoiding the blame for therapeutic failures!

The overriding power of God in all things medical results in the ubiquitous caveat applied to all therapies: *in Allah ya yarda,* "If God agrees." Just as the spirits must have God's tacit or overt approval to strike down an individual, so the medicine must have God's permission in order to work. Sometimes the medicine may work and sometimes it may not; the same medicine may cure some cases of the same ailment

4. Thus, the common expression *Allah sarki ne!* "God is king," and the ubiquitous slogan painted on Hausa lorries in slightly obscure English, "No King as God."

but still fail in others. In cases where God has ordained environmental causes for minor afflictions, the cures may work most of the time; in more serious cases they may work only occasionally. Therapy in this sense is almost like bringing a proposal before a judge, who either accepts or rejects it. This is why prayer and supplication (ro'kon Allah, "beseeching God") are so important for the sick. God may have overlooked their cases in the shuffle of running the universe and needs to be reminded of their plight. The judgment, however, whatever it may be, should not be questioned, for it is God who makes it. The power of life and death lies in His hands. As the proverb expresses it, Allah maganin kome, "God is the medicine for everything."

Since, however, Hausa thought also holds that there should be a remedy sanctioned by God for every ill, the suspicion of the chronically ill patient must be that the particular healer who has been treating him doesn't really know which medicines to use. One never knows if he has been sold false goods. Boka ba ya son mutuwa, ba ya son warkewa—ba ku'di. "The boka likes neither death nor recovery—there is no money in either [because treatment stops]," as one cynical villager expressed it. Thus, the patient may travel for miles from town to town and village to village seeking for the herbalist who knows the secret remedy that will unlock the fetters of his suffering. As the illness becomes more severe, more crippling, the secrets become harder to obtain, and hence only a chosen few are thought to possess them. Recovery depends upon the coming together of the proper medicine with its specific illness, a process that may be exceedingly difficult to bring about.

Knowledge of the proper medicine is hard to attain. It must be won through some combination of long study of the sacred books (Muslim traditions say that Muhammed sanctioned many cures), by communication with the spirits, by inheritance of remedies known to the ancestors, or by intellectual speculation that seeks to unravel the many threads of these secrets and then reweave them in the treatment of illness. The components of medicines are found in nature and are seen as coming from God. Herbalists call them maganin Allah, "medicine from God." As with that enigmatic genius of the early Renaissance, Paracelsus, the idea is strong among Hausa herbalists that for every ill God has created a remedy and that by admission to the circle of those who know how to observe the "signatures" of illness in nature, one can find the proper remedies.[5] Once these ideas are grasped the practice of herbal medicine becomes a matter that allows considerable scope for a creative imagination.

A number of themes that recur in Hausa medical practice will now be followed, pointing out the associations of ideas, symbolic motifs, and intellectual correspondences that characterize the Hausa approach to therapy. In this way we may come to understand something of the functioning of the minds of Hausa medical practitioners, and to appreciate the many permutations that may be generated by their modes of thought in the course of their practice.

■ Themes in Hausa Medicine

Secrets and Power. If one were forced to sum up the central idea of Hausa medicine in one word, that word would be power. The essence

5. Pagel (1958:148–49) has explained it thus:

> The doctrine of "Signatures" is based on a morphological principle: A herb reveals by a certain configuration of the colour of its leaves, flowers, or roots an affinity with a certain star, organ or disease.
>
> The root Satyrion (orchid) is it not formed like a man's private parts? Hence it promises through magic and has been found by magic to restore manhood and sexual desire to man. Also the thistle—do not its leaves prick like needles? Hence there is no better remedy against internal stitches. Eyebright (*Eufragia*) shows the image—signature—of eyes, hence it is led by sympathy towards and cures the eye. Iris (*Dactyletus, Aristolochia*) cures cancer, for "its image locates itself in the body at the place to which it belongs by form."
>
> It is the shape of a medicine that directs it to the appropriate place of action without any further guide. For Nature by virtue of its "alchemy" has carved out this shape from formless "prime matter," converting it into "ultimate" matter endowed with a specific "form." This is closely connected with the "virtue" of a remedy and hence its chemical composition. There is thus no real contradiction between the morphological principle of "signatures" and Paracelsus' chemical theory of the "quintessence"—the effective extract of a plant or mineral without shape or form. Both principles culminate and ultimately agree in the specificity which they attribute to herbs and remedies—a specificity of form as well as of chemical essence.

It should not be assumed that Hausa medical practitioners refine their thinking quite this much, but the systematic elaboration of these ideas by Paracelsus sheds much light upon the type of thought processes involved in medical theories of this kind.

of Hausa medicine is the search for power, power to cure sickness, increase bodily strength, eliminate vulnerability, gain popularity, increase sexual potency or attractiveness, obtain financial success, eliminate a rival, or attain some other desired social end. In political thought power is linked with authority, with official position; but in medical and religious thought it is linked with knowledge, especially the knowledge of secrets. The major pathways to such secrets are through Islam, through intercourse with the spirits, and through access to inherited secrets (see Chapter 6). In particular, the revelations of God in the form of the Koran are important, for these revelations are a direct pathway to divine power. Study of the word of God leads one to a knowledge of the divine essence, a source of considerable power. Hence, Koranic verses are widely used for medical purposes, specially the prevention of illness and the warding off of malevolent influences. One famous Islamic medical treatise, the *Tibb-ul-Nabbi* of the fifteenth-century Egyptian medical writer al-Suyuti, states:

> But mark you, there are some words which do indeed have some intrinsic property which helps by the permission of Almighty God. To the truth of this there is the testimony of many learned men. For what do you think about the very words of God and the reported saying of 'Ali: "The Quran is the best of all medicines." Bin Maja reports this saying. . . . The Umm-ul-Quran is the most useful verse of all to recite because it contains the magnification of God together with the purity of His worship and the calling upon Him for help. It is said that the exact point of curing by verse recitation is at the words "Thee do we serve and Thee do we beseech for help." (Elgood 1962:131)

Of particular interest in this regard is the number ninety-nine, which in Islam refers to the ninety-nine names of God. These ninety-nine names are descriptive, indicative of the power and majesty of God. The list of names composed from the Koran is used as the basis for Islamic meditations, and the rosary is based upon three cycles of thirty-three beads which together total ninety-nine. In the Islamic mysticism of the Sufis, these names are of extreme importance and hold a prominent place in their rituals. Through constant "recollection" or "remembrance" (in Arabic, *dhikr*) of God, the aspiring mystic seeks to immerse himself in the divine essence. As Trimingham has written (1971:194):

The early Sufis found in *dhikr* a means of excluding distractions and of drawing near to God, and it has come to mean a particular method of glorifying God by the constant repetition of His name, by rhythmic breathing either mentally (*dhikr khafi*) or aloud (*dhikr jahri* or *jali*). *Dhikr*, the manuals tells us, is the "pivot" of mysticism. Supreme importance is given to the Names and Words (= phrases), for by means of their recital divine energy transfuses the reciter's being and changes him.

Small wonder, then, that many herbal recipes are based upon ninety-nine different ingredients: not only are the powers of the ingredients directed toward the desired end, but the power of God transfuses itself through the potion as well.[6] The ninety-nine names of God and His word—in its form as the Koran—recited, written, and worn as a charm or washed off a slate and drunk down as a prophylactic or cure are thus important sources of divine power.

Another important source of power surrounded by an aura of sacred-ness in Islam is the water of the Well of Zamzam. According to Muslim traditions the Well of Zamzam was opened by the angel Gabriel to succor the patriarch Abraham's concubine Hagar and their son Ishmael when he cast them out of his camp into the wilderness (von Grunebaum 976:24; see also Genesis 21:1–21). This well is located within the sacred precincts of Mecca and its level is supposed to remain miraculously constant no matter how much water is drawn from it (Burton 1893, II:164; von Grunebaum 1976:24). The waters of the well form an important part of the ritual of pilgrimage and it is incumbent upon the pilgrim to drink this water and to bathe with it in the course of his devotions (von Grunebaum 1976:30, 34–35). As with the Koran, the waters of the Well of Zamzam are thought to be charged with miraculous curative powers. As Robinson wrote, observing its use in Hausaland at the end of the last century (1900:201): "The water, which is somewhat heavy to the taste, and of a milky colour, is believed to be

6. Other numbers are also important in Hausa medicine. Among these are the number four, which is associated in Hausa thought with femininity; three, a masculine number; and seven, the sum of three and four, a number combining both masculine and feminine principles. These numbers may be important in preparing medicines for use by men or women, or in the way in which they are administered. This system of numerical symbolism has been described in detail by Guy Nicolas (1968).

an infallible cure for all diseases, provided the patient is only prepared to imbibe a sufficient quantity." This water is controlled by a hereditary guild of water dispensers known as the Zamzami and is purveyed throughout the Islamic world (Burton 1893, II:163–64; von Grunebaum 1976:24). It is common for pilgrims to take it home with them at the end of their travels in Mecca for use during illness or for ablutions after death. Hausa healers who have made the *hajj* to Mecca often profess to use it as an ingredient in their herbal recipes. Alhaji Audu Boka, for example, had an entire eighteen-liter kerosene tin full of it, which he used in treating difficult cases.[7]

The waters of Zamzam and the verses of the Holy Koran are two items in Islamic medicine that come directly from God. Knowledge of Arabic opens the pathway to a considerable amount of other esoteric lore pertaining to astrology, divination, and medicine, and these are popular sources of information (Abdalla 1979). Another pathway to secret knowledge is claimed by the *'yam bori*, whose special relationship with the spirits is said to bring about the revelation of medical secrets unknown to the uninitiated.

Hints of other secrets may be found in nature, where reservoirs of power exist that may be tapped for their curative properties. Nearly every plant may be used for some medical purpose, for example, if only its proper application can be known. There are also other, more powerful forces which, if only they could be harnessed, could be put to medical use. A great deal of ingenuity is used in trying to find ways to accomplish this. In chapter 6 it was noted how 'Dam Baba applied fire to a tree in order to "charge" its medicinal bark with the power of the

7. Sir Richard Burton was considerably more skeptical of its curative properties. In his *Personal narrative of a pilgrimage to Al-Madinah and Meccah*, he wrote (1893, II:163):

> The produce of Zemzem is held in great esteem. It is used for drinking and religious ablution, but for no baser purposes; and the Meccans advise pilgrims always to break their fast with it. It is apt to cause diarrhoea and boils, and I never saw a stranger drink it without a wry face. Sale is decidedly correct in his assertion: the flavour is salt-bitter, much resembling an infusion of Epsom salts in a large tumbler of tepid water. Moreover, it is exceedingly "heavy" to the digestion. For this reason Turks and other strangers prefer rain-water, collected in cisterns and sold for five farthings a gugglet. It was a favourite amusement with me to watch them whilst they drank the holy water, and to taunt their scant and irreverent potations.

fire in hope that it would then act to "burn out" the illness in the
patient who was to take the medicine. Charles Robinson recorded a
similar example during his sojourn in Kano in 1894 (1900:141–42):

> I have brought back with me a charm, the general use of which,
> unless its reputed powers have been exaggerated, would cause a
> considerable diminution in the world's population. The charm is
> to be written out in the first instance on a board; the ink is then to
> be washed off. In the mixture of water and ink thus obtained is
> to be soaked a piece of wood taken from a tree that has been
> struck by lightning. The mixture is then to be used for washing
> the human body, the result being that the enemy of the man who
> has thus washed himself will die.

As with fire, the force of the lightning is thought to animate the medicine, charging it with power. Similar thinking no doubt lies behind the
observation made by Clapperton as he penetrated Hausaland in the
first quarter of the nineteenth century that "gunpowder was much
sought after as a medicine" (Denham and Clapperton 1826, II:6).
Medicinal power will be obtained wherever it can be found.

Hot and Cold. As was pointed out in chapter 5, the interplay of hot
and cold is a major force in the environmental determination of the
day-to-day illnesses suffered in ordinary living. Cold, in particular, is
insidious in this regard, causing a vast number of complaints by increasing the phlegm in the body, producing head and chest colds, killing
the blood, sapping a man's strength, and causing a variety of internal
ailments. Heat, on the other hand, is a source of pain, rashes, skin
irritations, and afflictions of the superficial body. Although cold affects
the internal organs, it may also lead to external swellings as it works
its way outward. Not surprisingly, the way to prevent the effects of
cold is to apply hot substances, while the way to treat the ill effects of
too much heat is to apply cooling substances. The excess phlegm or
"dead blood" that may result from too much cold or heat is removed
from the body by purgation or cupping. The major method of treating
colds is by the use of *kayan yaji,* "spicy, aromatic substances," which
are hot. These include black pepper (*masoro, Piper guineense*), red
peppers (*barkono, Capsicum annuum* and *C. frutescens*), ginger (*cittar
aho, Zingiber officinale*), Ethiopian pepper (*kimba, Xylcoia aethiopica*),
garlic (*tafannuwa, Allium sativum*), Melegueta pepper (*citta, Amomum*

melegueta), potash (*kangwa*), and onions (*albasa, Allium cepa, A. ascalonicum*). These may be prepared in beverages, or mixed together and eaten. A very popular use of such hot substances is as aphrodisiacs to increase sexual potency. In the aftermath of childbirth, when women are thought to be more susceptible to environmental cold, they are fed large amounts of hot, spicy foods, heavily laced with potash, and are forced to take extremely hot bathes, beating themselves with bundles of leaves dipped in near scalding water to drive the heat into their bodies. Rheumatic and joint pains seen as stemming from the penetration of cold may be treated with washings of hot water laced with hot, spicy substances. Fevers, which are seen as stemming from the effects of cold penetrating the body are treated with hot, spicy foods, as well as with herbal infusions made from a wide variety of plants and roots. Swellings of the body attributed to cold may be treated with either plasters or poultices made of the leaves of plants which are hot or irritating. One such plant is the Mexican prickly poppy (*Argemone mexicana*), known in Hausa as *'kan'kamarka ta bi ka*, "may your evil wish recoil on you," a reference to its prickly leaves. The prickly leaves of this plant make it an excellent counter-irritant (thus, a "hot" substance), and it has the extra property of appearing in the dry season in the borrow pits of the village, which are filled with water in the rainy season. Its appearance is thus associated with dryness and hotness at a location normally associated with wetness (hence coldness), which reinforces its reputation as a remedy for swellings caused by cold. Boils, which may also be seen as cold working its way out of the body, are often treated by lancing with a hot metal arrowhead, a process called *sakiya*.

Scorpion stings and other hot, painful injuries may be treated by cooling them with a tomato, often the bitter tomato (*gauta, Solanum melongena*). Rashes, ulcers, and similar sores are seen as the effects of heat, and the pain associated with them is also known as *zafi* ("heat"). Such afflictions are commonly treated with poultices supposed to have a soothing (cooling) effect on them, made by using honey, pulpy bandages from the African bowstring hemp (*moda, Sanseviera* sp.), the leaves of the horseradish tree (*zogalagandi, Moringa pterygosperma*), and other ingredients. Clapperton, for example, reported the following treatment for smallpox (1829, II:76):

Small-pox is at present very prevalent. The patient is treated in
the following manner:—When the disease makes its appearance,
they anoint the whole body with honey, and the patient lies down
on the floor, previously strewn with warm sand, some of which
is also sprinkled upon him. If the patient is very ill, he is bathed
in cold water early every morning, and is afterwards anointed with
honey, and replaced on the warm sand. This is their only mode of
treatment; but numbers died every day of this loathsome disease,
which had been raging for the last six months.

Sweet, Sour, Bitter, and Salt. As with the balance of hot and cold, the
balance of the qualities of sweet, sour, bitter, and salt are important in
Hausa medicine. A disproportion of any of these is thought to predispose one to a number of internal ailments. Excessive sweetness may
cause an expansion of phlegm, and should be treated with astringent
substances such as potash. Excessive salt or sweet may lead to the
overgrowth of the vaginal orifice with a film in pregnant women,
necessitating surgical intervention in the course of difficult labor. Excessive bitterness may disrupt pregnancy; sourness may predispose to
bloody urine, and so on.

The general treatment of gastrointestinal distress centers on the use
of these four qualities to alleviate the symptoms. In particular, sweetness and sourness are thought to cause these ailments (no doubt because it is much easier and more pleasant to eat sweet or sour foods
than those which are bitter or excessively salty), and they are treated
by infusions of bitter or salty substances. Stomach disorders are commonly treated with the bitter *gauta* tomato or by bitter infusions made
from any of a large number of plants such as the vine *garahuni* (*Momor-
dica balsamina*); the bark of the African mahogany tree (*Khaya senegalensis*), whose Hausa name (*ma'daci*) means "the bitter one"; the
roots of the plant *duman dutse* (*Aristolochia albida*); the plant *shiwaka*
(*Vernonia amygdalina*); the "African peach" *tafashiya* (*Sarococephalus
esculentus*)—to name but a few of those present in the Hausa pharmacopoeia.

A wide variety of salts are used medicinally. Ordinary salt (*gishiri*)
is sometimes used to clean wounds and may be rubbed into swollen
lymph nodes in the armpits or groin, a condition known as *kaluluwa* in

Hausa, and seen as stemming from a wound distal to the node on an extremity. Other varieties of salt are used as universal ingredients in stomach remedies and health tonics. The most common of these ingredients is *kanwa*, or potash. *Kanwa* is divided into two kinds: white potash (*farar kanwa*), which is used in cooking, soapmaking, and is given to animals, and red potash (*jar kanwa*), which is used medicinally. In addition, other types of salts such as *urgunu* and *manda* have a wide variety of medicinal uses, the latter being especially valued as a blood tonic because of its dark red coloring. *Mangul*—a dark Borno salt sold in cakes (*kaskwam mangul*), cones (*lela*), or blocks (*kanta*)— is highly prized by the Fulani as a medicine for cattle. Hausa traders have long been interested in the varieties of salts as medicinal substances and have classified them according to their properties. On salts and their uses Lovejoy (1978a:635) has written, in reference to the development of the Borno salt industry:

> The medicinal uses were numerous: *ungurnu* natron from Lake Chad itself, white natron from Mangari and Kawar, and red natron from Mangari and Kawar contained high concentrations of sodium carbonates and hence were excellent for stomach ailments. Local medicinal knowledge credited the different types of natron with specific properties: some were milder and better for children and elders, while others were useful in pregnancy. Because Mangari salt was so similar to natron, it, too, could be used as medicine. In addition, natron and varieties of Mangari salt were used in various mixtures to treat dandruff, problems related to pregnancy, eye disorders, to enhance virility, and as an ingredient in curative potions or mixtures.

As with bitter herbs, salts appear to be charged with a general medicinal power that makes them useful in the treatment of a wide variety of ailments, if only one knows the proper ingredients with which to combine them.

Strength and Toughness. In Hausa medical thought proper health depends upon having adequate strength (*'karfi*). Lack of strength is often one of the first signs of illness, and this lassitude can progress to the point where the patient is prostrated by fatigue and gradually declines into one of the Hausa sicknesses characterized by wasting and severe weakness, such as "white fever" (*farin mashashara*) or jaundiced fatigue ("yellow fever," *shawara*). Loss of strength can be averted by using purgatives periodically to blow out excess phlegm and by prophylactic cupping to remove "dead blood." A more positive approach, however, is to prepare and use herbal tonics, which increase bodily strength and thus make the body less susceptible to illness.

In Hausa such herbal tonics are called *tsimi* and are made by steeping various combinations of herbs, roots, and bark in large pots to extract their medicinal properties. As Dalziel wrote in the introduction to his important volume, *The Useful Plants of West Tropical Africa*, (1937:VIII): "In West Africa, as elsewhere, there are probably few plants which have not at some time or place been credited with medicinal properties." The observation of these tonics confirms this view. In the vast store of Hausa botanical lore there are a multitude of plants which, for lack of a better category, can be referred to simply as "medicinal." They are regarded as having the capability of infusing strength and warding off sickness, especially sickness due to cold, when prepared properly. Prepared according to individual recipes, these tonics are gulped down in large draughts, often laced with hot, spicy additives, and are thought to possess properties that increase the body's energy and allow a man to work in the fields all day without growing tired—and also to perform sexually all night without weariness. Bodily strength (*'karfin jiki*) and penis strength (*'karfin bura*) are closely linked concepts in Hausa medicine.

Also related to strength is the idea of toughness (*tauri*) of the body. Strength is associated with energy and vigor; toughness is associated with invulnerability to injury. Both are aspects of preventive medicine. Invulnerability to injury can take many forms. Koranic and herbal charms are used to ward off evil influences, to prevent the attacks of witches and spirits. Other kinds of medicines are used to protect against physical injury. These medicines are known as *maganin 'karfe*, or "medicine for metal," believed to make the body tough enough to withstand the attack of a cutting blade—a sword, a knife, or a hoe. As such they are understandably popular with farmers who work in the fields and may wound themselves while cultivating, with butchers who work with sharp knives, with hunters, and with soldiers. Considerable fortunes were made during the Nigerian civil war by herbalists who purveyed remedies of this sort in the army camps. Extremely powerful medicines of this kind are thought to be possessed by the sword dancers ('yan tauri), who make public displays of their invulnerability by slashing at themselves with their weapons without doing injury. Most Hausa snakebite medicines (maganin maciji) are of this type: the emphasis is not so much on taking care of the bite after the fact— although medicines do exist for this—but rather in driving the snakes away or making one's skin so hard that they cannot penetrate it with their fangs should they attack. (The fact that all snakes are regarded as poisonous and that any snakebite is thus a potentially fatal event means that these medicines are highly regarded.) In the course of bori initiation the devotees learn the secrets of such herbal remedies— known among the bori as maganin jifa, "throwing medicine"—which render them impervious to the violent falls they undergo in the course of possession, and also render them less susceptible to serious illness induced by the spirits. Maganin 'karfe is thus a way of increasing one's immunity to sickness by preventing the penetration of the body by objects capable of causing wounds: spirits, snakes, knives, or bullets. Similarly, the added toughness of the body increases the toughness and durability of a man's penis, enabling it to stay firm and erect for longer periods during intercourse. Toughness, energy, and sexual performance are closely linked. If a man's body cannot be cut, the thrusting and jabbing of his penis during sexual relations should be enhanced to a similar degree. A good example of maganin 'karfe is the plant faskara toyi (Blepharis linearifolia), whose name means "resistant to burning." It is said to be the only plant that can survive a brush fire, and will be the first one to appear in the midst of the charred grasses in the wake of such an event.

Shape and Texture. Not surprisingly, the physical characteristics of substances, such as their shape, color, and texture, have an important bearing on their uses in Hausa medicine (color is discussed in detail below). Many medicinal uses depend on the observed physical properties of substances, such as stickiness. The seeds of the plant fid da hakukuwa ("remove spicules of grass," Dyschoriste perrottetii) have a mucilaginous coat. When these seeds are placed in the eye, irritating bits of chaff cling to them and are more easily removed. Remedies against diarrhea contain powdered earth (farar 'kasa, "white earth," also used in plastering) or the sticky sap of the gutta-percha tree (gamji, Ficus platyphylla). The resins from various acacia trees are used as counter-irritants in treating scabies and other skin diseases. Cotton and the leaves of the bowstring hemp (*moda, Aloe barteri*) are used in bandaging and poulticing, for example. Pastes made of other kinds of leaves, animal fat, shea butter, cattle dung, or cows' butter are also used as poulticing agents and plasters.

Other medicinal associations are based on physical shape or form. The thorns of a number of acacia trees (for example, *dakwara, Acacia senegal*) resemble fangs and are ingredients in a number of snakebite remedies for this reason. The association of physical shape with medicinal use is best seen, however, in the wide variety of substances sold as aphrodisiacs, particularly those designed to increase the performance of the penis. These may be small, prickly or burr-covered plants that are useful for their "catching" properties—even as they catch and cling onto one's clothing, so they are thought to be helpful in attracting or catching women. One such thorny shrub (*Carissa edulis*) is known as *ciza'ki* or "eating sweetness," both for its paired, sweet berries and also, one presumes, for the rewards expected after using it. More commonly, however, these aphrodisiacs are hard, phallus-shaped roots or tall, straight grasses. Among these medicinal plants one may mention elephant grass (*tofa, Imperata cylindrica*) with its long, straight stalks and sharp, hard tops, and the grasses known as *tsintisyar maza* or "men's brooms" (*Loudetta phragmitoides*), whose stalks are used in making arrow shafts and whose thick, hard roots are sold all over the Sudan as aphrodisiacs. The germinating shoots of the deleb palm (*muruci, Borassus aethiopum*) are thought to be especially potent. They look like a large, erect penis standing out between two thighs, and the impressive stalk of the palm tree that ultimately results from such a shoot needs no further comment as to its phallic associations. The roots of one plant, known as *ruwan zabi* "guinea fowls' water" contain a slick, white fluid which bears a striking resemblance to semen and is thought by some herbalists to be an excellent cure for impotence.

Location. In addition to their physical characteristics, the location at which medicinal substances are found is often important.[8] Most herbal medicines come from the bush, the place of wild, uncontrolled power. While it is tempting to suggest that it is for this reason that herbalists search the bush for medicines, in order to tap the power of the undomesticated lands surrounding the villages, the practical reason is simply

8. A detailed discussion of location and concepts of space in Hausa cosmology may be found in the article by Guy Nicolas (1966).

that that is where the plants are found. The bush contains a vast array of plants and other substances compared to the small number of trees and shrubs that can be found within the precincts of the village. But if medically desirable herbs are found close to home they are used without distinction as to origin. Most herbalists have favorite locations in which to look for their medicines, and may have located a specific tree or clump of shrubs in the bush that forms a ready source for their ingredients, and which they know they can depend upon. Some of these areas are sanctioned by family tradition, and are thus important for this reason: Alhaji Audu Boka and 'Dam Baba came to southern Katsina from their ancestral home in Sokoto. They always maintained that one thing which hampered their practice was the fact that the best medicines grew around their home community, and that the local medicinal plants were second-rate. On several occasions they made trips back to their family community and returned with large bags stuffed with medicinal bark, roots, leaves, and other substances to improve the quality of their practice.

While the overall efficacy of herbal medicines may thus depend upon the part of the country from which they come, some medicines are enhanced by the exact location from which they are taken. In particular, medicines used against attacks by spirits and other evil forces are best when they come from high places. The spirits, being related in nature to the winds from which their name derives, are naturally linked with the sky. Thus, better medicines against the spirits are found upon high rocks out in the bush or atop the rocky inselbergs that rise up from the bush. Medicinal barks are enhanced for such use if they are hacked from the trees near the top, rather than at the bottom. For this reason vultures' nests are highly prized ingredients of herbal remedies, being located high in the trees and difficult to collect. One of the most important ingredients in the fumigants used against the spirits is the parasite *kauci*, or "African mistletoe" (*Loranthus* spp.), which grows on a wide variety of trees and shrubs and sends its suckers into the bast and inner wood to draw out nutrients. *Kauci* is classified according to the tree on which it is found: as *kaucin tsamiya*, "*kauci* of the tamarind tree" or *kaucin ka'danya*, "*kauci* of the shea butter tree," etc. Its medicinal properties are supposed to vary according to the tree on which it is found, but in all cases it forms an important ingredient of medicines against the spirits.

In the vicinity of the village one particular location was thought to be especially favorable for aiding fertility in barren women. In a field a few miles west of the village there was a large phallus-shaped rock known locally as *dutsin ro'ko* or "pleading rock." It was said to be inhabited by powerful spirits who could be persuaded to help infertile women become pregnant. The woman was supposed to approach the rock, plead with the spirits to aid her in her plight, and leave a few coins as "greeting money" or "money of persuasion" at the base of the rock in order to obtain their assistance.

Some plants are associated with wet coldness and the illnesses it causes. Plants found in swampy or marshy areas may be important in this regard. The yellow Mexican prickly poppy, *'kan'kamarka ta bi ka*, which grows in the dried-up borrow pits during the hot season has already been noted in this regard. The white thorny acacia (*farar kaya*, *Acacia sieberiana*) is found frequently near streams and stagnant water holes, and for this reason is often used in remedies against guinea worm, which is white and is commonly known to result from drinking stagnant water out in the bush. Grasses which have grown through a crack in a rock or which have actually split a rock in the course of their growth are highly prized ingredients of aphrodisiacs, it being hoped that the same sort of power can be transferred to the penis of the man. A highly prized remedy for failing lactation (*ciwon nono*) described by one herbalist was made with the bark of the tree *ka'dan-yar rafi* ("shea butter tree of the watercourse," *Manilkara lacera* or *Adina microcephala*). The association of this tree with flowing water was supposed to help stimulate the flow of milk in the mother. Its effects were enhanced if mixed with sour milk and the white, milky sap of a fig tree. If one could add to this compound part of the skin of a crocodile—a powerful animal whose natural Nigerian habitat is, of course, the river—the medicine would be sure to succeed.

Parallels of location may also be important in the preparation of sorcery poisons. Tremearne recorded the following recipe in which animal intestines are used to create abdominal pains in the victim (1914b:166–67):

The following charm can be used by a man against any woman who has rejected or even insulted him. Take the intestines of a goat and blow them out. Then put a medicine prepared from the roots of certain trees inside, mentioning the woman's name, and again blow, and tie the intestines up. Then put them in the fire, and they will fizzle and pop, and as they do this so will the female be seized with internal pains, and lose control over herself. So bad will she become that when the parents or other relatives know that your feelings have been hurt, they will guess what is happening, and will rush to you, and promise you anything if you let her get well again. Then, if you take the intestines off the fire, the illness will leave her at once.

The Power of Animal Associations. Along with the crocodile a number of other animals are associated in Hausa thought with special powers or unique properties that can be tapped for medical purposes. The skins of many of these animals are made into coverings for Koranic or herbal charms, for they are thought to act as catalysts, accelerating and potentiating the effects of the medicines they enclose. The hides of elephants, crocodiles, and hyenas are valued for this if they can be obtained, but that of any other wild, powerful beast is thought to have similar effects. Fish scales or hedgehog skins may be used for counter-irritation in treating scabies and other skin ailments, and some say fish heads are a good cure for headaches (although most people would be likely to use aspirin tablets). The droppings of elephants have a wide variety of medical uses—supposedly being effective in treating elephantiasis, for example. Dried and powdered hyena and mongoose feces are a welcome ingredient in the incense used in treating insanity. Mud from the nests of dauber wasps is especially useful in the treatment of chest pains, especially the sharp, stabbing, superficial pains of pleurisy, which may be likened to the sting of a wasp. The lion is preeminently associated with power,[9] and lion fat is said to be a powerful medicine to keep thieves away if smeared around the doorway of one's hut. The heart of a lion, if it can be obtained, is said to be a powerful medicine which induces courage; here, as in other cases, the scarcity of the material contributes to its reputation for powerful effects.

The medicinal associations of other animals are derived from specific observations about their behavior and are related to the conditions they are supposed to treat. For example, there is a small, scarlet, velvety

9. A traditional Hausa salutation to a European or other highly placed individual is *Za'ki, babban dodo!* "Lion, big *dodo*-spirit!"

spider known in Hausa by a number of names, the most common of which is *damina* or "rainy season," for that is when this creature appears, making its way over the seedlings and furrows in the fields. It may be captured, carefully wrapped up, and sewn into a charm worn by children to ward off the effects of damp cold, which causes the infantile convulsions also known as *damina* or *tafiyar ruwa*, "going away in the rainy season." A species of black ants known in Hausaland as *tururuwa* are noted for their industrious efforts in collecting grain. These ants—or the earth from their nests—are used in the preparation of medicines that are supposed to increase one's business, drawing it to one's market stall or shop as effectively as the ants carry home their stores of corn. Tremearne noted (1915:52) that "the head and feet of an ostrich or gazelle enable the eater to run as fast as the bird or animal concerned, and so escape from foes in war." On the same page he also reported that Hausa warriors used the body of an electric eel, dried and made into a girdle, as a medicine that reputedly would cause the paralysis of any enemy attempting to strike them. The white feathers of the pied crow (*hankaka, Corvus scapulatus, Corvus albus*) are sewn into a leather belt (*guru*) and worn around the waist by barren women as medicines to enhance fertility, partly because the color white is associated with fertility and reproduction, but also because the crow is thought to steal eggs or the offspring of other birds to raise as its own: *Hankaka mai da 'dan wani ya zama naka*, "Crow, converter of another's children into your own," as the proverb says, an expression that may also be applied to an exceptionally generous person. The skin of a black donkey is said by some herbalists to be a strong medicine for treating epilepsy, because of the relationship between the grand mal type of seizure and the donkey's penchant for throwing himself to the ground and wallowing in the dust: *Jaki ba ya wuce toka*, "The donkey doesn't pass the ashes [because he likes to roll in them]," according to the proverb. The suffering patient is tied into the skin and taken to the foot of a tamarind tree (a favorite abode of spirits) and treated with medicinal incense.

Tremearne reported the following remedies for the treatment of prolonged or difficult labor (1915:33): "But when a case of painful labour is expected, take the dried after-birth of a cat, put it into a vessel of water, and give it to the woman. At the third mouthful she will give birth. A somewhat slower method, but really efficacious, is to make her

inhale the fumes of a burning snake slough." The relationship between
a sloughed snakeskin and a medicine to accelerate labor is easy to see.

Because of its ability to change colors the chameleon is regarded as a
very powerful animal by the Hausa. In describing the more esoteric
Hausa medicinal recipes, the chameleon often figures prominently. It
is especially useful in the preparation known as *baduhu*, "giver of
darkness," a charm for invisibility reputedly very popular among
thieves (who use it in conjunction with invulnerability medicines), and
adulterers, who use it as an aid in meeting their partners unobserved.
One recipe for *baduhu*, obtained from a man who confided that he had
never revealed it to anyone before for less than fifty naira, is as follows.
First one must capture a chameleon. Then he must take a small pot and
fill it with the milk of a black goat. The chameleon must be put in the
milk and the pot sealed over. Then, on the night before a big market
day, one must go to a big shelter in the market—the kind where large
crowds of men gather—and bury it an arm's length in the ground. One
should return at night after the market has ended and dig up the pot.
The chameleon should have disappeared (presumably having dissolved
or otherwise entered into the milk). The solution should then be drunk,
imbibing its powers. This should be done three times, or, for extra
strength, nine times. The power of invisibility is thus conferred, to be
used at the discretion of its owner.[10]

Color Symbolism. In addition to associations with animal power, another important set of concepts in Hausa medicine pertains to color
relations. In a well-known article published in 1965, Victor Turner
called attention to the widespread importance in African symbolism of
a color triad of white, red, and black. Other authors have since studied
and confirmed this fact for a variety of African cultures.[11] Among the

10. An alternate method of attaining the same end involves writing the proper
Koranic verses on a slate with the blood of a chameleon, washing them off, and
drinking down the solution; or writing a Koranic charm on a slate and then washing it into a bowl full of chameleon blood. The power of God's word is combined
with the powers of the chameleon. Many such recipes use Koranic writing as the
"energizer" which sets off the reaction. Other recipes for *baduhu* are given in
Tremearne (1914b:169–70).
11. For example, Buxton (1973:382–40) on the Mandari of the southern Sudan;
Ngubane (1977:113–39) on the Nyuswa-Zulu of South Africa; and Janzen (1978:
199–203) on the BaKongo of the lower Zaire. Jacobson-Widding (1979) is an extensive study of color symbolism among the peoples of the lower Congo.

Hausa, too, there is a similar system of symbolism important in medical thought that is based upon associations between values, colors, and body substances involving white, red (under some circumstances yellow), and black.[12]

White (Fari). The color white is associated with breast milk (*nono*) and semen (*maniyyi*). Its general symbolic associations include life, popularity, happiness, goodness, attraction, and light, as may be noted in the following kinds of usages:

1. *farin ciki*, "white inside," meaning happiness or contentment
2. *farar zuciya*, "white heart," referring to a person with a pleasant disposition or equable temperament
3. *farin rai*, "white life," a good, pleasant, or successful life
4. *farin jini*, "white blood," popularity
5. *farin sani* "white knowledge," something known exceedingly well
6. *farar gwana*, "white expertise," that is, foresight
7. *farin kai*, "white head," a learned or educated person
8. *farin labari*, "white news," or good news
9. *farin gamo*, "white meeting/luck," or good luck
10. *farin hannu*, "white hand," the hand of divination

Medicines based on white substances are used as love potions, to attract more business to one's market stall, and especially to insure fertility, prevent sterility, and enhance the flow of milk from the mother's breast or to prevent or cure the illnesses of young children. Since the under-five mortality rate in many parts of Hausaland approaches 50 percent, these are extremely important associations in terms of traditional medical practice. The most common ingredients in these medicines are things such as the white feathers of the pied crow referred to above, sugar, sour milk, and particularly the fruit, sap, and bark of the numerous kinds of fig trees found throughout the countryside, such as the *dullu* tree (*Ficus capensis*) whose other Hausa name, *uwar yara*, means "mother of children," from its production of large clusters of fruit.

Red (Ja). The color red is associated with blood, *jini*, a word that may refer to "blood" in general or, depending on the context, to menstrual blood or the shedding of blood, i.e., murder. The symbolic associations

12. Hausa color symbolism is treated in more lengthy fashion in Ryan (1976). A more general survey of Hausa symbolism in literary sources is Ryan (1974).

of the color red are centered around the concepts of power, force, severity, and strength, as may be seen in the following usages:

1. *Ja* by itself may be used to mean "a superior," in reference to the rule of darker-skinned peoples by those of lighter color, as in the case of the darker Hausa being governed by the lighter-skinned Fulani and the white man, whose skin is "red" in Hausa

2. *jan zuciya,* "red heart," a person of stout heart; an enduring, courageous, or obstinate person

3. *jan ciki,* "red inside," exertion or extreme effort

4. *jar wahala,* "red trouble," severe trouble

5. *hauka ja* "red madness," severe madness

6. *jan aiki,* "red work," hard or difficult work

7. *jan hali,* "red character," a person of forceful character

8. *jad dariya,* "red laughter," laughter that covers up extreme anger or mortification

9. *jam baki,* "red mouth," picking a fight or quarrel, unfounded bragging or boasting

10. *jan 'kashi,* "red bones," referring to great endurance

11. *jan gwarzo,* "red warrior," an exceptionally brave and successful warrior

The use of red substances in Hausa medicine is limited almost exclusively to ailments associated with the blood—tiredness due to "dead," "watery," or "weak" blood, menstrual disorders (which may be seen as linked to fertility problems)—and to paralysis and withered limbs, which in the Hausa view result from the loss of blood to a vampire spirit which drinks it out of a limb, resulting in its atrophy and loss of function. Most of these blood medicines are trees or plants that produce red flowers or have a red juice: the flowers of the coral tree *minjiriya* (*Erythrina senegalensis*); the plant *ba-jini* ("giver of blood," *Ostryoderris chevalieri,* also called *jina-jina*); the plant *jinin mutum* ("man's blood," *Arnebia hispidissima*), whose roots are blood red and produce a reddish-purple dye; and a tuberous plant referred to as *bi-jijiyoyi,* or "follower of the blood vessels," which has a pink root with a dark red center and is supposed to be useful in treating illnesses caused by disturbances of the blood and its vessels, such as *jiri,* the pounding temporal headache thought to result from turbulence in the blood.

Yellow (*rawaya*) is used medically almost exclusively for the treatment of *shawara,* a greatly feared Hausa disease characterized by jaun-

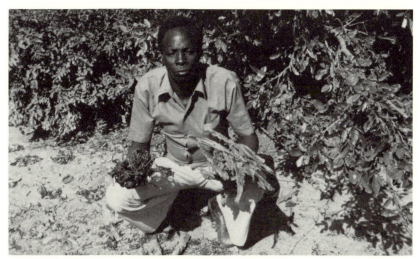

17. *'Dam Baba holding the flowers and bark of the* minjiriya *tree,* Erythrina senegalensis.

dice, extreme fatigue, and dark urine—a triad associated with hepatitis. This disease is seen, in Hausa thought, as stemming from disorders of the blood. The blood may die off, turning black, may fade away into nothingness or turn white, or turn pustulent yellow, giving the resultant yellow discoloration of the whites of the eyes (sometimes also described as scarlet, *jawur*, or even green, *kore*). Medicines made for the treatment of this ailment, which is not thought curable by hospital medicine,[13] are invariably yellow. Ingredients include turmeric roots (*zabibi, Curcuma longis*); the yellowish bark of the coral tree; the roots of the plant *rawaya* (*Cochlospermum tinctorium*), whose name means "yellow" in Hausa and whose roots are actually used in preparing yellow dye; the bark of the chew-stick tree (*marke, Anogneissus leiocarpus*); and the root of the tree *Swartzia madagascarensis*, known in Hausa as *bayama*, a word closely related to *bayamma*, an alternate term for *shawara*.

13. There is no specific treatment for typical acute viral hepatitis in the arsenal of scientific medicine as yet. A high-calorie diet and prolonged rest are about the best that can be offered. People who approached me for medicines for this disease were usually satisfied if they were given a supply of folic acid tablets, which are yellow and can be accurately (though not completely) described as a "blood medicine."

Black (Ba'ki). The color black is associated with excrement (*kashi*). Its symbolic associations are with death, evil, sorrow, darkness, and repulsion, as can be noted in the following usages:

1. *ba'kin ciki*, "black inside," meaning unhappiness or sorrow
2. *ba'kar zuciya*, "black heart," someone with a foul temper or evil disposition
3. *ba'kin rai*, "black life," a life of misfortune, evil deeds, or failure
4. *ba'kin kai*, "black head," an ignorant person
5. *ba'kin daji*, "black bush," dense, formidable bush
6. *ba'kin kishi*, "black jealousy," bitter jealousy
7. *ba'kar magana*, "black words," angry, bitter words
8. *ba'kin labari*, "black news," bad news
9. *ba'kar aniya*, "black intentions," evil intentions
10. *ba'kin shege*, "black bastard," as in English, a thoroughly rotten person
11. *ba'kin bunu*, "black thatch," that is, old thatch, the kind that stands out against the lighter, newer thatch; hence, a bad person among a number of decent ones
12. *ba'kin jini*, "black blood," in moral terms referring to unpopularity; in physiological terms, referring to dead, useless blood that can cause sickness
13. *ba'kar gaskiya*, "black truth," an unpleasant or unpalatable truth
14. *ba'kar haja*, "black merchandise," that is, unsalable goods that remain week after week in the market, finding no buyers
15. *ba'kin karuwa*, "black prostitute/profligate," a burglar, thief, or blackguard
16. *ba'kin kumallo*, "black nausea," actually referring to vomiting (possibly originally associated with the foul, dark vomit of yellow fever), in contrast to *farin kumallo*, "white nausea," which refers only to biliousness, gas, and an upset stomach—a less severe condition, as befits "whiteness"
17. *ba'kin zafi*, "black heat/pain," in reference to a dark patch of leprosy

In Hausa medicine black substances are ingredients in the more occult medicinal recipes that are supposed to cause the death of an enemy through sorcery or to bring invisibility to the owner. One such recipe involving the chameleon was discussed previously. Ingredients in other compounds may include such items as the ashes of a black cat, the hair of a black dog, the hooves of a black goat, the blood of a black chicken, the entrails of a black donkey, or earth taken from a grave (Tremearne 1914b:165–66, 170; 1915:48). This latter ingredient is supposedly sprinkled by thieves on sleeping householders, causing them to fall into a deep, trance-like sleep from which they will not awaken until their compounds have been ransacked and all their valuables stolen. Such medicines are reported to be popular among adulterous wives, who can thus cause their husbands to sleep soundly while entertaining partners (made invisible by these remedies) who may enter their huts unseen and unmolested. Black ingredients associated with evil and danger—black cobras and black scorpions, for example—are common ingredients in sorcery poisons, but more important, they are found in medicines that have a positive therapeutic effect in driving away offending spirits who are causing illness.

Attraction-Repulsion, Intrusion-Expulsion. One area of Hausa medical practice in which many of the themes discussed above find expression is that dealing with the concepts of attraction and repulsion or expulsion. Many Hausa medical nostrums are concerned with attracting good fortune, securing the attentions of a male or female sexual partner, garnering popularity, or increasing one's business—these prescriptions are attractive, seeking to draw good things toward the person who uses them. Conversely, the desire to ward off sickness and evil is also great and there are consequently a large number of other medicaments designed to repel malevolent forces or expel noxious substances from the body.

Attractive medicines are generally composed of pleasant substances. It has been seen previously, for example, how spirit possession adepts eager to attract their friendly spirit helpers keep rooms in their compounds that are heavily loaded with perfumes, sweets, sugar water, and other substances because spirits are attracted to these things. Because of the association of white with prosperity, pleasantness, and happiness, the herbal ingredients used in such attractive medicines are also often white: the bark and sap of fig trees (which, in addition to being white, is also sticky); the white-flowered herb *rimin samari* ("silk-cotton tree of the youths," *Oldenlandia senegalensis*); the white sap of plants such as *nonon kuriya* ("dove milk," *Euphorbia convolvuloides* and *E.* spp.) or *tumfafiya* (*Calotropis procera*). Orchids, either terrestrial or epiphytic, are ingredients in medicinal washing solutions believed to increase one's attractiveness, particularly if applied to the face and eyes. Because of their resemblance to the germinating radicle of the deleb palm (*muruci*, regarded as a powerful aphrodisiac) the terrestrial orchid is known as *murucin daji* ("bush *muruci*") and the epiphytic orchid as *murucin sama* ("*muruci* high-up," in reference to its arboreal habitat). Plants of the latter type have the suggestive name in Hausa of *manta uwa*, "forget mother," in reference to its supposedly disinhibitory effects and aphrodisiacal properties. It is also used in some medicines that are supposed to increase the speed of weaning. The plant *ka fi boka* ("you are better than a herbalist," *Ipomoea argentaurata*) has whitish flowers which make it an important ingredient in "attractive" medicines, and the plant *ka fi mallam* ("you are better than a Koranic scholar," *Evolvulus alsinoides*), with light blue flowers, is reputed to have similar properties. Many of these substances are used as fertility medicines, seeking to attract new life, or as medicines to increase the flow of breast milk.

Other "attractive" medicines have somewhat more vulgar components, believed to be effective simply because of their place of origin. Tremearne has recorded two such recipes for attractive medicines. These instances, both involving women who wished to attract lovers or to ensure the faithfulness of their husbands, are illustrative of the general principles. In the first recipe, "she takes a small piece of meat, places it high up between her legs and sleeps with it there all night. In the morning, she cuts it up very fine, dries and powders it, and gets it into the food of the one whom she admires, and a similar result follows. It should have been stated that in all of these love charms, the name of the person desired must be spoken aloud at each stage" (Tremearne 1914b:163–64). The wife using the second recipe "takes some small pieces of hair cut from various parts of her body, nail-paring, drops of spittle, eye-matter, ear-wax, and *mantowa*[14] with her husband's food. In this case, she puts deteriorated parts of herself into his system, and so is enabled to rule him" (Tremearne 1915:47). Recipes of this kind may include water in which the individual has bathed his or her genitals, a procedure directly evocative of the desired ends. A Koranic

14. The plant *mantowa* referred to is probably the same as *manta uwa* mentioned previously.

scholar can also create a written prescription to be worn or drunk down for any of the aforementioned purposes.

More important than any of these "white" medicines, love philtres, and potions for good luck are those medicines with a negative aspect designed to repel evil or get rid of harmful substances in the body. These may be prophylactic medicines, such as a Koranic or herbal charm worn to ward off attacks by witches, sorcerers, and spirits, or a purge taken to rid the body of excess phlegm; or they may be thera-peutic: incense used to drive evil spirits out of a suffering maniac, or violent emetics, cathartics, or diuretics taken in an attempt to rid the body of sickness.

Medicines designed to combat evil forces such as black spirits once they have attacked someone are designed to operate by forcing the spirit to relinquish his hold on the patient by making life as miserable as possible for the spirit. Generally, this is accomplished in two ways. One is by the preparation of medicinal incense (*turare na aljannu* or *hayakin iskoki*). The afflicted person, usually mentally deranged, is kept in a small, closed room. A fire is built at one end, and to it is added the powdered medicine. Once placed on the fire these medicines begin to burn, giving off noxious, thick smoke. This smoke, which as a kind of medicinal "air" or "scent" possesses some of the same ethereal qualities as the offending spirit, is inhaled by the patient and acts to make the spirit resident in his body uncomfortable (it certainly causes the patient considerable discomfort). The substances that go into these medicines are many, and partake of qualities that bring themselves to bear on the spirits from several directions. Common ingredients include West African mistletoe which, because of its association with high places in trees, is thought to be particularly efficacious against spirits; twigs from the nests of vultures, who are considered dirty, disgusting birds due to their carrion-eating habits; dried and powdered hyena, mongoose, or wildcat droppings—especially prized and often hard to find, located only after considerable searching along the trails and rocky outcroppings in the bush; pulverized bodies of the *ja'ba*, or stinking West African shrew mouse; the crushed and dried bodies of black scorpions; and any number of herbal components derived mainly from fragrant or foul-smelling plants and grasses such as *bunsurun fadama* ("billy-goat of the marshland," *Eragrostis cilianensis*), *jema* (*Vetiveria nigritana*), and that ubiquitous medicinal ingredient, the roots of the

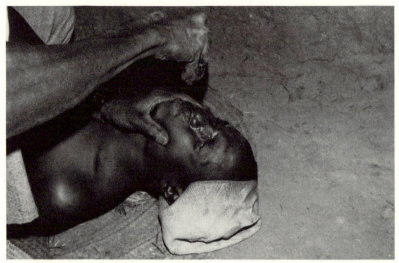

18. *Administering a herbal compound through the nose for treatment of a mental disorder.*

plant called *uwar magunguna* ("mother of medicines," *Securidaca longipedunculata*). This sooty regimen is continued as long as the patient can stand it, frequently combined with medicinal snuff (*sha'ke*). As a verb form *sha'ke* means "to throttle, to choke, to fill to utmost capacity." In medical terms this means infusing as much medicine into the nasal cavities as possible, in powdered or liquid form. The powdered ingredients of *sha'ke* are usually finely pulverized pieces of medicinal bark combined with generous doses of spices and peppers designed to provoke violent sneezing, in which they succeed. The liquid form, made from a combination of medicinal leaves, is squeezed as a runny paste or dripped as a thick liquid into the patient's nose. In both cases the object is to cause the patient to expel the offending spirit by sneezing, or to cause him to gag and blow the spirit out in the streams of mucus this treatment induces. Although some spirits are said to have special relations with and susceptibilities to certain species of trees, in practical experience close correlations between individual spirits and specific herbal ingredients are not seen. These remedies are used against all spirit-induced illnesses and function as "broad spectrum" antibiotics rather than highly selective therapeutic agents. The foundation of this kind of treatment, like our own, is allopathic. It aims to create a set of conditions incompatible with or antagonistic to the condition being treated, i.e., possession by a spirit.

The other therapeutic strategy involves the removal or expulsion of physical (as opposed to spiritual) substances that are thought to have caused or may—if left untreated—cause sickness or discomfort. Such procedures may include the excision of the uvula to prevent its over-growth, with resulting blockage of the oropharynx; surgical trimming of the hymen to correct hypertrophy which, it is feared, may lead to closure of the vagina; cupping to remove black "dead blood" which has been killed by heat or cold; vaginal cutting to remove "obstruc-tions" to delivery; or the administration of herbal medicines to elimi-nate the causal agents of illness by inducing vomiting, diarrhea, or diuresis. These medicines are given to expel "excess phlegm" (*majina*), intestinal worms, venereal diseases, jaundice (*shawara*), and other agents of sickness. Within the Hausa pharmacopoeia are many sub-stances that possess diuretic, emetic, or cathartic properties. Among these plants are *filasko* (*Cassia obovata*, Senegal senna); *tafasa* (*Cassia tora*); *rafasa* (*Euphorbia aegyptiaca*), which is used especially for tape-worm; *nannaho* (*Celosia laxa*), also used for tapeworm; *bi ni da zugu* (the "Physick nut," *Jatropha curcas*), whose name in Hausa means "follow me with a towel" in reference to its reputedly swift cathartic effects; *marga* or *gama fa'da* ("bringer of quarreling," *Cassia siebe-riana*); *malmo* (*Syzygium guineese*); prepared indigo (*shuni*), which is well known as an abortifacient; henna (Hausa *lalle*, *Lawsonia iner-mis*); *bayama* (*Swartzia madagascariensis*); the poisonous *tururibi* (*Lasiosiphon kraussianus*), which also serves as a fish poison; the white thistle, *dayi* (*Centaurea* spp.), and many others. Nearly all these medi-cines are prepared with generous amounts of potash, which is thought to serve as an astringent to reduce the amount of phlegm in the body. Remedies for venereal disease, drunk in large quantities, are deemed es-pecially valuable if they produce marked diuresis, it being thought that the illness will be flushed away in the process. Hausa medical thought holds that many internal ailments can be passed out in the urine or feces, or expelled by vomiting, and therefore attempts to promote these acts are common modes of therapy. Robinson (1900:270) advised travelers to take large numbers of croton oil pills with them to Hausa-land, as they were the most popular of any of his medicines, and Denham (1826, I:201–2) recorded the astonishment and pleasure of one patient to whom he administered a small dose of tartar emetic in treating a fever.[15] Unfortunately, this kind of therapy may result in an already ailing patient being subjected to severe strains in the course of his "cleansing," which serve to worsen rather than help his prognosis.

■ Empiricism, Experimentation, and Efficacy:
Hausa Traditional Medicine and Western Science

The aim of medicine, as the great French physiologist Claude Bernard once wrote (1927:1), is "to conserve health and to cure disease." Both Hausa traditional medicine and Western bioscientific medicine have this as their ultimate aim. In attempting to reach this common goal, however, they travel quite different paths and use very different methods, and in these differences lie the reasons why scientific medicine has made so much greater progress toward the ultimate destination than has its more rudimentary Hausa counterpart. Some of the differences in methods are obvious: Hausa therapeutic practice is almost devoid of significant surgical techniques and, conversely, scientific medical practitioners are not in the habit of subduing their patients in rooms full of medicinal incense derived from vultures' nests and hyena dung, or forcing compounds made with red peppers up their patients' noses.[16] These, however, are relatively secondary differences. The major separation, the "great divide" as Ernest Gellner calls it (1974:150), lies at a deeper level and involves differing views of the world and different techniques of thought stemming from those worldviews. The implications of these differences are far from insubstantial.

Both medical systems are attempts to solve problems, to correct imbalances, to establish some sort of control over human experience based on an underlying view of the world. As Gellner has written (1974:125): "No society, no culture or language, either does or can exist, which

15. Croton oil is a drastic cathartic which is no longer used in Western medicine due to its violent effects on the bowel. Tartar emetic (antimony potassium tartrate) is sometimes still used to induce vomiting in cases of poisoning, but its main use is now intravenous infusion in the treatment of schistosomiasis.
16. There are, however, some uncomfortable parallels in the cases of convulsive electroshock therapy and the heavy sedation of mental patients with psychoactive drugs. Western medicine can do some awful things to people in the course of therapy, as critics such as Ivan Illich (1977) have pointed out.

operates on the assumption of a chaotic nature, of a world not amenable to conceptual order." In the sense that modern science and traditional African thought both produce coherent pictures of the world, there would seem to be some striking parallels between them.[17] The assumption of an underlying system or order in the world makes it possible to take actions that follow logically, according to the dictates of the system, in hopes of attaining a desired end. The crucial difference between science and traditional Hausa thought, however, lies in the way "reality" is depicted by each system.

The world as described by Western science is a self-contained unity which operates along impersonal, mechanistic lines. Its operation is regular and it contains forces that can be observed and measured to obtain uniform standards which can be used for prediction. It is because of this regularity of possibilities generated by the paradigm that scientists are able to speak (albeit rather presumptuously) of "natural laws" which may be described in mathematical terms. The assumption of unity, of a regularity that does not vary in a random manner is the foundation stone on which scientific progress is based, for it allows the generation of hypotheses that can be tested under controlled experimental conditions, and ultimately supported or falsified and abandoned.

Such a view of the world leads to a very tough-minded attitude concerning human knowledge. If reality is regular in its operation, the factor limiting human knowledge is therefore the ability (or lack of it) to reason clearly and to wrest from nature the details of its inner workings through the application of rigorous, unyielding logic and experimentation. In the field of medicine nobody expressed this view more forcefully than Claude Bernard, whose famous book *An Introduction to the Study of Experimental Medicine,* first published in 1865, still stands as an important statement of the scientific method as applied to medicine (Bernard 1927:2–3).

> Scientific medicine, like the other sciences, can be established only by experimental means, i.e., by direct and rigorous application of

17. In a series of thought-provoking articles, Robin Horton (1964, 1967, 1976) has even gone so far as to describe African traditional thought as a theory-generating process akin to science and has described "ritual man" in Africa as a subspecies of "theory-building man." This position has been criticized by many writers, notably Beattie (1966, 1970, 1973), Ross (1971), and Gellner (1974:154–67).

reasoning to the facts furnished us by observation and experiment. Considered in itself, the experimental method is nothing but reasoning by whose help we methodically submit our ideas to experience,—the experience of facts. . . . Reasoning will always be correct when applied to accurate notions and precise facts; but it can lead only to error when the notions or facts on which it rests were originally tainted with error or inaccuracy. That is why experimentation, or the art of securing rigorous and well-defined experiments, is the practical basis and, in a way, the executive branch of the experimental method as applied to medicine. If we mean to build up the biological sciences, and to study fruitfully the complex phenomena which occur in living beings, whether in the physiological or the pathological state, we must first of all lay down principles of experimentation, and then apply them to physiology, pathology and therapeutics. Experimentation is undeniably harder in medicine than in any other science; but for that reason, it was never so necessary, and indeed so indispensable. The more complex the science, the more essential is it, in fact, to establish a good experimental standard, so as to secure comparable facts, free from sources of error. Nothing, I believe, is to-day so important to the progress of medicine.

The *duniya* (world) of Hausa thought is much different. One proverb says *Duniya ba ta tabbata*, "Nothing in the world is certain." Instead of an impersonal world of matter, the universe is populated by spirits, witches, souls, and sorcerers. The spirits, with all the capriciousness of unruly pranksters, strike whomever they choose. In Hausa thought, as in most African traditional thought, the world is thus seen in personalistic rather than impersonal terms, and above everything and controlling the world is Allah. Unlike the Newtonian clockmaker, who set the world in motion and then withdrew from its affairs, Allah is active in its every working. He controls its operations through His will, determining things as He sees fit. The ultimate way in which the world runs is therefore very much like the court of a chief. The Hausa proverbial exclamation *Allah sarki ne!* or "God is Chief!" encapsulates this view. The world is God's kingdom, to be run as He sees fit in the manner in which a chief rules his lands, and human beings are mere "commoners," subject to His bidding.

It stands to reason, therefore, that Hausa medicine is not based upon experimental foundations. A world that operates through the will of God is always subject to that will, and thus an element of unpredictability, of capriciousness, is built into the description of reality. *In Allah ya yarda*—"if God agrees"—is the rider attached to all medical practice, all plans for the future. Detailed observations leading to tightly propounded hypotheses, which can then be tested under carefully controlled circumstances, are of little use if this one, permanent variable cannot be controlled. The will of God acts as a metaphysical safety valve to cut out possible crises engendered by failure. The foundations of Hausa medicine are removed from the realm of falsifiability and thus assume the status of metaphysical axioms (cf. Ross 1971; Popper 1972.)

The results of this are quite profound. As Ernest Gellner has written (1974:176):

> What really makes the criterion of falsifiability so powerful is this: if you insist that a believer specifies the conditions in which his faith would cease to be true, you implicitly force him to conceive a world in which his faith is *sub judice*, at the mercy of some "fact" or other. But this is precisely what faith, total outlooks, systematically avoid and evade. They fill out the world of their adherents, the world they in a way create, and they interpret the processes of cognition in such a way that all verdicts must, in the end, be returned in their favour. Note that they have little to fear from a requirement that they be "verifiable": generally speaking, they pervade the world they create so completely that verifications abound—here a verification, there a verification, everywhere a verification.

We are back to Uwarture's statement that curable diseases are caused by spirits, while incurable diseases remain so due to the will of God.

What this means, finally, is that Hausa medicine, like Galenic medicine, has remained qualitative in nature. Without specific criteria to differentiate disease and well-defined standards by which to gauge treatment and its effects; the Hausa healer often engages in practices that are essentially expressive of the ends he desires for his patient, rather than causally effective in bringing them about. A series of generally superficial observations about disease processes and their result-

ing signs and symptoms, metaphysical assumptions about the structure
of reality, and some perceived correlations between the botanical world
and human illness are all taken together to produce therapeutic strategies for the treatment of sickness: yellow roots and flowers are used
to treat jaundice; red substances to produce strength and cure disorders
of the blood; white sap and clusters of fruit to remedy infertility or
promote popularity, and so on. The Koranic scholar works by similar
means, using Muslim scripture and traditions. The drinking of Koranic
writing which has been washed off a slate, the wearing of a protective
amulet to ward off witches or evil spirits, or the administration of a
herbal tonic may all be seen as expressions of the desire to recover from
sickness, to avoid misfortune, or to attain a desired social end. Hausa
medicines are thus often affirmative of ends desired, rather than controlling or determinative of the course of illness.

The absence of a well-defined nosology based on careful observation
of illness, the absence of any detailed knowledge of the anatomical
structure and physiological function of the human body (not to mention a total unawareness of the microbial world), coupled with a lack
of critical method means that Hausa medicine lacks the firm foundations it would need to develop into a well-integrated system capable of
progressing in knowledge and therapeutic effectiveness. But does this
mean that Hausa therapeutic practices are without merit? Among many
educated Africans today there is a strong feeling that traditional medicine is grounded in a firm foundation of empirical fact, gathered by
experience and trial and error over time. For example, A. Bouquet, in
a paper presented at the First Inter-African Symposium on Traditional
Pharmacopoeias and African Medicinal Plants held in Dakar, Senegal,
in 1968, boldly stated (1968:56): "Traditional medicine is the result
of a long heritage of empiricism based upon the close observation of
sickness and transmitted orally from one generation to the next." Similarly, M. Hanbali, in an article on Hausa medicinal plants stated
(1973:9): "We should emphasize the necessity for an urgent investigation into our flora. The fruitful result of this research will permit us to
save huge amounts of money, eradicate many if not all of our maladies
with our plants and preserve our cultural heritage."

One suspects that a good deal of this feeling is based on the understandable desire to defend African culture against the frequently disrupting impact of European civilization and the legacy of inferiority

that was often left as the last remnants of colonialism. Indeed, if one examines the history of pharmacology one finds an impressive list of drugs derived from herbal origins, the most famous of which is perhaps digitalis—still the mainstay of treatment in congestive heart failure— which was discovered by the English physician William Withering as an ingredient in a tonic for dropsy prepared by an old Shropshire woman according to a traditional family recipe.[18] Other such drugs include curare, cinchona, and reserpine. The latter, used in the treatment of psychiatric disorders and obtained originally from plants of the genus *Rauwolfia*, is also used by Yoruba herbalists in their treatment of mental illness (Prince 1960). Considering the enormous variety of plants that grow in the tropics, it is to be expected that certain of them would contain alkaloids that exhibit pharmacological activity and that by happenstance, an unsophisticated rough-and-ready empiricism, and tradition, some of these activities should be known—after all, vomitories do cause emesis and purgatives do purge—and, indeed, some investigations of traditional remedies have given rather surprising results.[19] But generally, if one examines the large compilations of herbal remedies and lists of medicinal uses of West African plants made by such authors as Dalziel (1937), Traore (1965), and Ayensu (1978), one finds an enormous number of remedies for all sorts of ailments utilizing a wide range of botanical (and other) ingredients—but little consensus as to what medicines are specific for what ailments. Large numbers of plants in the Hausa pharmacopoeia are regarded simply as "medicinal," as ingredients in tonics to be used for the general preservation of health.

The extent to which traditional remedies contain active pharmacological principles that are effective in curing disease and preserving

18. "In the year 1775, my opinion was asked concerning a family receipt for the cure of dropsy. I was told that it had long been kept a secret by an old woman in Shropshire, who had sometimes made cures after the more regular practitioners had failed. I was informed also, that the effects produced were violent vomiting and purging; for the diuretic effect seemed to have been overlooked. This medicine was composed of twenty or more different herbs; but it was not very difficult for one conversant in these subjects, to perceive, that the active herb could be no other than the Foxglove" (Withering 1785:2).

19. Ampofo (1977), for example, describes the clinical investigation of traditional remedies in Ghana which apparently revealed a plant highly effective in aiding in the expulsion of guinea-worm, and another that had antidiabetic properties.

health is still unknown. The pharmacological investigation of Nigerian medicinal plants is still in its infancy. Although some work has been done (e.g., Rowson 1965; Parrott 1970; Etkin 1980, 1981; Etkin and Ross 1982), a great deal more research must be undertaken if the composition and range of pharmacologically active agents in the traditional Hausa pharmacopoeia are to be determined. In one of the few pharmacological studies of Hausa medicinal plants that has been undertaken,[20] Parrott stated (1970:36):

> During the study of over 300 local herbal treatments used by native practitioners in the Emirates of Kano, Katsina, Katagum and Hadejia in Northern Nigeria, it was found that some 45 contained a known active principle which could be related to their therapeutic effects. A few more had religious overtones and a considerable number depended on the powers of sympathetic magic to achieve the patients' relief. The vast majority, however, appeared to have no specific activity that could be assigned to any one principle or group of principles.

There are many reasons for this generally unimpressive showing. Hausa concepts of illness describe symptoms that may be presented by any number of disease processes. Hausa medical thought has not developed a nosology of disease that can be compared systematically with scientific pathology. Since different underlying pathogenetic mechanisms can produce similar signs and symptoms, and because Hausa medicine possesses no way of identifying and discriminating among these processes, therapy is very often a hit-or-miss proposition,[21] and

20. The study of the biochemical properties of Hausa medicinal plants is in its infancy. See Etkin (1980, 1981) and Etkin and Ross (1982) for recent research in this area.

21. A good example of this in the history of Western medicine is the treatment of "dropsy" by the use of the foxglove, which contains digitalis. "Dropsy" is an antique medical term defined by the Oxford English Dictionary as "A morbid condition characterized by the accumulation of watery fluid in the serous cavities or the connective tissue of the body." William Withering was able to cure some cases of dropsy with his foxglove preparation, but some remained intractable. Because treatment resulted in diuresis with a reduction in edema, Withering reasoned that it was primarily a diuretic and used it as such, but no explanation was forthcoming for the irregular nature of the cures. In fact, digitalis exerts a diuretic effect

even if a pharmacologically active agent with specificity for the condition under treatment is used, the traditional practitioner faces enormous problems in the standardization of dosages, regularity of administration, and maintenance of an effective therapeutic level of the drug (see Parrott 1970). Since the vast majority of human illnesses are self-limited in any case, any treatment followed by recovery can easily be attributed to the actions of the medicine given, rather than the natural resolution of the disease process. "Relief" and "cure" are often highly subjective interpretations which the therapist has a vested interest in defining in terms favorable to himself. Even in cases where there is an obvious element of therapy based on solid knowledge (such as bone-setting), the "cures" obtained by the practitioner are often far below what a Western physician would find acceptable.

In the Hausa case the absence of wide, kin-based groups and clan traditions means that medical knowledge is transmitted within very narrow family traditions, or to apprentice adepts, and that there is no clearly defined "Hausa medical tradition" standardized, taught, and generally accepted throughout Hausaland—only a range of ideas and accepted therapies that exist in many different forms in many different areas.[22] Although there is a medical literature in Hausa, generally written in Arabic script, these writings appear to be nothing more than uncritical compilations of Islamic "Prophetic" medicine with admixtures of Hausa medical recipes (Abdalla 1979). Rural traditional practitioners, who are often functionally if not actually illiterate, make little use of these writings, and certainly do not carry on exchanges of medical knowledge through any kind of correspondence. Medical traditions, although partaking of a common range of ideas and assumptions, tend to be very local, even individual, in nature.

---

only as a secondary effect of its improvement of myocardial contractility in cases of congestive heart failure. Since congestive heart failure produces edema through the accumulation of fluid, which backs up due to the poor contractility of the heart, it would have been an unrecognized subcategory of the disease "dropsy." Eighteenth-century medicine simply did not have categories refined enough to solve the puzzle presented to them by digitalis. See note 18 above and Withering (1785).

22. This aspect of medicine has been commented on at some length by Murray Last in a recent stimulating paper (1980).

Although one may certainly find medical practitioners of unusual skill and insight, rustic thinkers of genius,[23] the absence of carefully controlled, rigorous, critical thought means that empirical findings are often compounded with and may be obscured by the addition of ingredients used for their symbolic, rather than pharmacological, input. A good example of this is to be found in L. W. LaChard's article on the arrow poisons of northern Nigeria. His investigations turned up a list of some seventeen plants used as ingredients in making arrow poisons, one of which belonged to the toxin-producing genus *Strophanthus*. He believed, as do most others, that this was the active basis of the arrow poisons, which were known to work. In addition to this vegetable compound, however, the arrows were also subjected to a second coating with a concoction made of animal materials.

> Prior to a "big palaver" the arrows are dipped first into the vegetable poison and allowed to dry, then they are smeared with this animal virus. This latter is made in various ways, but generally by mixing portions of the entrails of a dead monkey, heads of snakes, quantities of menstrual fluid, pus emanating from ulcers and guinea-worm sores and other materes morbi. . . . The natives assert that the vegetable poison alone, if used upon arrows, is insufficient to kill a man. (LaChard 1905:26–27)

LaChard was sufficiently aghast at the composition of this mixture to think that either it or the vegetable poison could be fatal, but one gets the distinct feeling that it is the symbolic associations with putrefaction, blackness, impurity, sickness, evil, and death that are supposed to be the animating forces of this recipe.

If the matter were merely one of determining the presence or absence of active pharmacological principles, it would perhaps not be so difficult to render a verdict on the efficacy of Hausa traditional medicines. Unfortunately, the matter is much more complicated than this. In his analysis of the Hausa pharmacopoeia he collected, Parrott stated that in spite of his failure to isolate active substances in most of the preparations, "the effectiveness of many of these could not be doubted" (1970:36). If one is to come to an accurate opinion about the value of

23. One thinks of Muchona the Hornet described by Victor Turner (1964), Marcel Griaule's conversations with the Dogon thinker Ogotemmeli, or the Ugandan surgeon, described by Felkin (1884), who successfully performed a caesarean section.

traditional medicine, one must investigate much more than the mere nature of the plants which contribute to medicine recipes. The actual substance taken by the patient, the manner in which the medicine is administered, and the social setting in which the therapeutic encounter takes place must all be evaluated. To do this in a controlled, "double-blind" situation, as would be the case in a sophisticated scientific drug study, would be next to impossible in Hausaland.

The social setting is particularly important, for there are many "non-specific forces" that surround illness and its treatment (Beecher 1962). The patient's expectations and perceptions of his situation have an important bearing on the outcome of his illness (Bootzin 1985; Hahn 1985). The attitudes inculcated by the patient's culture can have a dramatic influence on his response to illness, as has been shown in the case of cultural variations in the response to pain (Zabrowski 1952; Wolff and Langley 1968). The severity of a wound as perceived by a patient, for example, has a far greater impact on the amount of pain that results than the amount of actual physical damage incurred (Beecher 1956a). Morphine administered in large doses has relatively little effect on brief episodes of pain produced experimentally, but almost never fails to alleviate suffering in cases of actual pathology (Beecher 1956b); thus the reaction or information-processing phase of pain appears to be extremely important, perhaps more so than the incoming physical sensations. Worry, fear, fright, and anxiety can produce ill health; loss of the will to live can even cause death (Finney 1934; Cannon 1942; H. A. Davidson 1949; Lex 1974); and the reaction to illness can be an illness itself (Gliedman et al. 1958).[24]

The importance of the "placebo effect" in medicine is well known, and is related to the environmental factors surrounding illness (Houston 1938; Pepper 1945; Wolff et al. 1946; Wolf 1950; Findley 1953; Beecher 1955, 1962; Shapiro 1960, 1964; White et al. 1985). The word "placebo" stems from Latin roots and means literally "I will please," referring to the positive therapeutic results expected from the administration of an inert substance or one that does not have specific activity

24. A recent summary of work in the field of psychosomatic medicine, edited by Lipowski, Lipsitt, and Whybrow (1977), contains considerable material that is relevant to the points made above. The current status of research on placebos is summarized in White, Tursky, and Schwartz (1985); of special note are the contributions by Hahn (1985) and Bootzin (1985).

for the condition for which it is given. The beneficial results come from the psychological and psychophysiological relief which stems from reassurance and the alleviation of anxiety in the patient. Shapiro has offered a medical definition of the placebo and its effects as follows (1968:682):

> A *placebo* is defined as any therapy (or that component of any therapy) that is deliberately used for its non-specific psychologic or psychophysiological effect, or that is used for its presumed specific effect on a patient, symptom or illness, but which unknown to therapist and patient is without specific activity for the condition being treated. A *placebo*, when used as a control in experimental studies, is defined as a substance or procedure that is without specific activity for the condition being evaluated. The *placebo effect* is defined as the non-specific psychologic or psychophysiological effect produced by the placebo.

The placebo and its effects are powerful forces not to be discounted in medical practice. For example, in the treatment of angina pectoris even today the placebo effect remains an important aspect of therapy (Benson and McCallie 1979), as it undoubtedly does in the administration of *all* medicines (Hahn 1985). Evans and Hoyle noted and demonstrated this in a drug therapy study as early as 1933, when they wrote (1933:335): "It is remarkable that placebo treatment gave better results than most of the active drugs, and appeared statistically to be the better form of treatment." The effects produced by placebos have been shown to increase as the stress and anxiety felt by the patient increase (Beecher 1960) and, depending upon the personality structure of the patient and his fears and expectations concerning therapy, placebos may even produce toxic effects or addiction in some individuals (Leslie 1954:858; Wolf and Pinsky 1954; Pogge 1963; Mintz 1977). Placebo effects may even be so strong as to overshadow the pharmacological effects of the drug given (Wolf 1950).

The Harvard anesthesiologist Henry K. Beecher summed up the general therapeutic impact of placebos thus (1955:1606):

> It is evident that placebos have a high degree of therapeutic effectiveness in treating subjective responses, decided improvement,

interpreted under the unknown technique as a real therapeutic effect, being produced in 35.2 ± 2.2% of cases. This is shown in over 1,000 patients in 15 studies covering a wide variety of areas: wound pain, the pain of angina pectoris, headache, nausea, phenomena related to cough and to drug-induced mood changes, anxiety and tension, and finally the common cold, a wide spread of human ailments where subjective factors enter. The relative constancy of the placebo effect over a fairly wide assortment of subjective responses suggests that a fundamental mechanism in common is operating, and that it deserves more study.

At the center of the placebo effect lies the relationship between the healer and his patient. Adler and Hammett (1973:596) suggested that "regardless of period or culture, those defined as patients—distressed or disabled—have always been helped by two aids of incalculable importance: participation in a shared cognitive system that made otherwise chaotic symptoms understandable and access to a relationship with a culturally sanctioned parental figure." This shared cognitive system and the formation of the therapeutic partnership between healer and patient conveys important symbolic information to the patient that is often crucial for his recovery (Hahn 1985). "The giving of a pill by the physician to the patient is the symbol for the statement 'I will take care of you' and the very force of the statement gives support and reassurance and often relief from pain" (Wolff in Wolff et al. 1946:1719). The Hausa herbalist who prescribes a remedy for his patient invariably says *za ka warke*, "you will recover" as he hands over the medicines (with, of course, the stated or implied caveat that God must agree). Such assurance helps to alter the patient's perception of his situation, transmitting the message "You *can* get better" or "You *can* be cured," results which not infrequently follow. "The reaction to illness may be such that the healthy or non-illness–involved aspects of the personality are prevented from functioning adequately. Relief of this secondary reaction may well free the effective aspects of the person's capacity, so that what appears to be only symptomatic relief may express itself in a more general restoration of effective functioning" (Gliedman et al. 1958:350).

The important point is that the social setting of medical practice, and especially the relationship between the patient and the healer, exerts a powerful influence on the recovery from sickness. The mere act of seeking help from an established and socially sanctioned medical authority—such as a *mallam*, a *bori* adept, a market medicine seller, or a *boka*—can have a significant therapeutic impact. Even the act of surgery—perhaps the cupping done by a Hausa barber—can often bring significant palliation even where no demonstrable physical repair has been wrought (Beecher 1961). The simple feeling that something is being done to correct one's condition helps bring relief. The more tangible the evidence that something is happening, the greater the placebo effect (Leslie 1954; Beecher 1960)—for example, in treating cuts and wounds in the village it was noted that the antiseptics that burned and stung the most were always the most preferred. Everyone agreed that these were strong medicines—they could feel them at work. In the treatment of snakebite in particular the placebo effect is of great importance. Since the Hausa regard all snakes as poisonous until proven otherwise, administration of any medicine will accomplish a remarkable reduction in anxiety, and the generally low incidence of mortality in snakebite cases serves to enhance the reputation of the local therapist.[25]

Especially in the treatment of psychiatric disorders it would seem that traditional medical therapy can play a role in the treatment and reintegration of mental patients into society. Traditional healers may have an excellent understanding of the social milieu in which their patients live and the social forces which act upon them. Their insights may provide valuable therapeutic help for the emotionally and mentally distressed, healing through reassurance and persuasion, major components in most schemes of psychotherapy (Frank 1973; Bootzin 1985). Largely as a recognition of these facts, much of the work on African healing systems has stressed their psychiatric aspects. With the woe-

25. "The common symptom in human snakebite is *fright and fear of rapid death*. But the danger of poisonous snakebite in human victims has been greatly exaggerated: one-half of the people bitten by poisonous snakes such as cobras, vipers and sea snakes develop no significant poisoning (because little or no venom is injected). Serious poisoning is rare in man and death is *highly exceptional*—particularly if adequate medical treatment is received within a few hours of the bite" (Reid 1972:810). This author recommends vitamin B complex as a placebo injection in cases where no significant systemic poisoning is observed.

fully inadequate facilities available for the care of the mentally ill, indigenous practitioners will continue to play an important role in the
provision of psychiatric care (Forster 1962:44; Swift and Asuni 1975:
200–201). As Geoffry Tooth remarked in his study of mental illness in
the Gold Coast over thirty years ago (1950:67):

> A visit to the Gold Coast Asylum should convince an impartial
> observer that the African's lack of confidence in the European
> management of this branch of medicine is well founded. More-
> over, it seems unlikely that an alien psychiatrist could ever suc-
> ceed in assimilating the complexities of the West African back-
> ground in time to make an appreciable contribution in this field.
> So that, until African psychiatrists can be trained, it would seem
> better to allow the care of the majority of the insane to remain in
> lay hands.

Among the Yoruba in southern and western Nigeria attempts have
been made to integrate local culture and village life into a system for
the treatment of mental patients, with some success (Lambo 1956;
Anonymous 1964; Osborne 1969). In countries where financial resources are few and where the task of providing complete Western
scientific medical care for the entire population is clearly impossible in
the foreseeable future, consideration is now being given to the attempt
to integrate traditional practitioners into the health care delivery system in order to bring their insights and social influence to bear on the
health problems of their societies (e.g., Dunlop 1974–75; Harrison
1974–75; Imperato 1974–75). Whether or not these attempts will be
successful remains to be seen. There are considerable practical—as well
as ethical—problems involved in such attempts. As yet no significant
attempts have been made to incorporate practitioners of traditional
Hausa medicine into the Nigerian health care system, although many
Hausa herbalists are eager for such attempts to be made (but largely,
it would appear, for reasons of increased prestige and personal ag-
grandizement).

As more effective medical and surgical treatment becomes available
to rural Hausa villagers it may be that traditional medicine will fade in
importance. There are some signs that this is already happening, particularly in cases where immediate and dramatic relief can be provided
by simple therapeutic procedures; but Hausa traditional medicine is not

likely to vanish entirely. For all its uncritical components it is firmly grounded in the social life and cultural expectations of the Hausa people. John Beattie has remarked (1966:67) that "in so far as magical and religious rites contain an essentially expressive element, they may, so far, be satisfying and rewarding in themselves." The human dimensions of illness cannot be treated sufficiently by the rudimentary dispensing of tablets to long queues of sick people. As long as the Hausa quest for *lafiya* continues, with all its implications, there will still be those who search for a special kind of *magani* to solve their emotional, spiritual, and physical problems, whatever they may be.

Conclusion

In za a yi tuka a yi mata hanci domin kada ta warware.

(If you are going to make rope, knot the threads so they don't unwind.)

HAUSA PROVERB

One of the fundamental problems facing clinicians practicing bioscientific medicine in industrialized Western countries is the complexity of the medical system. High technology raises enormous questions about the proper utilization of expensive resources, who gets access to various tests or procedures, and who should control them and act as "gate-keepers" (Jennett 1986). Concurrent with the often spectacular successes that scientific medicine has achieved in such fields as acute care, the control of infectious diseases, and the development of artificial organs, there has been a slow but progressive erosion of community consensus on many major moral issues. The medical community in industrialized countries no longer has a common moral view or shared moral order within which to make decisions. Society, as well as medicine, has grown increasingly complex and the patient and physician may have vastly different views of the moral framework in which their encounter takes place. Indeed, one of the most difficult problems facing medical ethicists in the industrialized West is this: What is the basis for medical ethics in a pluralistic society? An entire field of "bioethics" has sprung up to help answer this and related questions, providing not a new set of moral rules by which to live, but rather attempting to provide a common language and a common method of reasoning to help sort through this awesome tangle of moral and ethical dilemmas (Spicker and Engelhardt 1977).

While it would be simplistic to assume that the Hausa do not face moral dilemmas or wrestle with difficult moral questions, their situation is far different from that which

exists in our society. This book has been an attempt to outline the nature of life in rural Hausa society and to sketch the moral parameters
within which their medical system operates, for the Hausa moral
order is indeed more unified than ours and much of their medical practice reflects this fact. The patient-healer relationship proceeds more
smoothly when there is a shared world of assumptions among the parties involved.

I have described in this book the basic outlines of an African peasant
society, centered around family and the village, supported by an agricultural economy with a strong emphasis on vigorous petty trading,
and enveloped by a more or less universal Muslim worldview which is
only partly penetrated by residual and persistent beliefs about the
powers of evil spirits, witches, and sorcerers. Within this relatively
ordered world a variety of traditional medical practitioners ply their
crafts against a background of shared assumptions and expectations,
improvising therapy for the individual patient by selecting from the
appropriate cultural themes.

The most important of these themes is *lafiya*, a fundamental concept
in Hausa thought. As we have noted, *lafiya* is usually translated simply
as "health," but in reality it is a much broader term which denotes balance, order, stability, peacefulness, tranquility, prosperity, normality—
well-being in a broad sense. It denotes not only a state of bodily
health, but also a state of domestic tranquility, environmental balance,
social order, and moral propriety which is highly valued by the Hausa
in all things. *Lafiya* is "health," therefore, in the sense of the word suggested by the World Health Organization nearly forty years ago: "a
state of complete physical, mental and social well-being and not merely
the absence of disease or infirmity" (Engelhardt 1975:125). No wonder,
then, that the Hausa proverb states *Zama lafiya ya fi zama sarki*, "Being
well is better than being chief"—physical, emotional, spiritual, and
domestic tranquility are far superior to material goods or political
power. *Lafiya ta fi dukiya*, "Health is better than wealth."

Since *lafiya* connotes the fundamental, proper order of things, be it a
physiological or social equilibrium, *magani*, or "medicine," denotes the
means by which disordered states may be returned to their proper
order. *Magani* is a "remedy" in the broadest sense and medicine therefore is as concerned with the return of social propriety and balance as
it is with the treatment of disordered physiology. Rudolf Virchow, that

towering giant of nineteenth-century European medicine, maintained that medicine was a social science, pure and simple, and wrote that "the last task of medicine is the constitution of society on a physiological basis. . . . Medicine is a social science and politics nothing else but medicine on a large scale" (Ackerknecht 1953:46). While medicine has never achieved this lofty status in Western scientific circles, the Hausa concept of *magani* carries many of these connotations, for *lafiya* includes social and political well-being as well as physical health.

This explains why, for example, Koranic charms can be called "medicine" while directed toward ensuring the health of one's horse, promoting the growth of crops, keeping evil spirits away from one's compound, or gaining the favors of a desired young woman. They all serve to promote the attainment of *lafiya*, well-being in its largest sense. This also explains why many of the ingredients in Hausa medicine seem nonpharmacologic or unrelated to simple physiologic processes.

While there has been much talk (especially among those on the medical "fringe") in Western society about promoting the "holistic" practice of medicine, the great, unresolved question still remains how to treat the "whole person"—mentally, physically, and spiritually—in a fragmented, pluralistic society. Hausa traditional medicine is more "holistic" largely due to the greater moral cohesiveness of Hausa society, and this is reflected in the pharmacopoeia of Hausa traditional medicine.

The last chapter explained in some detail how Hausa medicines select their therapeutic effects by drawing upon a complex indigenous symbol system of colors, shapes, locations, tastes, textures, religious power, animal images, and numerological beliefs, in addition to inherent biochemical properties. In using such medications Hausa practitioners and patients draw upon an enormous reservoir of cultural power in addition to whatever culturally discovered pharmacological agents they may have at their disposal. This can explain why a Hausa patient may be more comfortable with a *boka* who fumigates him with medicinal smoke and fills his food with hot, spicy substances than he is standing in line for hours at a dispensary only to receive a sharp word and a handful of pills from an unhappy and overworked attendant, in spite of the fact that the latter may actually be more effective for his ailment in the long run.

The Hausa patient, like his American or European counterpart, craves much more than the administration of medicines when he or she is ill. There is an ever-present need for sympathy, for reassurance, for security in the face of illness. Hausa traditional medicine makes extensive use of familiar objects from Hausa life and through them calls upon an intricate symbol system to aid in the healing process. Perhaps the healing effects of Hausa therapeutics lie not so much in what goes into the patient as in the milieu which supports that medication, the intricate system of symbols interwoven with Hausa life which infuses Hausa medicine with its power and meaning. Until bioscientific medicine can provide the rural Hausa villager with the same intimacy of care and the same supportive environment in which to face the challenges of illness, Hausa traditional medicine will find a place in the lives of the Hausa people, for they also crave a fullness of life, a personal peace, and a domestic tranquility which exceeds the ability of mere scientific medicine to provide.

Bibliography

Abdalla, Ismail H. 1979. "Medicine in nineteenth century Arabic literature in northern Nigeria: A report." *Kano Studies* (n.s.) 14:91–99.

Abraham, R. C. 1959. *The language of the Hausa people.* London: University of London Press.

———. 1962. *Dictionary of the Hausa language.* 2d ed. London: University of London Press.

Abubakar, Sa'ad. 1974. "The emirate type of government in the Sokoto Caliphate." *Journal of the Historical Society of Nigeria* 7:211–29.

———. 1977. *The Lami'be of Fombina: A political history of Adamawa, 1809–1901.* Zaria: Ahmadu Bello University Press and Oxford University Press.

Ackerknecht, Erwin H. 1943. "Primitive autopsies and the history of anatomy." *Bulletin of the History of Medicine* 13:334–39.

———. 1953. *Rudolph Virchow: Doctor, statesman, anthropologist.* Madison: University of Wisconsin Press.

———. 1971. *Medicine and ethnology: Selected essays,* edited by H. H. Walser and H. M. Koelbing. Baltimore: Johns Hopkins University Press.

Adam, J. G., N. Echard, and M. Lescot. 1972. "Plantes medicinales Hausa de l'Adar (Republique du Niger)." *Journal d'Agriculture Tropicale et de Botanique Appliquée* 19:259–399.

Adamu, Mahdi. 1976. "The spread of Hausa culture in west Africa, 1700–1900." *Savannah* 5:3–13.

———. 1978. *The Hausa factor in west African history.* Zaria: Ahmadu Bello University Press and Oxford University Press.

Adeleye, R. A. 1971. *Power and diplomacy in northern Nigeria, 1804–1906: The Sokoto Caliphate and its enemies.* London: Longmans.

Adler, Herbert M., and Van Buren O. Hammett. 1973. "The doctor-patient relationship revisited: An analysis of the placebo effect." *Annals of Internal Medicine* 78:595–98.

Africanus, Leo [Al-Hassan Ibn-Mohammed Al-Wezaz Al-Fasi]. 1896. *History and description of Africa.* Translated by John Pory in 1600; edited, with an introduction, by Robert Browne. 3 vols. London: Hakluyt Society.

Al-Maghili, Sheikh Mohammed, of Tleman. 1932. *The obligations of princes: An essay on Muslim kingship.* Translated by T. R. Baldwin. Beirut: Imprimerie Catholique.

Ames, David W., and Anthony V. King. 1971. *Glossary of Hausa music and its social contexts.* Evanston, Ill.: Northwestern University Press.

Ampofo, Oku. 1977. "Plants that heal." *World Health,* November 1977, pp. 26–30.

Anonymous. 1964. "The village of Aro." *Lancet* 2:513–14.

Anonymous. 1968. *Labaru na da da na yanzu.* 2d ed. Zaria: Northern Nigerian Publishing Company.

Arberry, Arthur J. 1950. *Sufism: An account of the mystics of Islam.* New York: Harper and Row. Paperback, 1970.

————. 1964. *The Koran interpreted*. London: Oxford University Press.

Arnett, E. J. 1922. *The rise of the Sokoto Fulani, being a paraphrase and in some parts a translation of the infaku'l maisuri of Sultan Mohammed Bello*. Kano.

Awe, Bolanle. 1965. "Empires of the western Sudan: Ghana, Mali and Songhai." In *A thousand years of west African history*, edited by J. F. Ade Ajayi and Ian Espie, pp. 55–71. Ibadan: University of Ibadan Press.

Ayensu, Edward S. 1978. *Medicinal plants of west Africa*. Algonac, Mich.: Reference Publications.

Azarya, Victor. 1976. *Dominance and change in north Cameroun: The Fulbe aristocracy*. Beverly Hills, Calif.: Sage Publications.

————. 1978. *Aristocrats facing change: The Fulbe in Guinea, Nigeria and the Cameroun*. Chicago: University of Chicago Press.

Balogun, Ismail A. B. 1975. *The life and works of 'Uthman Dan Fodio*. Lagos: Islamic Publications Bureau.

Bargery, George P. 1934. *A Hausa-English dictionary and English-Hausa vocabulary*. London: Oxford University Press.

Barkow, Jerome H. 1971. "The institution of courtesanship in northern Nigeria." *Geneva-Africa* 10:58–73.

————. 1972. "Hausa women and Islam." *Canadian Journal of African Studies* 6:317–28.

————. 1973. "Muslims and Maguzawa in North Central State, Nigeria: An ethnographic comparison." *Canadian Journal of African Studies* 7:59–76.

————. 1974. "Evaluation of character and social control among the Hausa." *Ethos* 2:1014.

Barth, H. 1859. *Travels and discoveries in north and central Africa from the journal of an expedition undertaken under the auspices of H.B.M.'s government in the years 1849–1855*. Philadelphia: J. W. Bradley.

Beattie, John. 1966. "Ritual and social change." *Man* (n.s.) 1:60–74.

————. 1970. "On understanding ritual." In *Rationality*, edited by Bryan R. Wilson, pp. 240–68. Oxford: Basil Blackwell.

————. 1973. "Understanding traditional African religion: A comment on Horton." *Second Order* 2:3–11.

————. 1977. "Spirit mediumship as theatre." *Royal Anthropological Institute Newsletter*, June 1977, no. 20, pp. 1–6.

Becker, C. H. 1961. "Djizya." In *Shorter encyclopedia of Islam*, edited by H. A. R. Gibb and J. H. Kraemer, pp. 91–92. Leiden: E. J. Brill.

Beecher, Henry K. 1955. "The powerful placebo," *Journal of the American Medical Association* 159:1602–6.

————. 1956a. "Relationship of significance of wound to pain experience." *Journal of the American Medical Association* 161:1609–13.

————. 1956b. "The subjective response and reaction to sensation: The reaction phase as the effective site for drug action." *American Journal of Medicine* 20:107–13.

————. 1960. "Increased stress and effectiveness of placebos and active drugs." *Science* 132:91–92.

————. 1961. "Surgery as placebo: A quantitative study of bias." *Journal of the American Medical Association* 176:1102–7.

————. 1962. "Nonspecific forces surrounding disease and the treatment of disease." *Journal of the American Medical Association* 179:437–40.

Bello, Alhaji Sir Ahmadu. 1962. *My life*. Cambridge: Cambridge University Press.

Benson, Herbert, and David P. McCallie. 1979. "Angina pectoris and the placebo effect." *New England Journal of Medicine* 300:1424–29.

Berg, C. C. 1974. *"Sawm."* In *Shorter encyclopedia of Islam*, edited by H. A. R. Gibb and J. H. Kramers, pp. 504–7. Leiden: E. J. Brill.

Bernard, Claude. [1865] 1927. *An introduction to the study of experimental medicine*. Reprint, translated by Henry Copley Greene. New York: Macmillan and Co.

Besmer, Fremont E. 1975. *"Boorii:* Structure and process in performance." *Folia Orientalia* 16:101–30.

————. 1983. *Horses, musicians, and gods: The Hausa cult of possession-trance*. South Hadley, Mass.: Bergin and Garvey.

Bierce, Ambrose. [1911] 1958. *The devil's dictionary*. Reprint. New York: Dover Publications.

Birks, J. S. 1978. *Across the savannas to Mecca: The overland pilgrimage route from west Africa*. London: Frank Cass.

Bisilliat, Jeanne. 1976. "Village diseases and bush diseases in Songhay: An essay in description and classification with a view to a typology." In *Social Anthropology and medicine*, edited by J. B. Loudon, pp. 553–94. London: Academic Press.

Bivar, A. D. H., and Mervyn Hiskett. 1962. "The Arabic literature of Nigeria to 1804: A provisional account." *Bulletin of the School of Oriental and African Studies* 25:104–48.

Boahen, A. Adu. 1962. "The caravan trade in the nineteenth century." *Journal of African History* 3:349–59.

Bootzin, Richard R. 1985. "The role of expectancy in behavior change." In *Placebo: theory, research and mechanisms*, edited by Leonard White et al., pp. 196–210. New York: Guilford Press.

Bouquet, A. 1968. "The traditional pharmacology of Congo-Brazzaville knowledge and practice." In *First Inter-African Symposium on Traditional Pharmacopoeias and African Medical Plants, Dakar, 1968*, pp. 56–61. Lagos: Organization of African Unity, Scientific, Technical, and Research Committee, Publication no. 104.

Bovill, E. W. 1970. *The golden trade of the Moors*. 2d ed. Paperback, revised, with additional material by Robin Hallett. London: Oxford University Press.

Browne, E. G. 1921. *Arabian medicine*. Cambridge: Cambridge University Press.

Bryant, Alfred T. 1970. *Zulu medicine and medicine men*. Cape Town: C. Struick.

Buchanan, K. M., and J. C. Pugh. 1955. *Land and people in Nigeria: The human geography of Nigeria and its environmental background*. London: University of London Press.

Buckley, Anthony. 1985. *Yoruba medicine*. London: Oxford University Press.

Buntjer, B. J. 1971. "The changing structure of *gandu*." In *Zaria and its region*, edited by M. J. Mortimore, pp. 157–69. Zaria: Ahmadu Bello University, Department of Geography, Occasional Paper no. 4.

Burgel, J. Christoph. 1977. "Secular and religious features of medieval Arabic medicine." In *Asian medical systems: A comparative study*, edited by Charles Leslie, pp. 44–62. Los Angeles: University of California Press.

Burton, Sir Richard. 1893. *Personal narrative of a pilgrimage to Al-Medinah and Meccah*. 2 vols. London: Tylston and Edwars.

Burtt, E. A. 1932. *The metaphysical foundations of modern physical science: A historical and critical study*. London: Routledge and Kegan Paul.

Buxton, Jean. 1973. *Religion and healing in Mandari*. Oxford: Clarendon Press.

Callaway, Barbara J. 1984. "Ambiguous consequences of the socialisation and seclusion of Hausa women." *Journal of Modern African Studies* 22:429–50.

Campbell, Donald E. H. 1926. *Arabian medicine and its influence on the Middle Ages*. 2 vols. London: Kegan Paul, Trench, Trubner and Co.

Cannon, Walter B. 1942. "Voodoo death." *American Anthropologist* 44:169–81.

Chelhod, Joseph. 1973. "A contribution to the problem of the pre-eminence of the right, based upon Arabic evidence." In *Right and left: Essays on dual symbolic classification*, edited by Rodney Needham, pp. 239–62. Chicago: University of Chicago Press.

Clapperton, Hugh. 1829. *Journal of a second expedition into the interior of Africa from the bight of Benin to Soccatoo*. London: John Murray. Reprint. London: Frank Cass, 1969.

Cohen, Abner. 1965. "The social organization of credit in a west African cattle market." *Africa* 35:8–19.

———. 1966. "Politics of the kola trade." *Africa* 36:18–36.

———. 1969. *Custom and politics in urban Africa: A study of Hausa migrants in Yoruba towns*. London: Routledge and Kegan Paul.

Collingwood, R. G. 1940. *An essay on metaphysics*. Oxford: Clarendon Press.

Coulson, Noel J. 1964. *A History of Islamic law*. Edinburgh: Edinburgh University Press.

Cragg, Kenneth. 1969. *The house of Islam*. Belmont, Calif.: Dickinson.

Dalby, David. 1964. "The nourn garii in Hausa: A semantic study." *Journal of African Languages* 3:273–305.

———. 1975. "The concept of settlement in the west African savannah." In *Shelter, sign and symbol*, edited by P. Oliver, pp. 197–205. London: Barrie and Jenkins.

Dalziel, John. 1916. *A Hausa botanical vocabulary*. London: T. Fisher Unwin.

———. 1937. *The useful plants of west tropical Africa*. London: Crown Agents for Overseas Governments and Administrations, HMSO.

Darrah, Allan, and John Froude. n.d. *Hausa medicine for western doctors*. Zaria: Departments of Sociology and Medicine, Ahmadu Bello University, mimeographed, 35 pp.

Davidson, Henry A. 1949. "Emotional precipitants of death." *Journal of the Medical Society of New Jersey* 46:350–52.

Davidson, N. McD., Lorna Trevitt, and E. H. O. Parry. 1974. "Peripartum cardiac failure: An explanation for the observed geographic distribution in Nigeria." *Bulletin of the World Health Organization* 51:203–8.

Davies, J. N. P. 1965. "Primitive autopsies and background to scientific medicine in central Africa." *New York State Journal of Medicine* 65:2830–36.

Denham, Major Dixon, and Captain Hugh Clapperton. 1826. *Narrative of travels and discoveries in northern and central Africa in the years 1822, 1823, and 1824.* London: John Murray.

Dry, D. P. L. 1950. "The family organization of the Hausa of northern Nigeria." B.Sc. thesis, on deposit in Rhodes House Library, Oxford.

———. 1952. "The Hausa attitude to authority." In *Proceedings of the West African Institute for Social and Economic Research*, Ibadan, April 15–19, 1952.

———. 1953. "The place of Islam in Hausa society." D.Phil. thesis, Institute of Social Anthropology Library, Oxford.

———. 1956. "Some aspects of Hausa family structure." In *Proceedings of the Third International West African Conference*, Ibadan, December 12–21, 1949, pp. 158–63. Ibadan: Nigerian Museum.

Dry, Elizabeth. 1956. "The social development of the Hausa child." In *Proceedings of the Third International West African Conference*, Ibadan December 12–21, 1949, pp. 164–70. Ibadan: Nigerian Museum.

Dudley, Billy J. 1968. *Parties and politics in northern Nigeria.* London: Frank Cass.

Dunlop, David W. 1974–75. "Alternatives to 'modern' health-delivery systems in Africa: Issues for public policy consideration on the role of traditional healers." *Rural Africana* 26:131–40.

Dusgate, Richard H. 1985. *The conquest of northern Nigeria.* London: Frank Cass.

East, Rupert, and Abubakar Imam. 1949. *Ikon Allah.* Zaria: Gaskiya.

Elgood, Cyril. 1962. "Tibb-ul-nabbi or medicine of the Prophet; being a translation of two works of the same name: I. The tibb-ul-nabbi of Al-Suyuti; II. The tibb-ul-nabbi of Mahmud bin Mohamed al-Chaghhayni." *Osiris* 14:33–192.

———. 1970. *Safavid medical practice, or, the practice of medicine, surgery and gynaecology in Persia between 1500 A.D. and 1750 A.D.* London: Luzac and Co.

El-Masri, F. N. 1963. "The life of Shehu Usuman dan Fodio before the *jihad.*" *Journal of the Historical Society of Nigeria* 2:435–48.

Engelhardt, H. Tristram, Jr. 1975. "The concepts of health and disease." In *Evaluation and explanation in the biomedical sciences*, edited by H. T. Engelhardt, Jr. and S. F. Spicker, pp. 125–41. Boston: D. Reidel.

Erlmann, Veit. 1982. "Trance and music in the Hausa boorii spirit possession cult in Niger." *Ethnomusicology* 26:49–58.

Etkin, Nina L. 1980. "Indigenous medicine among the Hausa of northern Nigeria." *Medical Anthropology* 3:401–29.

———. 1981. "A Hausa herbal pharmacopoeia: Biomedical evaluation of commonly used plant medicines." *Journal of Ethnopharmacology* 4:75–98.

Etkin, Nina L., and P. J. Ross. 1982. "Food as medicine and medicine as food: An adaptive framework for the interpretation of plant utilization among the Hausa of northern Nigeria." *Social Science and Medicine* 16:1559–73.

Evans, William, and Clifford Hoyle. 1933. "The comparative value of drugs used in the continuous treatment of angina pectoris." *Quarterly Journal of Medicine* (n.s.) 2:311–38.

Evans-Pritchard, E. E. 1937. *Witchcraft, oracles and magic among the Azande.* Oxford: Clarendon Press.

Faber, Knud. 1930. *Nosography: The evolution of clinical medicine in modern times.* New York: Paul B. Hoeber.

Fage, J. D. 1969. *A History of west Africa: An introductory survey.* Cambridge: Cambridge University Press.

Faulkingham, Ralph H. 1970. "Political support in a Hausa village." Ph.D. diss., Michigan State University, East Lansing, Mich. Ann Arbor, Mich.: University Microfilms.

———. 1975. *The spirits and their cousins: Some aspects of belief, ritual and social organization in a rural Hausa village in Niger.* Amherst, Mass.: University of Massachusetts, Department of Anthropology, Research Report no. 15.

Felkin, Robert W. 1884. "Notes on labour in central Africa." *Edinburgh Medical Journal* 29:922–30.

Ferguson, Douglas E. 1973. "Nineteenth-century Hausaland, being a description by Imam Imoru of the land, economy, and society of his people." Ph.D. diss., University of California at Los Angeles. Ann Arbor, Mich.: University Microfilms.

Field, Margaret J. 1937. *Religion and medicine of the Ga people.* London: Oxford University Press.

———. 1960. *Search for security: An ethno-psychiatric study of rural Ghana.* London: Faber and Faber.

Fika, Adamu Mohammed. 1978. *The Kano civil war and British over-rule.* Ibadan: Oxford University Press.

Findley, Thomas. 1953. "The placebo and the physician." *Medical Clinics of North America* 37:1821–26.

Finney, J. M. T. 1934. "Discussion on shock." *Annals of Surgery* 100:746–47.

Fisher, Allan G. B., and Humphrey J. Fisher. 1970. *Slavery and society in Muslim Africa: The institution in Saharan and Sudanic Africa and the trans-Saharan trade.* London: C. Hurst.

Fisher, Humphrey J. 1973. "Hassebu: Islamic healing in black Africa." In *Northern Africa: Islam and modernization,* edited by Michael Brett, pp. 23–47. London: Frank Cass.

———. 1977. "The eastern Maghrib and the central Sudan, ca. 1050–1600. In *The Cambridge history of Africa, III: From ca. 1050 to ca. 1600,* edited by Roland Oliver, pp. 232–330. London: Cambridge University Press.

Fleischer, N. K. F. 1975. "A study of traditional practices and early childhood anaemia in northern Nigeria." *Transactions of the Royal Society of Tropical Medicine and Hygiene* 69:198–200.

Forde, Daryll. 1946. "The north: The Hausa." In *The native economies of Nigeria*, edited by Margery Perham, pp. 119–80. London: Faber and Faber.

Forster, E. B. 1962. "The theory and practice of psychiatry in Ghana." *American Journal of Psychotherapy* 16:7–51.

Foster, George M. 1953. "Relationships between Spanish and Spanish-American folk medicine." *Journal of American Folklore* 66:201–17.

Foy, H. Andrew. 1915. "Inoculation of small-pox as a prophylactic measure as practised by the natives at Djen in Nigeria." *Journal of Tropical Medicine and Hygiene* 18:255–57.

Frank, Jerome D. 1973. *Persuasion and healing: A comparative study of psychotherapy*. Rev. ed. Baltimore: Johns Hopkins University Press.

Frobenius, Leo. [1913] 1963. *The voice of Africa, being an account of the travels of the German inner African exploration expedition in the years 1910–1912*. 2 vols. Reprint. New York: Benjamin Blom.

Fry, David R. 1965. "Some complications of illicit injections." *West African Medical Journal* 14:167–69.

Fuglestad, Finn. 1978. "A reconsideration of Hausa history before the jihad." *Journal of African History* 19:319–39.

Gardet, Louis. 1958. "Al-Asna al-Husna." In *Encyclopedia of Islam*, I, pp. 714–17. 2d ed. Leiden: E. J. Brill.

Gelfand, Michael. 1956. *Medicine and magic of the Mashona*. Cape Town: J. C. Juta.

———. 1964a. *Medicine and custom in Africa*. Edinburgh: Churchill and Livingston.

———. 1964b. *Witch doctor, traditional medicine man of Rhodesia*. London: Harvill Press.

Gellner, Ernest. 1974. *Legitimation of belief*. Cambridge: Cambridge University Press. Paperback, 1979.

Gibb, H. A. R. 1975. *Islam*. London: Oxford University Press. Retitled version of *Mohammedanism*, 2d ed. 1965.

Gilles, H. M. 1978. "Dr. A. W. Williamson, M.B., B.S., M.R.C.P., D.T.M.&H." *Annals of Tropical Medicine and Parasitology* 72:303.

Gillies, Eva. 1976. "Causal criteria in African classifications of disease." In *Social anthropology and medicine*, edited by J. B. Loudon, pp. 358–95. London: Academic Press.

Gilliland, Dean Stewart. 1971. "African traditional religion in transition: The influence of Islam on African traditional religion in north Nigeria." Ph.D. diss., Hartford Seminary Foundation. Ann Arbor, Mich.: University Microfilms.

Gliedman, L. H., E. H. Nash, Jr., S. Imber, A. R. Stine, and J. Frank. 1958. "Reduction of symptoms of pharmacologically inert substances and by short-term psychotherapy." *Archives of Neurology and Psychiatry* 79:345–51.

Goddard, A. D. 1973. "Changing family structures among the rural Hausa." *Africa* 43:207–18.

Goddard, A. D., J. C. Fine, and D. W. Norman. 1971. "A socio-economic study of three villages in the Sokoto close-settled zone. I. Land and people." Zaria and Samaru: Institute for Agricultural Research, Samaru, Miscellaneous Paper no. 34.

Goodwin, Donald, and Samuel B. Guze. 1979. *Psychiatric diagnosis.* 2d ed. New York: Oxford University Press.

Gouffé, Claude. 1966. " 'Manger' et 'boire' en Haoussa." *Revue de L'Ecole des Langues Orientales* 3:77–111.

Gray, Robert F. 1969. "The Shetani cult among the Segeju of Tanzania." In *Spirit mediumship and society in Africa,* edited by J. Beattie and J. Middleton, pp. 171–87. London: Routledge and Kegan Paul.

Greenberg, Joseph H. 1941. "Some aspects of Negro-Mohammedan culture-contact among the Hausa." *American Anthropologist* 43:51–61.

———. 1946. *The influence of Islam on a Sudanese religion.* Seattle: University of Washington Press, American Ethnological Society Monographs, no. 10.

———. 1947a. "Islam and clan organization among the Hausa." *Southwestern Journal of Anthropology* 3:193–211.

———. 1947b. "Arabic loan words in Hausa." *Word* 3:85–97.

———. 1963. *Languages of Africa.* Bloomington: Indiana University Research Center in Anthropology, Folklore, and Linguistics, Publication no. 25. (*International Journal of American Linguistics* 29:1–173.)

Greenwood, Bernard. 1980. "Ambiguity and illness classification in a pluralistic medical system—A Moroccan example." Paper presented at the Conference on African Medical and Health Systems as Systems of Thought, Causality, and Taxonomy, Cambridge, England, June 23–26, 1980.

Griaule, Marcel. 1965. *Conversations with Ogotemmeli: An introduction to Dogon religious ideas.* New York: Oxford University Press. Paperback, 1970.

Gruner, A. Cameron. 1930. *The canon of medicine of Avicenna.* London: Luzac.

Guillame, Alfred. 1956. *Islam.* Harmondsworth, Middlesex: Penguin Books.

Hahn, Robert A. 1985. "A sociocultural model of illness and healing." In *Placebo: Theory, research and mechanisms,* edited by Leonard White et al., pp. 167–95. New York: Guilford Press.

Hallam, W. K. R. 1966. "The Bayajida legend in Hausa folklore." *Journal of African History* 7:47–60.

Hanbali, M. 1973. "Research notes: Hausa traditional medicine and pharmacy." *Lagos Notes and Records* 4:9–10.

Harley, George W. 1941. *Native African medicine, with special reference to its practice in the Mano tribe of Liberia.* Cambridge: Harvard University Press.

Harris, P. G. 1930. "Notes on Yauri (Sokoto Province), Nigeria." *Journal of the Royal Anthropological Institute* 70:283–334.

Harrison, Ira E. 1974–75. "Traditional healers: A neglected source of health manpower." *Rural Africana* 26:5–16.

Hart, Conn V. 1969. *Bisayan Filipino and Malayan humoral pathologies: Folk medicine and ethnohistory in Southeast Asia.* Ithaca, N.Y.: Cornell University, Department of Asian Studies, Southeast Asia Program, Data Paper no. 76.

Harwood, Alan. 1971. *Witchcraft, sorcery and social categories among the Safwa.* London: Oxford University Press for the International African Institute.

Hassan, Alhaji, and Malam Shuaibu Na'ibi. 1962. *A chronicle of Abuja.* Rev. enl. ed. Translated by Frank Heath. Lagos: African Universities Press.

Heathcote, David H. 1974. "A Hausa charm gown." *Man* (n.s.) 9:620–24.

Hill, Polly. 1969. "Hidden trade in Hausaland." *Man* (n.s.) 4:392–409.

———. 1972. *Rural Hausa: A village and a setting.* Cambridge: Cambridge University Press.

———. 1977. *Population, prosperity and poverty: Rural Kano 1900 and 1970.* London: Cambridge University Press.

Hill, Polly, and R. H. T. Smith. 1972. "Spatial and temporal synchronization of periodic markets: Evidence from four emirates in northern Nigeria." *Economic Geography* 32:345–55.

Hilton-Simpson, M. W. 1922. *Arab medicine and surgery: A study of the healing art in Algeria.* London: Oxford University Press.

Hiskett, Mervyn. 1957. "Material relating to the state of learning among the Fulani before their jihad." *Bulletin of the School of Oriental and African Studies* 19:550–78.

———. 1960. "Kitab-al-farq: A work on the Habe kingdoms attributed to 'Uthman dan Fodio'." *Bulletin of the School of Oriental and African Studies* 23:558–79.

———. 1962. "An Islamic tradition of reform in the western Sudan from the sixteenth to the eighteenth century." *Bulletin of the School of Oriental and African Studies* 25:577–96.

———. 1965. "The historical background to the naturalization of Arabic loanwords in Hausa." *African Language Studies* 6:18–26.

———. 1971. "The 'song of the Shaihu's miracles': A Hausa hagiography from Sokoto." *African Language Studies* 12:71–107.

———. 1973a. *The sword of truth: The life and times of Shehu Usuman Dan Fodio.* London: Oxford University Press.

———. 1973b. "The development of Islam in Hausaland." In *Northern Africa: Islam and modernization,* edited by M. Brett, pp. 57–64. London: Frank Cass.

———. 1975. *A history of Hausa Islamic verse.* London: School of Oriental and African studies, University of London.

Hogben, S. J., and A. H. M. Kirk-Greene. 1966. *The emirates of northern Nigeria: A preliminary survey of their historical traditions.* London: Oxford University Press.

Hopen, C. Edward. 1958. *The pastoral Fulbe family in Gwandu.* London: Oxford University Press for the International African Institute.

Hopkins, A. G. 1973. *An economic history of west Africa.* London: Longmans.

Hore, P. N. 1970. "Weather and climate." In *Zaria and its region,* edited by M. J. Mortimore, pp. 41–54. Zaria: Ahmadu Bello University, Department of Geography, Occasional Paper no. 4.

Horton, Robin. 1964. "Ritual man in Africa." *Africa* 34:85–104.
———. 1967. "African traditional thought and western science." *Africa* 37:50–71, 155–87.
———. 1976. "Understanding African traditional religion: A reply to Professor Beattie." *Second Order* 5:3–29.
Houston, W. R. 1938. "The doctor himself as therapeutic agent." *Annals of Internal Medicine* 11:1416–25.
Hudson, Robert P. 1974. "Disease and illness: In quest of the Hippocratic grail." *Dialogue*, December 1974, pp. 24–30.
———. 1975. "Perspectives." In *Major's physical diagnosis*. 8th ed. Edited by M. H. Delp and R. T. Manning, pp. 1–19. Philadelphia: W. B. Saunders.
Huisman, A. J. W. 1974. "*Djinaza*." In *Shorter encyclopedia of Islam*, edited by H. A. R. Gibb and J. H. Kramer, pp. 89–90. Leiden: E. J. Brill.
Hull, Richard William. 1968. "The development of administration in Katsina Emirate, northern Nigeria, 1887–1944." Ph.D. diss. Columbia University, New York. Ann Arbor, Mich.: University Microfilms.
Hunwick, J. O. 1976. "Songhay, Bornu and Hausaland in the sixteenth century." In *History of West Africa*. Volume I, edited by J. F. Ade Ajayi and M. Crowder, pp. 152–95. London: Longman.
Hutchinson, J., and J. M. Dalziel. 1954. *Flora of west tropical Africa*. Volume I, part I. 2d ed. Revised by R. W. J. Keay. London: Crown Agents for Overseas Governments and Administrations.
———. 1958. *Flora of west tropical Africa*. Volume I, part II. 2d ed. Revised by R. W. J. Keay. London: Crown Agents for Overseas Governments and Administrations.
———. 1963. *Flora of west tropical Africa*. Volume II. 2d ed. Edited by F. N. Hepper. London: Crown Agents for Overseas Governments and Administrations.
———. 1968. *Flora of west tropical Africa*. Volume III, part I. 2d ed. Revised and edited by F. N. Hepper. London: Crown Agents for Overseas Governments and Administrations.
———. 1972. *Flora of west tropical Africa*. Volume III, part II. 2d ed. Revised and edited by F. N. Hepper. London: Crown Agents for Overseas Governments and Administrations.
Illich, Ivan. 1977. *Limits to medicine* (*Medical nemesis: The expropriation of health*). Harmondsworth, Middlesex: Penguin Books.
Imperato, Pascal James. 1974–75. "Traditional medical practitioners among the Bambara of Mali and their role in the modern health-care delivery system." *Rural Africana* 26:41–53.
———. 1977. *African folk medicine: Practices and beliefs of the Bambara and other peoples*. Baltimore: York Press.
Ingham, John M. 1970. "On Mexican folk medicine." *American Anthropologist* 72:76–87.
Jacobson-Widding, Anita. 1979. *Red-white-black as a mode of thought: A study of triadic classification by colours in the ritual symbolism and cognitive*

thought of the peoples of the lower Congo. Stockholm: Almqvist and Wiksell International (Uppsala Studies in Cultural Anthropology, no. 1).

Jansen, G. 1973. *The doctor-patient relationship in an African tribal society*. Assen, The Netherlands: Van Orcum.

Janzen, John, with William Arkinstall. 1978. *The quest for therapy in lower Zaire*. Berkeley: University of California Press.

Jennett, Bryan. 1986. *High technology medicine: Benefits and burdens*. London: Oxford University Press. New edition.

Johnston, H. A. S. 1966. *A selection of Hausa stories*. London: Oxford University Press.

————. 1967. *The Fulani Empire of Sokoto*. London: Oxford University Press.

Kennedy, John G. 1967. "Nubian Zar ceremonies as psychotherapy." *Human Organization* 26:185–94.

King, A. V. 1966. "A boori liturgy from Katsina: Introduction and Kiraarii texts." *African Language Studies* 7:105–25.

————. 1967. "A boori liturgy from Katsina, cont." *Supplement to African Language Studies* 7. London: School of Oriental and African Studies, University of London.

Kirk-Greene, A. H. M. 1965. *The principles of native administration in Nigeria, selected documents 1900–1947*. London: Oxford University Press.

————. 1966. *Hausa ba dabo ba ne: A collection of 500 proverbs*. Ibadan: Oxford University Press.

————. 1967. "The linguistic statistics of northern Nigeria: A tentative presentation." *African Language Review* 6:75–101.

————. 1974. *Mutumin Kirki: The concept of the good man in Hausa*. Bloomington: African Studies Program, Indiana University. (Third Hans Wolff Memorial Lecture.)

Konner, Melvin, and Carol Worthman. 1980. "Nursing frequency, gonadal function and birth spacing among !Kung hunter-gatherers." *Science* 207:788–91.

Kraft, Charles H., and A. H. M. Kirk-Greene. 1973. *Teach yourself Hausa*. London: English Universities Press.

Kretchmer, Norman, O. Ransom-Kuti, R. Hurwitz, C. Dungy, and Wole Alakija. 1971. "Intestinal absorption of lactose in Nigerian ethnic groups." *Lancet* 2:392–95 (August 21, 1971).

Krusius, Paul. 1915. "Die Maguzawa." *Archiv für Anthropologie* 42:288–315.

Kuhn, Thomas S. 1970. *The structure of scientific revolutions*. 2d enl. ed. Chicago: University of Chicago Press.

LaChard, L. W. 1905. "The arrow-poisons of northern Nigeria." *Journal of the African Society* 5:22–27.

Lambo, T. A. 1956. "Neuropsychiatric observations in the western region of Nigeria." *British Medical Journal* 2:1388–96.

————. 1960. "Further neuropsychiatric observations in Nigeria." *British Medical Journal* 2:1696–704.

Lane, Edward William. 1860. *An account of the manners and customs of the modern Egyptians*. London: John Murray.

Last, D. Murray n.d. "Tradition in Hausa medicine." 11 pp, mimeographed.
———. 1967a. *The Sokoto Caliphate*. London: Longman.
———. 1967b. "A note on attitudes to the supernatural in the Sokoto jihad." *Journal of the Historical Society at Nigeria* 4:3–13.
———. 1970a. "Some Hausa ideas concerning sickness." Text of a talk given to the clinical meeting of the teaching hospital, Ahmadu Bello University, Zaria, May 8, 1970, 9 pp., mimeographed.
———. 1970b. "Aspects of administration and dissent in Hausaland, 1800–1968." *Africa* 40:345–57.
———. 1976. "The presentation of sickness in a community of non-Muslim Hausa." In *Social anthropology and medicine*, edited by J. B. Loudon, pp. 104–49. London: Academic Press.
———. 1979. "Strategies against time." *Sociology of Health and Illness* 1:306–17.
———. 1980. "The importance of not knowing." Paper presented at the Conference on African Medical and Health Systems as Systems of Thought, Causality, and Taxonomy, Cambridge, England, June 23–26, 1980.
Last, D. Murray, and M. A. Al-Hajj. 1965. "Attempts at defining a Muslim in nineteenth century Hausaland and Bornu." *Journal of the Historical Society of Nigeria* 3:231–40.
Law, R. C. C. 1967. "The Garamantes and trans-Saharan enterprise in classical times." *Journal of African History* 8:181–200.
Leslie, Alan. 1954. "Ethics and practice of placebo therapy." *American Journal of Medicine* 16:854–62.
LeVine, Robert A. 1966. *Dreams and deeds: Achievement motivation in Nigeria.* Chicago: University of Chicago Press.
LeVine, Robert A., and D. R. Price-Williams. 1974. "Children's kinship concepts: Cognitive development and early experience among the Hausa." *Ethnology* 13:25–44.
Levtzion, Nehemia. 1976. "The early states of the western Sudan to 1500." In *The History of west Africa*. Volume I. 2d ed. Edited by J. F. Ade Ajayi and M. Crowder, pp. 114–51. London: Longman.
Levy, Reuben. 1957. *The social structure of Islam.* Cambridge: Cambridge University Press.
Lewis, Gilbert. 1976. "A view of sickness in New Guinea." In *Social anthropology and medicine*, edited by J. B. Loudon, pp. 49–103. London: Academic Press.
Lewis, I. M. 1966. "Introduction." In *Islam in tropical Africa*, edited by I. M. Lewis, pp. 1–125. London: Oxford University Press.
———. 1969. "Spirit possession in northern Somaliland." In *Spirit mediumship and society in Africa*, edited by J. Beattie and J. Middleton, pp. 188–219. London: Routledge and Kegan Paul.
———. 1971. *Ecstatic religion: An anthropological study of spirit possession and shamanism.* Harmondsworth, Middlesex: Penguin Books.
Lex, Barbara. 1974. "Voodoo death: New thoughts on an old explanation." *American Anthropologist* 76:818–23.
Lipowski, Z. J., Don R. Lipsitt, and Peter C. Whybrow, Eds. 1977. *Psychosomatic*

medicine: Current trends and clinical applications. New York: Oxford University Press.

Lovejoy, Paul E. 1971. "Long distance trade and Islam: The case of the nineteenth-century Hausa kola trade." *Journal of the Historical Society of Nigeria* 5:537–47.

———. 1978a. "The Borno salt industry." *International Journal of African Historical Studies* 11:629–68.

———. 1978b. "The role of the Wangara in the economic transformation of the central Sudan in the fifteenth and sixteenth centuries." *Journal of African History* 19:173–93.

Low, Victor. 1972. *Three Nigerian emirates: A study in oral history*. Evanston, Ill.: Northwestern University Press.

Lugard, Lord. 1970. *Political memoranda*. 3rd ed. London: Frank Cass.

Luning, H. A. 1965. "The impact of socio-economic factors on the land tenure pattern in northern Nigeria." *Journal of Local Administration Overseas* 4:173–82.

MacDonald, D. B., and H. Masse. 1965. "*Djinn*." In *The encyclopedia of Islam*. Volume II, pp. 546–50. Leiden: E. J. Brill. New edition.

McDowell, C. M. 1969. "The breakdown of traditional land tenure in northern Nigeria." In *Ideas and procedures in African customary law*, edited by Max Gluckman, pp. 266–78. London: Oxford University Press for the International African Institute.

Maclean, U. 1971. *Magical medicine: A Nigerian case study*. Harmondsworth, Middlesex: Penguin Books. Paperback, 1974.

Madauci, Ibrahim, Yahaya Isa, and Bello Dura. 1968. *Hausa customs*. Zaria: Northern Nigerian Publishing Company.

Madsen, William. 1955. "Hot and cold in the universe of San Francisco Tecospa, valley of Mexico." *Journal of American Folklore* 68:123–39.

Maugham, W. Somerset. 1963. *The razor's edge*. Harmondsworth, Middlesex: Penguin Books.

Mauss, Marcel. 1954. *The gift: Forms and functions of exchange in archaic societies*. Translated by Ian Cunnison. London: Routledge and Kegan Paul.

Means, John E. 1965. "A study of the influence of Islam in northern Nigeria." Ph.D. diss., Georgetown University. Ann Arbor, Mich.: University Microfilms.

Meek, C. K. 1925. *The northern tribes of Nigeria*. 2 vols. London: Oxford University Press. Reprint 1962. New York: Negro Universities Press.

Merrick, G. 1905. *Hausa proverbs*. London: Kegan Paul, Trench, Trubner and Co. Reprint 1969. New York: Negro Universities Press.

Messing, Simon. 1958. "Group therapy and social status in the Zar cult of Ethiopia." *American Anthropologist* 60:1120–26.

Middleton, John, and David Tait. 1958. *Tribes without rulers: Studies in African segmentary systems*. London: Routledge and Kegan Paul.

———, and E. H. Winter. 1963. "Introduction." In *Witchcraft and sorcery in East Africa*, edited by John Middleton and E. H. Winter, pp. 1–26. London: Routledge and Kegan Paul, 1963.

Miller, Walter R. S. 1936. *Reflections of a pioneer.* London: Church Missionary Society.

Miner, Horace. 1965. "Urban influences on the rural Hausa." In *Urbanization and migration in west Africa,* edited by Hilda Kuper, pp. 110–29. Los Angeles: University of California Press.

Mintz, Ira. 1977. "A note on the addictive personality: Addiction to placebos." *American Journal of Psychiatry* 134:327.

Moughtin, J. C. 1964. "The traditional settlements of the Hausa people." *Town Planning Review* 35:21–34.

Muffet, D. J. M. 1964. *Concerning brave captains, being a history of the British occupation of Kano and Sokoto and of the last stand of the Fulani forces.* London: Andre Deutsch.

Nadel, S. F. 1942. *A black Byzantium: The Kingdom of Nupe in Nigeria.* London: Oxford University Press for the International African Institute.

———. 1954. *Nupe religion: Traditional beliefs and the influence of Islam in a west African chiefdom.* London: Routledge and Kegan Paul.

Newbury, C. W. 1966. "North African and western Sudan trade in the nineteenth century: A re-evaluation." *Journal of African History* 7:233–46.

Newman, Paul, and Roxana Ma Newman. 1977. *Modern Hausa-English Dictionary/Sabon 'kamus na Hausa zuwa Turanci.* Ibadan and Zaria: Oxford University Press.

Ngubane, Harriet. 1977. *Body and mind in Zulu medicine.* New York: Academic Press.

Nicolas, Guy. 1966. "Structures fondementales de l'espace dans la cosmologie hausa." *Journal de la Societe des Africanistes* 36:65–107.

———. 1968. "Un système numerique symbolique: le quatre, le trois et le sept dans la cosmologie d'une société hausa (vallee de Maradi)." *Cahier d'Études africaines* 4:566–627.

———. 1975. *Dynamique social et apprehension du monde au sein d'une société Hausa.* Paris: Institute d'Ethnologie, Musée National d'Histoire Naturelle.

Nicolas, Jacqueline Monfouga. 1967. *"Les juments des dieux:" Rites de possession et condition feminine en pays Hausa (Vallee de Maradi, Niger).* Niamey, Niger: IFAN-CNRS, Études Nigeriennes, no. 21.

———. 1972. *Amivalence et culte de possession: Contribution a l'étude de bori Hausa.* Paris: Editions Anthropos.

Nicolson, I. F. 1969. *The administration of Nigeria 1900 to 1960: Men, methods and myths.* Oxford: Clarendon Press.

Olderogge, D. A. 1960. "The origin of the Hausa language." In *Men and cultures: Selected papers of the Fifth International Congress of Anthropological and Ethnological Science, Philadelphia, September 1–9, 1956,* edited by A. F. C. Wallace, pp. 195–802. Philadelphia: University of Pennsylvania Press.

Olofson, Harold Andrus, Jr. 1976. "Funtua: Patterns of migration to a new Hausa town." Ph.D. diss., University of Pittsburg. Ann Arbor, Mich.: University Microfilms.

Onwuejeogwu, Michael. 1969. "The cult of the *bori* spirits among the Hausa." In

Man in Africa, edited by Mary Douglas and Phyllis M. Kaberry, pp. 279–305. London: Tavistock.

Organization of African Unity Scientific, Technical, and Research Commission. 1968. *First Inter-African Symposium on Traditional Pharmacopoeias and African Medicinal Plants, Dakar, 1968.* Lagos: OAUSTRC, Publication no. 104.

Orley, John. 1970. *Culture and mental illness: A study from Uganda.* Nairobi: East African Publishing House for the Makerere Institute of Social Research.

Orr, Sir Charles. 1911. *The making of northern Nigeria.* London: Frank Cass Reprint 1965.

Osborne, Oliver H. 1969. "The Yoruba village as a therapeutic community." *Journal of Health and Social Behavior* 10:187–200.

O'Shaughnessy, Thomas. 1948. *The Koranic concept of the word of God.* Rome: Pontifico Instituto Biblico (Biblica et Orientalia, Sacra Scriptura Antiquitatibus Orientalis Illustra, no. 11).

Paden, John N. 1973. *Religion and political culture in Kano.* Berkeley: University of California Press.

Pagel, Walter. 1958. *Paracelsus: An introduction to philosophical medicine in the era of the Renaissance.* Basel: S. Karger.

Palmer, H. R. 1913–15. "An early Fulani conception of Islam." *Journal of the African Society* 13:407–14; 14:53–59, 185–92.

———. 1914. "Bori among the Hausas." *Man* 14:113–17.

———. 1928. *Sudanese memoirs: Being mainly translations of a number of Arabic manuscripts relating to the central and western Sudan.* 3 vols. Lagos: Government Printer. Reprint 1967. London: Frank Cass.

Parrott, D. 1970. "A basis of a local pharmacopoeia for northern Nigeria." *Journal of Tropical Medicine and Hygiene* 73:36–38.

Pepper, O. H. Perry. 1945. "A note on the placebo." *American Journal of Pharmacy* 117:409–11.

Perham, Margery. 1937. *Native administration in Nigeria.* London: Oxford University Press.

Pogge, Raymond C. 1963. "The toxic placebo I: Side and toxic effects reported during the administration of placebo medicine." *Medical Times* 91:773–78.

Popper, Sir Karl R. 1972. "The demarcation between science and metaphysics." In *Conjectures and refutations: The growth of scientific knowledge.* 4th rev. ed. Pp. 253–92. London: Routledge and Kegan Paul.

Prince, Raymond. 1960. "The use of *Rauwolfia* for the treatment of psychoses by Nigerian native doctors." *American Journal of Psychiatry* 117:147–49.

Prothero, R. Mansell. 1962. "African ethnographic maps, with a new example from northern Nigeria." *Africa* 32:61–64.

Ramazzini, Bernardino. [1713] 1964. *Diseases of workers (De morbis artificum).* Translated by Wilmer Cave Wright from the Latin. New York: Hafner.

Rattray, R. Sutherland. 1913. *Hausa folk-lore, customs, proverbs, etc., collected and translated with English translation and notes.* 2 vols. Oxford: Clarendon Press. Reprint 1969. New York: Negro Universities Press.

Reading, Anthony. 1977. "Illness and disease." *Medical Clinics of North America* 61:703–10.

Redfield, Robert. 1953. "The natural history of the folk society." *Social Forces* 31:224–28.

———. 1960. "Peasant society and culture." In *The little community and peasant society and culture.* Chicago: University of Chicago Press.

Reid, H. A. 1972. "Clinical notes on snakebite." In *Manson's tropical diseases.* 17th ed. Edited by Charles Wilcoks and P. E. C. Manson-Bahr, pp. 801–5. London: Bailliere-Tindall.

Riesman, David. 1977. *Freedom in Fulani social life: An introspective ethnography.* Chicago: University of Chicago Press.

Rivers, W. H. R. 1924. *Medicine, magic and religion.* London: Kegan Paul, Trench, Trubner and Co.

Robbins, Stanley L., and Ramzi S. Cotran. 1979. *Pathologic basis of disease.* 2d ed. Philadelphia: W. B. Saunders.

Robinson, Charles Henry. 1900. *Hausaland, or, fifteen hundred miles through the central Soudan.* 3d ed. London: Sampson Low, Marston, and Co.

———. 1925. *Dictionary of the Hausa language.* 4th ed. 2 vols. Cambridge: Cambridge University Press.

Ross, Gillian. 1971. "Neo-Tylorianism: A reassessment." *Man* (n.s.) 6:105–16.

Rowson, J. M. 1965. "Recherches sur quelques plantes medicinales du Nigeria." *Annales pharmaceutiques francaises* 23:125–35.

Ruxton, F. H. 1916. *Maliki law.* London: Luzac and Co.

Ryan, Pauline M. 1974. "Aspects of Hausa symbolism with special reference to the literature." D.Phil. thesis, Rhodes House Library, Oxford.

———. 1976. "Color symbolism in Hausa literature." *Journal of Anthropological Research* 32:141–60.

St. Croix, F. W. de. 1945. *The Fulani of northern Nigeria: Some general notes.* Westmead, Hants.: Gregg International. Reprint 1972.

Salamone, Frank A. 1973. "Drug problem in a small emirate in northern Nigeria." *Human Organization* 32:322–25.

———. 1975a. "A Hausa bibliography." *Africana Journal* 6:99–163.

———. 1975b. "Becoming Hausa: Ethnic identity change and its implications for the study of ethnic pluralism and stratification." *Africa* 45:410–25.

Sarton, George. 1954. *Galen of Pergamon.* Lawrence: University of Kansas Press.

Schacht, Joseph. 1950. *The origins of Muhammadan jurisprudence.* Oxford: Clarendon Press.

———. 1957. "Islam in northern Nigeria." *Studia Islamica* 8:123–46.

———. 1964. *An introduction to Islamic law.* Oxford: Clarendon Press.

Shapiro, Arthur K. 1960. "A contribution to the history of the placebo effect." *Behavioral Science* 5:109–35.

———. 1964. "Factors contributing to the placebo effect: Their implications for psychotherapy." *American Journal of Psychotherapy* 18:73–88.

———. 1968. "Semantics of the placebo." *Psychiatric Quarterly* 42:653–95.

Shiloh, Ailon. 1965. "A case study of disease and culture in action: Leprosy among the Hausa of northern Nigeria." *Human Organization* 24:140–47.

Short, R. V. 1984. "Breast feeding." *Scientific American* 250(4):35–41.

Siegler, Miriam, and Humphrey Osmond. 1976. *Models of madness, models of medicine.* New York: Harper and Row. Paperback edition.

Simmons, Ozzie. 1955. "Popular and modern medicine in Mestizo communities of coastal Peru and Chile." *Journal of American Folklore* 68:57–71.

Skinner, Neil. 1965. *'Kamus na Turanci da Hausa: English-Hausa dictionary.* Zaria: Northern Nigerian Publishing Company.

———. 1968. "The origin of the name Hausa." *Africa* 38:253–57.

———. 1969. *Hausa tales and traditions: A translation of Frank Edgar's tatsuniyoyi na Hausa.* Volume I. London: Frank Cass.

———. 1977a. *Hausa tales and traditions: An English translation of tatsuniyoyi na Hausa, originally compiled by Frank Edgar.* Volume II. Madison: University of Wisconsin Press. Ann Arbor, Mich.: University Microfilms.

———. 1977b. *Hausa tales and traditions: An English translation of tatsuniyoyi na Hausa, originally compiled by Frank Edgar.* Volume III. Madison: University of Wisconsin Press. Ann Arbor, Mich.: University Microfilms.

Smaldone, Joseph P. 1977. *Warfare in the Sokoto Caliphate: Historical and socio-logical perspectives.* Cambridge: Cambridge University Press, African Studies Series, no. 19.

Smith, Abdullahi. 1970. "Some considerations relating to the formation of states in Hausaland." *Journal of the Historical Society of Nigeria* 5:329–46.

———. 1976. "The early states of the central Sudan." In *History of west Africa.* Volume I. 2d ed. Edited by J. F. Ade Ajayi and M. Crowder, pp. 152–95. London: Longman.

Smith, Mary F. 1954. *Baba of Karo: A woman of the Muslim Hausa.* London: Faber and Faber.

Smith, Michael G. 1952. "A study of Hausa domestic economy in northern Zaria." *Africa* 22:333–47.

———. 1954. "Introduction," and "Notes," to *Baba of Karo: A woman of the Muslim Hausa,* by M. F. Smith, pp. 11–36 and 257–90. London: Faber and Faber.

———. 1955. *The economy of Hausa communities of Zaria: A report to the Colonial Research Council.* London: HMSO, for the Colonial Office.

———. 1957. "The social functions and means of Hausa praise-singing." *Africa* 27:26–45.

———. 1959. "The Hausa system of social status." *Africa* 29:239–51.

———. 1960. *Government in Zazzau, 1800–1950.* London: Oxford University Press for the International African Institute.

———. 1961. "Kebbi and Hausa stratification." *British Journal of Sociology* 12:52–61.

———. 1964a. "The beginnings of Hausa society, A.D. 1000–1500." In *The Historian in tropical Africa,* edited by J. Vansina, R. Mauny, and L. V. Thomas, pp. 339–57. London: Oxford University Press.

————. 1964b. "Historical and political conditions of political corruption among the Hausa." *Comparative Studies in Society and History* 6:164–94.

————. 1965a. "Hausa inheritance and succession." In *Studies in the laws of succession in Nigeria*, edited by J. Duncan M. Derret, pp. 230–81. London: Oxford University Press for the Nigerian Institute of Social and Economic Research.

————. 1965b. "The Hausa: Markets in a peasant economy." In *Markets in Africa: Eight subsistence economies in transition*, edited by Paul Bohannan and George Dalton, pp. 130–82. Garden City, N.Y.: Doubleday. Paperback edition.

————. 1966. "The jihad of Shehu Dan Fodio: Some problems." In *Islam in tropical Africa*, edited by I. M. Lewis, pp. 408–24. London: Oxford University Press.

————. 1978. *The affairs of Daura: History and change in a Hausa state, 1800–1958.* Berkeley: University of California Press.

Spicker, Stuart F., and H. Tristram Engelhardt, Jr. 1977. "Introduction to medical ethics." In *Philosophical medical ethics: Its nature and significance*, edited by S. F. Spicker and H. T. Englehardt, Jr., pp. 3–17. Boston: D. Reidel.

Stenning, Derrick J. 1957. "Transhumance, migratory drift, migration: Patterns of pastoral Fulani nomadism." *Journal of the Royal Anthropological Institute* 87:57–73.

————. 1959. *Savannah nomads: A study of the Wo'daa'be pastoral Fulani of western Bornu Province, Northern Region, Nigeria.* London: Oxford University Press for the International African Institute.

Stock, Robert. 1979. "The effect of distance on illness behaviour: Evidence from rural Nigeria." Paper delivered at the Annual Conference of the Canadian Association of African Studies, Winnipeg, May 1–4, 1979.

Suarez, Maria Matilde. 1974. "Etiology, hunger, and folk disease in the Venezuelan Andes." *Journal of Anthropological Research* 30:41–54.

Sutton, J. E. G. 1979. "Towards a less orthodox history of Hausaland." *Journal of African History* 20:179–201.

Swift, C. R., and T. Asuni. 1975. *Mental health and disease in Africa.* Edinburgh: Churchill and Livingstone.

Taylor, F. W., and A. G. G. Webb. 1932. *Labarun al'adun Hausawa da zantata-kansu: Accounts and conversations describing certain customs of the Hausa.* London: Oxford University Press.

Temkin, Owsei. 1973. *Galenism: The rise and decline of a medical philosophy.* Ithaca, N.Y.: Cornell University Press.

Tooth, Geoffrey. 1950. *Studies in mental illness in the Gold Coast.* London: HMSO, Colonial Research Publication no. 6.

Traore, Dominique. 1965. *Comment le noir se soigne-t-il? Ou medecine et magie Africaines.* Paris: Presence Africaine.

Tremearne, A. J. N. 1912. *The tailed head-hunters of Nigeria.* London: Seeley, Service and Co.

————. 1913. *Hausa superstitions and customs: An introduction to the folk-lore and the folk.* London: John Bale, Sons, and Danielson.

———. 1941a. "Marital relations of the Hausas as shown in their folk-lore." *Man* 14:23–26, 137–39, 148–56.

———. 1914b. *The ban of the bori: demons and demon dancing in west and north Africa.* London: Frank Cass. Reprint 1969.

———. 1915. "Bori beliefs and ceremonies." *Journal of the Royal Anthropological Institute* 45:23–69.

Trevitt, Lorna. 1973. "Attitudes and customs in childbirth amongst Hausa women in Zaria City." *Savanna* 2:223–26.

Trimingham, J. Spencer. 1959. *Islam in west Africa.* Oxford: Clarendon Press.

———. 1962. *A history of Islam in west Africa.* London: Oxford University Press.

———. 1971. *The Sufi orders in Islam.* New York: Oxford University Press. Paperback 1973.

Tritton, A. S. 1934. "Shaitan." In *The encyclopedia of Islam.* Volume IV, pp. 286–87. Leiden: E. J. Brill.

Turner, Victor. 1964. "A Ndembu doctor in practice." In *Magic, faith and healing: Studies in primitive psychiatry today,* edited by Ari Kiev, pp. 230–63. Glencoe, Ill.: The Free Press.

———. 1965. "Color classification in Ndembu ritual: A problem in primitive classification." In *Anthropological approaches to the study of religion,* edited by Michael Banton, pp. 59–92. London: Tavistock.

———. 1968. *The drums of affliction: A study of religious process among the Ndembu of Zambia.* Oxford: Clarendon Press for the International African Institute.

Ullmann, Manfred. 1978. *Islamic medicine.* Edinburgh: Edinburgh University Press, Islamic Surveys no. 11.

Van Raay, H. G. T. 1975. *Rural planning in a savannah region.* Rotterdam: Rotterdam University Press.

Veith, Ilza. 1965. *Hysteria: The history of a disease.* Chicago: University of Chicago Press.

von Grunebaum, Gustave E. 1967. "The problem: Unity in diversity." In *Unity and variety in Muslim civilization,* edited by G. E. von Grunebaum, pp. 17–37. Chicago: University of Chicago Press.

———. [1951] 1976. *Muhammadan festivals.* London: Curzon Press.

Waldeman, Marilyn R. 1965. "The Fulani *jihad*: A reassessment." *Journal of African History* 6:333–55.

Watt, W. Montgomery. 1953. *Muhammed at Medina.* Oxford: Clarendon Press.

———. 1956. *Muhammed at Mecca.* Oxford: Clarendon Press.

———. 1967. *Companion to the Qur'an.* London: George Allen and Unwin.

———. 1968. *Islamic political thought: The basic concepts.* Edinburgh: Edinburgh University Press, Islamic Surveys no. 6.

———. 1969. *Islamic revelation in the modern world.* Edinburgh: Edinburgh University Press.

———. 1970. *Bell's introduction to the Qur'an.* Edinburgh: Edinburgh University Press, Islamic Surveys no. 8.

Wensinck, A. J. 1932. *The Muslim creed*. Cambridge: Cambridge University Press. Reprint 1965. London: Frank Cass.

Westermann, Dietrich, and M. A. Bryan. 1952. *The languages of west Africa*. London: Oxford University Press for the International African Institute, Handbook of African Languages, part II.

White, Leonard, Bernard Tursky, and Gary E. Schwartz, Eds. 1985. *Placebo: Theory, research and mechanisms*. New York: Guilford Press.

Whittaker, C. S., Jr. 1970. *The politics of tradition: Continuity and change in northern Nigeria, 1946–1966*. Princeton, N.J.: Princeton University Press.

Whitting, C. E. J. 1940. *Hausa and Fulani proverbs*. Lagos: Government Printer. Reprint 1967. Farnborough, Hants: Gregg International.

Whittle, H. C., and B. M. Greenwood. 1976. "Meningococcal meningitis in the northern savanna of Africa." *Tropical Doctor* 6:99–104.

Wightman, W. P. D. 1971. *The emergence of scientific medicine*. Edinburgh: Oliver and Boyd.

Willis, John Ralph. 1967. "*Jihad fi sabil Allah*: Its doctrinal basis in Islam and some aspects of its evolution in nineteenth-century west Africa." *Journal of African History* 8:395–415.

Winchester, Norris Brian. 1976. "Strangers and politics in urban Africa: A study of the Hausa in Kumasi, Ghana." Ph.D. diss. Indiana University. Ann Arbor, Mich.: University Microfilms.

Withering, William. 1785. *An account of the foxglove and some of its medical uses*. Birmingham: M. Swinney.

Wolf, Stewart. 1950. "Effects of suggestion and conditioning on the action of chemical agents in human subjects: The pharmacology of placebos." *Journal of Clinical Investigation* 29:100–109.

Wolf, Stewart, and Ruth H. Pinsky. 1954. "Effects of placebo administration and occurrence of toxic reactions." *Journal of the American Medical Association* 155:339–41.

Wolff, B. Berthold, and Sarah Langley. 1968. "Cultural factors and the response to pain: A review." *American Anthropologist* 70:494–501.

Wolff, Harold, et al. 1946. "The use of placebos in therapy." Presented at the Conference on Therapy, Cornell Medical College. *New York State Journal of Medicine* 46:1718–27.

Works, John A., Jr. 1976. *Pilgrims in a strange land: Hausa communities in Chad*. New York: Columbia University Press.

Yahaya, Ibrahim Yaro. n.d. "Kishi: Feeling among Hausa co-wives." *Kano Studies* (n.s.) 1:83–98.

Yeld, E. R. 1960. "Islam and social stratification in northern Nigeria." *British Journal of Sociology* 11:112–28.

Zabrowski, Mark. 1952. "Cultural components in responses to pain." *Journal of Social Issues* 8:16–30.

Zahan, Dominique. 1979. "Principes de medecine bambara." In *African therapeutic systems*, edited by Z. A. Ademuwagun et al., pp. 43–46. Waltham, Mass.: Crossroads Press (African Studies Association).

Index

Abdullahi, brother of Usman 'Dan Fodio, 124
Abortion, 229, 317
Abraham, 93, 94, 295
Acacia albida, 262
Acacia senegal, 303
Acacia sieberiana, 305
Adamawa, 124
Adar, 124
Adina microcephala, 305
Afterlife, 73, 98. *See also* Hell; Paradise
Agades, 121
Agriculture, 3, 13, 28–29, 35, 43, 51, 59, 71; cultivation of fields, 30–32; and the Fast of Ramadan, 90; harvest of crops, 30; among the Maguzawa Hausa, 131–32; planting of crops, 30; use of fertilizer in, 30, 133; use of oxen for plowing, 30, 95n
Ahmadu Bello, Alhaji Sir, 108
Ahmadu Bello University Hospital, 256, 282
Air, 124
Al-Maghili, Abd al-Karim, 119
Al-Majusi, 235
Al-Sayuti, 237
Albinism, 147, 191
Albizzia chevalieri, 262–63
Algeria, 223
Alhaji. See Pilgrimage
Alhaji Audu Boka (herbalist), 246, 258–77, 296, 304; case reports of, 261–76; family background of, 258; medical consultations of, 259–66; rivalry with Uwarture, 277–79
Allah: characteristics of, 76–77, 82–83, 88, 98, 133, 251, 290–91; fear of as a moral virtue, 99, 108; names of, 294–95; power and will of, 77–78, 100–101, 182–83, 288–91, 320–21; as the source of all blessings, 102–3, 212, 261; as a source of illness, 175, 183–92, 226, 261, 282–83, 289–92, 320; as a source of medicines, 212, 219–20,

252–54, 261, 288, 292–93; will of as a metaphysical safety valve, 321, 329
Allium ascalonicum, 298
Allium cepa, 298
Allium sativum, 297
Alms, 61n, 89, 101, 103, 192; and medicine, 220, 250, 254, 257, 260–61, 269; obligation to give, 82; relationship to sacrifice, 134
America. *See* United States
Ammomum melegueta, 297–98
Amosani (Hausa illness), 189–90. *See also* Cold
Anatomy, Hausa concepts of, 173, 175–83, 322
Animals, and Hausa traditional medicine, 304, 306–8
Anogneissus leiocarpus, 311
Antibiotics, 174, 227n, 282; compared to anti-witchcraft medicines, 195, 265, 317
Aphrodisiacs, 148n, 171n, 213, 215–16, 218, 222, 247, 298, 301–3, 305, 309, 313–15. *See also* Impotence; Infertility
Apostasy, 129
Arabia, 40, 75, 145n, 234
Arabic, 54, 75, 130, 195, 289, 325; as the language of God, 76, 86–87, 237–38, 296; political titles, 110
Argemone mexicana, 298
Aristolochia albida, 299
Arnebia hispidissima, 310
Arziki (special fortune), 39
Asante, 109
Atheism, 99
Authority, divine origins of, 88, 91–92, 111–12
Autopsy, 174–75
Avicenna, 223n, 234–35
Azande, xv, 289–90

Bacteriology, 174, 322; and spirits, 199n
Barbers, Hausa traditional (*wanzami*), 35, 36, 222–27; and circumcision, 54–

Prayer, spontaneous (*addu'a*), 2, 46,
55, 82, 188; and medicine, 237, 292
Preaching, Muslim, 88–90
Pregnancy, 50, 90, 182–83, 185, 190,
199, 229–30, 238, 299. *See also* Childbirth
Prestations, 102, 104
Presuppositions, unverified, 173
Priests, Muslim. See *Limam*
Prosperity, 79. *See also* Fate
Prostitutes (*karuwa*), 1, 21, 27, 39, 41,
97, 123, 259; arrangements with,
105, 154–55; behavior of, 147, 151,
155; and *bori*, 154, 156–57, 167;
definition of, 151–53; economics of,
154–55; and homosexuals, 153; male
justifications for, 50, 229; and
paganism, 156–57, 167; social organization of, 153–54, 158; as sources
of illness, 186–87; as sources of
social discord, 4–5, 156
Proverbs, Hausa (*karin magana*), ix, xi,
1, 17n, 19, 24–27, 29, 31–32, 35, 39,
41, 44, 48–49, 53, 59, 60–61, 65, 68–
73, 75, 78–79, 89–90, 96–97, 99–101,
103, 105, 112–14, 130–32, 139n, 144,
148, 155–56, 168, 170, 179, 191, 205,
211–12, 243, 245, 248, 254, 266, 279,
284, 291n, 292, 307, 320, 333–34
Puberty, 58–59. *See also* Circumcision
Purdah. See Wives, seclusion of
Purgatives, 188, 301, 315, 317, 323
Pus, 99, 227

Qadiriyya, 122. *See also* Sufism
Queen Elizabeth II, 221
Quryash, 145

Radio-Television Kaduna, 3, 89
Ramadan, Fast of, 29, 57, 63n, 82, 89–
91; celebration at the end of, 91–93;
importance of, 89–90; and the old,
98; origins of, 89–90; regulations
regarding, 89–91; and women, 143
Rationality, Hausa, xv, 284–332
Rauwolfia sp., 323
Redness, medical importance of, 309–
10. *See also* Blood
Research, foreign to Hausa culture, xiv
Reserpine, 323

Resurrection, 78; of Shehu Usman
'Dan Fodio, 109
Rhazes, 223n, 235
Rheumatism, 189, 263, 298. *See also*
Amosani; Cold
Rivers, W. H. R., 174, 285–86
Robinson, Charles Henry, 213–14, 239,
295, 317
Roofs, construction of, 16
Rosary, Muslim, 84, 294

Sacrifice, 95–96; to spirits, 133–34,
140, 166, 193–94, 197, 250
Sahara, 115, 235
Sahel, 6, 115
Sallah. See Festivals
Salt, 40; as a cause of illness, 185,
229, 299–300; medicinal uses of,
299–300; trade in, 115, 116n, 117,
300. *See also* Potash
Sanseviera sp., 298
Sarcocephalus esculentis, 299
Sardauna of Sokoto, 108
Sarki. See Chief
Savannah, 6, 29
Schistosomiasis, 185n, 318n
Schools: Koranic, 6, 33, 52–54, 58, 86–
87, 143; nature and organization of,
86–88; and village government, 3–4,
53, 59
Scorpions, stings of, 298
Seasons, 29, 71; Hausa names of, 29–
30. *See also* Dry season; Wet season
Secrets, 232, 238–39, 243, 289, 292, 293–
97, 325
Securidaca longipedunculata, 316
Semen, 181–82, 309
Senility, 178–79, 197, 206, 208
Sexual intercourse, 50, 60, 90, 148–49,
154–55, 168, 181, 182n, 198; and
illness, 147, 191, 261. *See also* Im-
potence; Venereal diseases
Shame (*kunya*), 24, 26, 50–52, 59, 62,
69, 104, 106, 132, 143–44, 145n, 147,
155
Shape and texture, in medicine, 302–3,
305
Shaving, of infant's head, 47. *See also*
Barbers
Shawara (Hausa illness), 188, 216, 221,

About the Author

Lewis Wall is Assistant Professor in the Department of Obstetrics and Gynecology, Duke University Medical Center, currently serving as
Honorary Clinical Research Fellow in the Uro-
dynamics Unit of the Department of Obstetrics
and Gynaecology, St. George's Hospital Medical
School, London. Fieldwork forming the basis for
this study was done as part of a doctoral thesis
for the Institute of Social Anthropology, Oxford
University, in association with the Department
of Community Medicine, Institute of Health,
Ahmadu Bello University.

Library of Congress Cataloging-in-Publication
Data
Wall, L. Lewis, 1950–
Hausa medicine.
Bibliography: p.
Includes index.
1. Hausa (African people)—Medicine.
2. Hausa (African people)—Social life and
customs. I. Title. [DNLM: 1. Medicine,
Arabic—Nigeria. 2. Medicine, Traditional—
Nigeria. WB 50 HN5 W12h]
DT515.45.H38W35 1988   306   87-30353
ISBN 0-8223-0777-4